Y0-CBC-961

Computers and Medicine

Bruce I. Blum, *Editor*

Computers and Medicine

Information Systems for Patient Care
Bruce I. Blum (Editor)

Computer-Assisted Medical Decision Making, Volume 1
James A. Reggia and Stanley Tuhrim (Editors)

Computer-Assisted Medical Decision Making, Volume 2
James A. Reggia and Stanley Tuhrim (Editors)

Expert Critiquing Systems
Perry L. Miller

Use and Impact of Computers in Clinical Medicine
James G. Anderson and Stephen J. Jay (Editors)

Selected Topics in Medical Artificial Intelligence
Perry L. Miller (Editor)

Implementing Health Care Information Systems
Helmuth F. Orthner and Bruce I. Blum (Editors)

Nursing and Computers: An Anthology
Virginia K. Saba, Karen A. Rieder, and Dorothy B. Pocklington (Editors)

A Clinical Information System for Oncology
John P. Enterline, Raymond E. Lenhard, Jr., and Bruce I. Blum (Editors)

J.P. Enterline   R.E. Lenhard, Jr.   B.I. Blum
Editors

A Clinical Information System for Oncology

With 103 Illustrations

Springer-Verlag
New York Berlin Heidelberg
London Paris Tokyo Hong Kong

John P. Enterline
Director, Information Systems
The Johns Hopkins Oncology Center
The Johns Hopkins Hospital
Baltimore, Maryland 21205
USA

Raymond E. Lenhard, Jr.
Vice President, Information Systems
The Johns Hopkins Hospital
Baltimore, Maryland 21205
USA

Series Editor
Bruce I. Blum
Applied Physics Laboratory
The Johns Hopkins University
Laurel, Maryland 20707-6099
USA

Library of Congress Cataloging-in-Publication Data
A clinical information system for oncology / edited by John P.
Enterline, Raymond Lenhard, and Bruce I. Blum.
    p.   cm. − (Computers and medicine)
  1. Oncology−Data processing.   2. Expert systems (Computer
science) I. Enterline, John P. II. Lenhard, Raymond. III. Blum,
Bruce I.   IV. Series: Computers and medicine (New York, N.Y.)
  [DNLM: 1. Cancer Care Facilities. 2. Hospital Information
Systems. 3. Hospitals, Special.   QZ 26.5 C641]
RC262.C532   1989
616.99′2′00285−dc19
DNLM/DLC   89-5909

Printed on acid-free paper.

© 1989 by Springer-Verlag New York, Inc.
All rights reserved. No part of this book may be translated or reproduced in any form without written
permission from Springer-Verlag, 175 Fifth Avenue, New York, New York 10010, U.S.A.
The use of general descriptive names, trade names, trademarks, etc. in this publication, even if the
former are not especially identified, is not to be taken as a sign that such names, as understood by
the Trade Marks and Merchandise Act, may accordingly be used freely by anyone.
While the advice and information in this book are believed to be true and accurate at the date of going
to press, neither the authors or editors nor the publisher can accept any legal responsibility for any
errors or omissions that may be made. The publisher makes no warranty, express or implied, with
respect to the material contained herein.

Typeset by Publishers Service, Bozeman, Montana.
Printed and bound by R.R. Donnelley & Sons, Harrisonburg, Virginia.
Printed in the United States of America.

9 8 7 6 5 4 3 2 1

ISBN 0-387-96956-X Springer-Verlag New York Berlin Heidelberg
ISBN 3-540-96956-X Springer-Verlag Berlin Heidelberg New York

We dedicate this book
to the faculty, staff, and patients
of The Johns Hopkins Oncology Center.

Without their dedication to excellence and desire to succeed,
the Oncology Clinical Information System
would not have been possible.

Series Preface

This series in Computers and Medicine had its origins when I met Jerry Stone of Springer-Verlag at a SCAMC meeting in 1982. We determined that there was a need for good collections of papers that would help disseminate the results of research and application in this field. I had already decided to do what is now *Information Systems for Patient Care*, and Jerry contributed the idea of making it part of a series. In 1984 the first book was published, and—thanks to Jerry's efforts—Computers and Medicine was underway.

Since that time, there have been many changes. Sadly, Jerry died at a very early age and cannot share in the sucess of the series that he helped found. On the bright side, however, many of the early goals of the series have been met. As the result of equipment improvements and the consequent lowering of costs, computers are being used in a growing number of medical applications, and the health care community is very computer literate. Thus, the focus of concern has turned from learning about the technology to understanding how that technology can be exploited in a medical environment.

This maturing of what is now called medical informatics caused me to reevaluate my objectives. I had a choice of learning more about the medical domain or building on my development experience to concentrate on the computer science aspects of system implementation. I chose the latter. I made many friends in my work with computers and medicine—at Johns Hopkins, in the professional community, and at Springer-Verlag. It has taken me longer that I expected just to say goodbye.

However, with this revised introduction I close out my last year as series editor. I must thank the authors and production people who made it all so easy for me. I am very pleased that Helmuth Orthner, of the George Washington University Medical Center, will succeed me as series editor. We have worked together for over a decade, and I am certain that he will bring the knowledge, insight, and background that will make this series respond to the dynamic needs of medical informatics.

By way of conclusion, let me observe that although many things have changed, the need for this series has not diminished. In the original Series Preface I wrote that there was a gap between current practice and the state-of-the-art. The three paragraphs that followed are equally true today, and I close out this final preface with them.

The lag in the diffusion of technology results from a combination of two factors. First, there are few sources designed to assist practitioners in learning what the new technology can do. Secondly, because the potential is not widely understood, there is a limited marketplace for some of the more advanced applications; this in turn limits commercial interest in the development of new products.

In the next decade, one can expect the field of medical information science to establish a better understanding of the role of computers in medicine. Furthermore, those entering the health care professions already will have had some formal training in computer science. For the near term, however, there is a clear need for books designed to illustrate how computers can assist in the practice of medicine. For without these collections, it will be very difficult for the practitioner to learn about a technology that certainly will alter his or her approach to medicine.

And that is the purpose of this series: the presentation of readings about the interaction of computers and medicine. The primary objectives are to describe the current state-of-the-art and to orient medical and health professionals and students with little or no experience with computer applications. We hope that this series will help in the rational transfer of computer technology to medical care.

Laurel, Maryland   Bruce Blum
1988

Preface

This book describes a clinical information system designed for a comprehensive cancer center. The Oncology Clinical Information System (OCIS) was developed at The Johns Hopkins Hospital and is of general interest for several reasons. It has been used in the management of a high volume of critically ill patients for over 10 years; during the past five years it has operated seven days a week, 24 hours a day (an indication of how closely it has been integrated into patient management activities); and, finally, it supports a variety of integrated decision making tools that comprise one of the most extensive medical information systems in general use today. Although OCIS was implemented in a cancer center, it is important to note that the principles used in its development and the functions that it supports are applicable to most medical environments. It is believed, therefore, that a description of this system and a discussion of its implementation history will be helpful to both the developers and users of future clinical information systems.

Work on the OCIS began in 1975. At that time there were relatively few clinical information systems in operation, and the cost of interactive computing was high. Studies of these early systems suggested that their half-lives were approximately equal to the publication cycle; by the time a journal article appeared about a system, there was a fifty-fifty chance that it was no longer in use. In the mid 1970s the Technicon Medical Information System, which since has been accepted as the prototypical hospital information system, was still under evaluation. When Henley and Wiederhold surveyed automated ambulatory medical record systems in 1975, they could identify only 16 worthy of evaluation. Even in this highly selective study, by the time that they reported their findings, one of these systems was no longer in operation. Thus, when we began work on the OCIS, the experience base in medical informatics was narrow.

In the decade that followed, the cost of computers fell and their capabilities improved. The personal computer revolution of the early 1980s played a major role in increasing the public's knowledge of computer technology. This computer literacy removed users' fear and uncertainty, and it became easier to introduce new automated functions. A user community had been trained to accept automated tools based upon their value and contribution to the task at hand.

Since the time that work on OCIS began, we have gained considerable experience with computer technology; the modes of health care reimbursement have changed; the volume of data which must be assessed to make sound medical decisions has grown; and computer applications have become ubiquitous in medicine. While familiarity with personal computers has facilitated a greater acceptance of automation, it has not altered the role of the computer in the process of care delivery. Most of the commercially available systems of the early and mid 1980s continue to respond to the perceived needs of the 1970s. They support administrative functions, seek to reduce labor costs, and perform clinically oriented activities only fortuitously. In general, clinical systems today are structured in an environment that was not designed to support medical decision making. Conversely, the OCIS is designed to facilitate medical decision making and the necessary administrative functions are built around this structure.

We believe that information systems, augmented with knowledge processing applications, offer a solution to the present information management burden faced by most health care facilities. This burden distracts from the delivery of quality medical care, encourages reactive (as opposed to anticipatory) responses to medical problems, and results in the imperfect collection and utilization of medical knowledge. Furthermore, it is certain that the next generation of comprehensive systems cannot be produced unless the lessons of the past are built upon. With this in mind, we have prepared this book. The successes of OCIS are presented so that they can be adopted by other systems. The failures of OCIS also are described so that others can avoid repeating our mistakes.

This book is organized in three parts: (I) introductory and overview material, (II) functional descriptions of the OCIS components, and (III) a summary evaluation of OCIS, directions for the future, and a description of experience in porting the system to other cancer treatment facilities. A brief description of these parts and their associated chapters follows.

The purpose of Part I is to provide some background together with the environmental and structural information necessary to understand OCIS. The chapters offer the general audience an insight into the need for decision support systems in medicine and, in particular, for the treatment of cancer. They also provide an understanding of how OCIS was developed and what it looks like today. There are three chapters prepared by the editors.

Chapter 1 describes the background, environment, functions, and structural operation of OCIS. It also contains a brief summary of the chapters which follow.

Chapter 2 presents the philosophical foundation for decision support systems as applied to the clinical management of oncology patients. This chapter includes both the rationale for OCIS and an example of how the system is used in the routine management of patients.

Chapter 3 reviews the development history of OCIS. Because this is largely a software development activity, the chapter includes a review of software engineering and the software tools used with OCIS as well as a narrative of the system's development.

Part II of the book contains a detailed description of OCIS. It presents the system from the perspective of its use in the Oncology Center; there are very few comparisons with other systems and no discussion of implementation details[1]. Each chapter contains a general introduction followed by a presentation of the OCIS tools in the context of their use. In most cases, the chapters have been written by the principal users of the applications. The material is organized as follows.

Chapter 4 (Clinical Data Management) presents the tools used to meet the clinical information needs described in Chapter 2. The primary author is the Manager of the OCIS and previous head of the clinical data coordinators, the group responsible for helping the physicians learn and use the system.

Chapter 5 (Protocol-Directed Care) presents the tools used to provide advice on patient management based upon the rules formalized in treatment and research protocols. This chapter was prepared by one of the initial developers.

Chapter 6 (Pharmacy System) describes a satellite oncology pharmacy run by the Department of Pharmacy. Although developed separately, the oncology pharmacy system is integrated with the other functions of OCIS. The authors are the past Director of the Oncology Pharmacy, a pharmacist, and the developer responsible for the implementation of this subsystem.

Chapter 7 (Hemapheresis System) describes the specialized tools required to manage the high volume of transfusions, product collection, and product-patient matching necessary in an oncology setting. The author is the Director of the Hemapheresis component of the Oncology Center.

Chapter 8 (General Administrative Functions) provides a description of the tools for patient scheduling, the management of a Tumor Registry, an OPD patient routing system, as well as a variety of other administrative functions. This chapter was prepared by the persons responsible for the various non-clinical activities.

Part III of the book contains two chapters.

Chapter 9 includes an evaluation summary and an overview of the future computing plans for the Oncology Center. The author is the Director of the Oncology Information Systems.

Chapter 10 recounts an experience in transporting OCIS functions to another cancer center. This chapter was prepared by an OCIS developer who installed the system in a second cancer center.

---

[1]A review of the OCIS data structures is in B.I. Blum, R.E. Lenhard, Jr., and E.E. McColligan, An Integrated Data Model for Patient Care, *IEEE Transaction on Biomedical Engineering*, BME-32:277–288, 1985.

In summary, we note that OCIS represents a viable approach to meeting modern medical computing needs. It is one of the most extensive medical decision support systems in use; it has a rich developmental history; it supports a unique and useful array of decision-making tools; and it provides administrative functions that are a necessary adjunct to patient care in today's medical environment. The success and long-term viability of OCIS are the result of both its initial orientation to patient management and its ability to adapt to a changing user demand.

We believe that our experience with OCIS will be useful for a variety of reasons. It illustrates how patient data can be managed to support medical decision making; it offers examples of information management tools that were developed inexpensively; it illustrates issues in both development and evaluation; and it demonstrates that the goal of a comprehensive clinical information system is realistic. Unfortunately, the development of OCIS (or any other large information system) takes time and is expensive. Consequently, a developer or user can have but limited hands-on experience. We hope, therefore, that the following chapters will assist the reader in expanding his conceptual view of clinical information systems. For the goal of this book is not to describe one system, rather it is to assist the medical community in better understanding how this type of system can aid in the primary mission of delivering and improving health care.

Naturally the development of a system as ambitious as the OCIS requires contributions from many people. In the material that follows, we must acknowledge that it was the interest, patience, and cooperation of the entire Oncology Center—faculty, clinical staff, administration, clerical personnel, the Information Systems' staff, and the patients—that helped us mold this system into its present form. We would like to thank Mike Fox, Dena Fulton, Darleen Rose, and Debbie Hutson for their tremendous help in preparing the text and many of the figures for this book. Special thanks is also extended to Gloria Stuart, who not only is one of the authors of this book, but provided help in proofing and coordinating the graphics for a majority of the book's chapters.

Most importantly, without the unwavering support of the Center's Director, Albert H. Owens, Jr., M.D., the OCIS would not have been possible. Dr. Owens not only had the initiative to create the Johns Hopkins Oncology Center, but had the foresight to integrate a clinical information system into its initial design.

The implementation of OCIS was supported primarily out of patient care revenues. We did receive a gift from the Educational Foundation of America for which we are grateful. Development of some of the research-oriented OCIS functions was supported through a Cancer Center Support Grant (# 5P30CA06973) from the National Cancer Institute. In closing this preface, we the editors also would like to thank our wives, Karen, Peggy, and Harriet, for their tolerance and understanding that compulsive husbands sometimes demand.

Contents

III. Evaluation and Future Directions

Contributors

Linda M. Arenth, M.S.
Adjunct Professor, The Johns Hopkins School of Nursing; Vice President for Nursing and Patient Services, The Johns Hopkins Hospital, Baltimore, Maryland, USA

Hayden G. Braine, M.D.
Associate Professor of Oncology, The Johns Hopkins University School of Medicine; Associate Professor of Laboratory Medicine, Department of Pathology, The Johns Hopkins University School of Medicine; Director, Hemapheresis Treatment Center, The Johns Hopkins Oncology Center, The Johns Hopkins Hospital, Baltimore, Maryland, USA

Jean P. Causey
Manager, Systems and Development, Department of Laboratory Medicine, The Johns Hopkins Hospital, Baltimore, Maryland, USA

Suanne Paulive Goldberger, B.S., R.Ph.
Formerly: Sr. Administrative Pharmacist, Oncology Pharmacy, The Johns Hopkins Oncology Center, The Johns Hopkins Hospital, Baltimore, Maryland, USA; *Currently*: Clinical Research Associate, Nova Pharmaceutical Corporation, Baltimore, Maryland, USA

Patricia M. Harwood, Pharm D.
Formerly: Research Associate, The Johns Hopkins University School of Medicine, Assistant Director, Department of Pharmacy, The Johns Hopkins Hospital, Baltimore, Maryland, USA; *Currently*: Assistant Director, Pharmacy, University of California, Irvine Medical Center, Orange, California, USA

Anne Kammer, A.R.T., C.T.R.
Manager, Oncology Medical Information, The Johns Hopkins Oncology Center, The Johns Hopkins Hospital, Baltimore, Maryland, USA

Catherine Kelleher, Sc.D., M.P.H., M.S.N.
Research Associate, The Johns Hopkins Oncology Center, The Johns Hopkins University School of Medicine, Baltimore, Maryland, USA

Gary Kinsey
Systems Programmer II, Oncology Information Systems, The Johns Hopkins Oncology Center, The Johns Hopkins Hospital, Baltimore, Maryland, USA

Lisa A. Lattal, M.H.A., J.D.
Ambulatory Service Manager, The Johns Hopkins Oncology Center, The Johns Hopkins Hospital, Baltimore, Maryland, USA

Elizabeth E. McColligan, M.S., M.P.H.
Director, Computer Center, Arthur G. James Cancer Hospital and Research Institute, The Ohio State University, Columbus, Ohio, USA

Farideh Momeni, M.S.
Systems Programmer III, Oncology Information Systems, The Johns Hopkins Oncology Center, The Johns Hopkins Hospital, Baltimore, Maryland, USA

Sara J. Perkel, M.B.A.
Administrator, The Johns Hopkins Oncology Center, The Johns Hopkins Hospital, Baltimore, Maryland, USA

Alan W. Sacker
Systems Programmer III, Oncology Information Systems, The Johns Hopkins Oncology Center, The Johns Hopkins Hospital, Baltimore, Maryland, USA

Gloria J. Stuart
Manager, Oncology Information Systems, The Johns Hopkins Oncology Center, The Johns Hopkins Hospital, Baltimore, Maryland, USA

I
Introduction and Overview

This section provides background information together with the environmental and structural information necessary to understand the OCIS. It is intended to provide a general insight into the need for decision support systems in medicine and in the treatment of cancer in particular. It also describes the development of the OCIS from its beginnings to what it is today.

1
The Oncology Clinical Information System

John P. Enterline, Raymond E. Lenhard, Jr., and Bruce I. Blum[1]

Introduction

The Oncology Clinical Information System (OCIS) at The Johns Hopkins Hospital is a computer-based decision support system for the clinical management of patients with cancer. It was developed in response to a need for more effective mechanisms to manage the large volume of clinical data used during the medical care of these patients. The goal of OCIS is to assist in providing an optimal clinical management, research, and educational environment for The Johns Hopkins Oncology Center through the automated collection, storage, and access of appropriate information. The major premise of the system is that timely access to complete and accurate clinical information will significantly improve the effectiveness and efficiency of the clinical management of cancer patients. Obviously, access to good information can only help if it is appropriately used. Consequently, considerable emphasis also is placed on providing the information in a format that conveys clinical meaning in a natural manner.

We believe that OCIS has achieved its objectives. It has made possible the effective use of large amounts of data in a timely manner for clinical care. It also supports many secondary tasks such as patient scheduling, admit/discharge

[1]John P. Enterline is presently Director of Information Systems at The Johns Hopkins Oncology Center. He joined the Center in 1983 as Director of Biostatistics and followed Bruce Blum as Technical Director of the OCIS. He assumed the role of Director of Information Systems later that year when Dr. Raymond Lenhard left to become Director of Information Systems for The Johns Hopkins Hospital.

Dr. Raymond E. Lenhard, Jr. was a professor of Oncology and head of Medical Oncology at The Johns Hopkins Oncology Center during the development of the OCIS. He was responsible for information systems, postgraduate medical training programs, and numerous clinical research projects. He is now Vice-President for Information Systems at The Johns Hopkins Hospital.

Bruce I. Blum was Technical Director of The Johns Hopkins Oncology Center's clinical information center when the Center opened in 1976. He played a major role in the design and implementation of the OCIS. He left the Oncology Center in 1983 and is now engaged in research in software engineering at The Johns Hopkins Applied Physics Laboratory.

functions, the ordering of procedures and blood products, clinical research protocol reporting, drug ordering and monitoring, charge capture, and a variety of administrative functions. Any comparable attempt to manage these OCIS tasks with manual techniques would be logistically difficult and financially prohibitive.

This chapter provides an overview of OCIS and the environment in which it operates. It begins with a brief description of the Oncology Center and its philosophy of patient management that led to the creation of OCIS. Following a brief development history, the basic functions of OCIS and its support organization are presented. Because the development process is dynamic, the chapter concludes with a brief overview of the Oncology Center's current activities and future plans.

Rationale for OCIS

Medical oncology is a relatively new discipline in internal medicine. Its origins in clinical pharmacology place a strong emphasis on drug development and have positioned the young specialty at the forefront of the design and conduct of clinical trials. The discipline of medical oncology requires both the fine categorization of specific clinical problems and quantitative methods to measure treatment outcome. Thus, there is a heavy emphasis on research protocols in the day-to-day management of cancer patients. The prospective collection of well-defined data items and the standardization of study results in time-oriented tabular format (flow sheets) have become necessary components of clinical care.

As would be expected, enormous volumes of laboratory, pharmacological, and clinical observations are needed to support the ongoing decision-making process and to determine the success of cancer treatment. Because of this, research-oriented data management tools have received general acceptance in clinical practice. Additionally, because most medical oncology training programs arose in a clinical research environment, the techniques learned in this setting have been adopted into clinical practice in both oncology and general internal medicine by graduates of these programs.

Given the overwhelming data management requirements of medical oncology, the opening of a new cancer facility at The Johns Hopkins Hospital in 1976 provided the opportunity to examine how an automated system might further patient care. After a detailed preliminary analysis, the Oncology Center administration committed itself to an automation project. They were convinced that the Center's proposed methods of patient care would be particularly well suited to the use of a computer-based system. Therefore, it chose to underwrite development of OCIS with internal funds.

Several key decisions regarding the OCIS philosophy were made early in the development process. First, the system was to be clinically oriented. It was to focus on the patient, then on the disease and other medical complications, and finally on specific treatments for diseases and complications. This meant that all treatments, whether primary or secondary, inpatient or outpatient, were to be integrated into one time-oriented database organized by patient. This implied that the system had to be concerned with the total patient history and not just particular disease and treatment episodes. There was an initial presumption that the system did not need to address either administrative or research tasks directly, except as they related to the clinical functions. Thus, OCIS could be designed around the information requirements for total patient care within the Oncology Center.

Another major decision leading to the philosophy and structure of OCIS was that it should be tightly coupled with the patient care process. As a system, all data and procedural support would be linked to ongoing patient care activities. This meant that there would be an analysis of the care process in the Oncology Center and, where appropriate, automated tools would be developed and integrated into the operational flow. As a result, early ties were formed with data-intensive ancillary functions, such as pharmacy and blood product support.

Of course, the development of these tools took time and the early computer resources were limited. Therefore, the third key decision and understanding was that the system would be phased into use gradually so that learning could be part of the design process; that is, the OCIS would not be a turnkey system but an evolutionary system prospectively sculpted to meet clinical needs.

The OCIS developers were fortunate in their initial choice of a database structure. If OCIS did not have a global patient orientation from its inception, development of any internal system would have logically centered around the administrative needs of the Oncology Center. In that case, it would have been necessary to integrate clinical functions with a system having an administrative architecture. This may have proved to be an impossible task owing to the relatively fixed nature of administrative structures and the dynamic nature of patient care. However, with the patient orientation, once the clinical functions were in place it was not difficult to add the necessary administrative tools and research links.

Further, if OCIS did not have a global patient management support orientation, the system might have become a series of specialized tools for the support of selected activities. All components of the OCIS are integrated because of this global structure. Every entity in the data model is either directly or indirectly linked to a patient record. One of the major benefits of this OCIS structure is that it permits the hosting of very simple features with broad utility (such as pain management tools, body surface area computations, and chemotherapy reaction monitoring) with only minor development activity.

Finally, we note that if there were not a willingness to underwrite a long-term commitment to automated support, the products of the early years of exploration and demonstration would have been scaled back to the limited number of applications that could be shown to save costs at that time. System growth might have been stunted at the level of what was efficient and essential in 1980.

In summary, the past success of OCIS is very dependent on the establishment of a favorable and flexible development environment within the Oncology

Center. Although such management vision may have been rare in the mid-1970s, one would hope that there are many who now share this perspective.

Building an Oncology Clinical Information System

The Johns Hopkins Oncology Center was organized in 1975 as part of the National Cancer Program sponsored by the National Cancer Institute. The basic goals of the Oncology Center are (1) specialized diagnosis and treatment management of patients with cancer, (2) conducting basic and clinical cancer research, and (3) education of medical specialists in the field of cancer.

The development of OCIS began just before the new Oncology Center building was opened. This created both opportunities and disadvantages. On the positive side, there was the freedom to organize the care process as the staff felt it ought to be organized, and there were few established precedents to inhibit change. On the other hand, this open structure implied that much learning would be required by both the clinical and development personnel. The experience base was narrow. A new system was to support a process that was not defined fully and that, by definition, had to operate effectively even before the system would be complete enough to provide it any assistance. The OCIS development team and the users were able to take advantage of the opportunities and overcome these difficulties. In the remainder of this section we describe our initial vision of OCIS and review its development history.

At this time (1988) the Oncology Center has over 200,000 square feet of space containing 84 inpatient beds, a large outpatient facility, several ancillary ambulatory care clinics, and a large basic research facility. A move to a new and much larger facility is planned for 1992. Presently, there over 750 full-time employees, including 80 clinical and research faculty, 40 fellows, and 150 nurses. The inpatient component of the Center admits over 800 individual patients per year, with an average of 2.1 admissions per patient, and an average length of stay of 25 days. The outpatient component of the Center has over 50,000 visits per year to its medical oncology and radiation oncology facilities.

The Decision Support Role of OCIS

The initial intent of OCIS was to help support the information essential for managing patients with complex, chronic medical problems who have repeated admissions to the hospital and frequent outpatient visits. When on the acute inpatient nursing unit, these patients present a special problem in data management. Much information is collected and reported. The physician finds it difficult to recall which tests have been ordered, which have been reported, and which are still pending. Moreover, when the test results return, they may not be delivered in the same chronological order in which they were sent.

As a result, physicians spend considerable time organizing clinical information. Frequently, they are required to telephone several laboratories to get the most recent information that may not have been returned to them. Additionally, they transcribe results by hand to flow sheets, which provide a more efficient tool for decision making. This time-consuming effort is driven by the level of illness of the patient and the urgency for retrieving and assessing information as quickly as possible. As physicians have only a limited amount of time to allocate to each patient, time spent correcting errors of omission and processing data must compete for time spent in direct patient care, family interactions, and making decisions on the basis of available (and often incomplete) information.

The goal of OCIS is to provide ready access to information that is not only reliable, complete, and timely, but that is also presented in a manner that leads most directly to the correct decision. Many models of computer-assisted decision support have been explored over the last several decades. Differences in these systems relate to the distribution of responsibility between man and machine. Artificial intelligence solutions attempt to capture the knowledge of experts in medical diagnosis and thereby automate some of the decision making. OCIS has taken a simpler path to decision support owing to its relatively narrow focus. Well-understood processes are automated. In all other cases the responsibility for assimilation of data into diagnostic and treatment plans is left to the physician. This implies that OCIS must be able to present its information in formats that the physicians will consider useful in patient management.

Naturally, OCIS was intended to operate in a specific institution. However, the concept can be applied both to other oncology environments and other medical subspecialties. The need to assess enormous volumes of data in a timely manner has become essential in many areas of health care.

We conclude this subsection by identifying some of the philosophic foundations and operational constraints that provided a context for its design.

Acutely ill patients should be clustered into treatment units organized by disease category. This implies that the assessment of information about a specific patient may be difficult.

The setting of limits and thresholds for action, along with the monitoring of data as these limits are approached is a prerequisite for the timely response to medical changes.

Care of cancer patients must be managed by a team of providers; the use of the system by nonphysician specialists to initiate and provide follow-up medical support of antibiotics, fluids, and platelets is necessary.

The senior supervisory staff must monitor the quality control and compliance with agreed-upon support standards. This is particularly important in a teaching environment in which the medical house staff spend one-third of their rotation in the Oncology Center.

There is a need to integrate senior staff knowledge into the system by establishing prospective treatment protocols for both research and individual therapy.

Graphic representation of data facilitates analysis by physicians and should be encouraged whenever feasible. For time-oriented information (both long and short term), displays that facilitate the recognition of subtle trends are required.

Information processing is aided by the clustering of data from various sources (hematology, laboratory, patient vital signs, pharmacy, blood bank) into meaningful disease-oriented displays that integrate several databases. Consequently, displays should group information into clusters by disease or treatment hypothesis, rather than by strict laboratory report groupings.

Because the Center staff rotates assignments frequently, any information system must provide considerable functionality to those who are not expert in its use. Such support may come from a very "friendly" interface or trained permanent staff members.

Development Chronology

The ten-year development, implementation, and evolution of OCIS are described in some detail in Chapters 3 and 9. The evolution of OCIS spans several generations of computer technology, and a short review of its history will be helpful toward understanding how OCIS fits into the Oncology Center's computer environment.

OCIS implementation has been organized as system phases.

Phase 0:   Development of an OCIS prototype began in 1975. It concentrated on determining general system requirements, demonstrating a rudimentary system, and selecting an appropriate hardware and software environment.

Phase I: This phase consisted of moving the prototype system to a PDP-11/70 operating under MUMPS and implementing the system on a broad scale. Virtually all OCIS features described in this book can be traced to the one-computer Phase I system.

Phase II: This phase of development consisted of two stages. The first was to translate the Phase I MUMPS applications into the newly released Standard MUMPS using a two-computer architecture. A special environment called TEDIUM[2] was developed to support this activity. The second stage entailed the integration of an evolving microcomputer environment with the OCIS database.

Phase III: The present phase of development integrates the essential OCIS functions both to take advantage of a rapidly evolving computing technology and to meet the other computational demands of the Oncology Center. This expanded environment includes local-area networks, user workstations, distributed processing, image access and analysis, and modular growth of the system.

Table 1 presents a summary of the development activities. Although the Phase I OCIS performed many useful functions, there were limitations that restricted its utility in a clinical setting. There was only a single computer, the

---

[2]TEDIUM is a registered trademark of Tedious Enterprises, Inc.

Table 1. Chronology of OCIS Developmental Efforts

July 1975	Analysis and prototype of clinical systems begun
October 1976	Oncology Center facility opened
August 1977	First PDP-11 delivered, Phase I development of clinical systems begun
December 1977	Prototype database moved to new system
April 1979	Limited clinical management system on line
August 1979	Second PDP-11 installed to provide needed power
June 1980	Phase I development of clinical system completed; conversion to Standard MUMPS begun (Phase II)
August 1982	Phase II conversion of clinical system completed
October 1982	IBM PC selected as Oncology Center standard
January 1983	Development of research component to OCIS begun
September 1983	Network with School of Hygiene statistical computer
August 1985	Conversion to MUMPS M11+ completed; threefold increase in throughput; additional on-line storage
August 1985	Prototype of clinical protocol management system completed
February 1986	High-speed access to newly developed Hospital network
September 1986	Final Phase III plans submitted for funding
August 1987	PDP-11/70s replaced by PDP-11/84s; MicroVAX II installed for hemapheresis system; data switch installed
May 1988	Two MicroVAX 3600s installed and port of selected OCIS functions begun; PDPs networked with MicroVAXs

data were not always timely, and not all the computer programs were complete. The Phase II system changed this. It provided a mature two-computer system that could support a 24-hour-a-day, 7-day-a-week operation. There also was a trained staff, a collection of proven programs, and a group of physicians that were anxious to increase their use of the system. All the necessary prerequisites for a timely information system were now in place.

Attention was now directed to operational, as opposed to functional, considerations. During the early period of use, data were manually collected and entered into the system. This was an expensive, error-prone activity that inhibited the timely display of information. As the technology matured, electronic links were implemented for both on-line and batch communication with other computer-based information systems in The Johns Hopkins Medical Institutions, that is Laboratory Medicine, Pathology, several Pharmacy charge capture systems, and the Hospital's Blood Bank.

As OCIS became an essential component in the care process, user demands for computer applications increased. Additional functions were added to or integrated with the system. These functions included

a unit-dose pharmacy system,
an in-house blood products system with order entry capabilities,
additional research and analysis capabilities,
additional administrative functions.

The query and report capabilities of the system were continuously enhanced, and a personal database that linked with data in the OCIS system was developed to assist with nonclinical data collection and analysis activities. Finally, moderate-level statistical tools, such as sample-size calculations, and low-level descriptive and analytic tools, were incorporated into the system in early 1983.

As the demand for data-processing applications increased beyond that initially intended for the central OCIS system, requirements for a broader applications environment became apparent. Fortunately, this need arose at approximately the same time the IBM PC was introduced (1982). Using the personal computers, the Oncology Center staff and faculty could address the specific computational needs that were not supported by OCIS. Of course, this trend was replicated in many medical and nonmedical environments at the same time. The advantage was that users had tools that required minimal external assistance for supporting their local needs. The obvious disadvantage was that the decentralization made the sharing of common resources and data more complex.

Within two years, there were over 80 PCs throughout the Oncology Center. Because it was unrealistic to expect OCIS to incorporate all the functions required by the Oncology Center, additional applications such as imaging, graphics, in-house publication, personal databases, and sophisticated statistical analysis tools were quickly incorporated into the Center's data-processing environment through PCs. Several local-area networks were developed in the administrative and laboratory areas. These networks presently incorporate approximately 40% of the Center's PC population.

Today, with over 140 PCs and 175 terminals, the Center is undertaking the task of integrating the prevalent PC MS/DOS[5] and MUMPS environments with additional environments, such as UNIX,[3] VAX/VMS,[4] OS/2,[5] Ethernet, TCP/IP, DECNet,[4] and the coming Open Systems Interconnect (OSI) architecture. Low-level communication between the OCIS/MUMPS system and the PC environment were established in early 1983. This level of communication between the two environments has increased gradually over the past four years, but has been restricted by a lack of integration tools and standards. Recently, the availability of such tools and standards has grown.

As shown in Figure 1, OCIS is now seen by users as one function or node in an Oncology Center network. It is the key clinical system, and its clinical database is used as a resource for the many research and administrative activities conducted at the Center. Because OCIS never was intended to meet all of the Center's computational needs, development efforts continue to be directed toward integrating the Oncology Center systems with each other and with other resources throughout The Johns Hopkins Medical Institutions. Present and future development activities are discussed in further detail in Chapter 9.

---

[3] UNIX is a trademark of AT&T Bell Laboratories.

[4] VAX/VMS and DECNet are Trademarks of the Digital Equipment Corp.

[5] OS/2 and MS/DOS are Trademarks of Microsoft, Inc.

Description of OCIS

The Oncology Center is a part of a larger system: The Johns Hopkins Hospital. Consequently, there is no need for OCIS is replicate functions that are available elsewhere. The Oncology Center relies upon the Hospital's admission–discharge–transfer system and its billing systems. As a part of the Hospital, the Oncology Center must also look to other departments to provide services or modify existing systems. For example, it is the responsibility of the Pharmacy Department to operate the pharmacy located in the Oncology Center and of the Clinical Laboratory Department to certify the laboratory located near the outpatient department.

Thus, OCIS should not be viewed as a complete system for a hospital unit. It is a patient-oriented information system, which complements the resources that others provide. Its mission is to establish a comprehensive, integrated information management facility for patient care. The remainder of this section describes the functions supported by OCIS. The following section provides an overview of Oncology Information Systems, which manages the operation of OCIS, and a description of the computing resources that support it.

OCIS Clinical Data Management Functions

The primary function of OCIS is to provide a subset of information from the medical record in an electronic form for both the generation of routine reports and on-line ad hoc access. In general, it is the intent of OCIS to minimize the need for the paper medical record in the day-to-day care of cancer patients. There are over 2500 variables for which data could be collected on each patient. These data can be used to generate reports on patient status or to provide ad hoc profiles on various patient parameters. Basic demographic and medical history data also can be easily viewed for all patients.

In addition to the primary clinical function of OCIS, there are several ancillary functions for which the system provides assistance. These include an inpatient pharmacy, a blood products matching and distribution system, an outpatient scheduling system, an in-house hematology system, an inpatient admit/discharge system, integrated treatment plans, and a clinical research protocol system.

The administrative spin-offs from OCIS include daily patient census, charge capture capabilities, a tumor registry, staff scheduling, and resource monitoring and forecasting capabilities. All of theses functions are summarized in Figure 2. As shown in the figure, virtually all computer-supported activities rely on information that is either directly related to the clinical status of a patient or related to the processing of such elements.

The patient data organization is structured as follows:

Summary patient information is linked to the unique identifier for all Johns Hopkins Hospital treatments (both inside and outside the Oncology Center). It includes a summary of Center treatments retained as short descriptive notes,

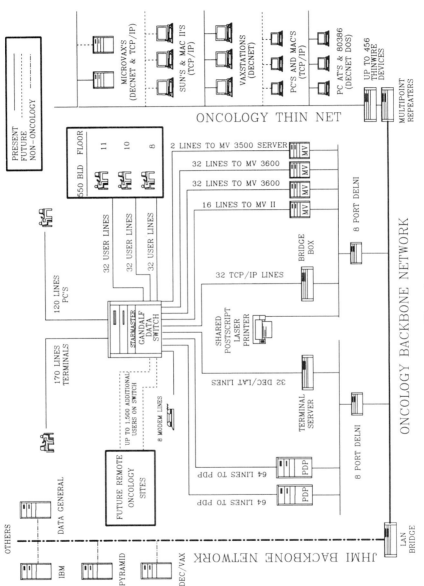

Figure 1.

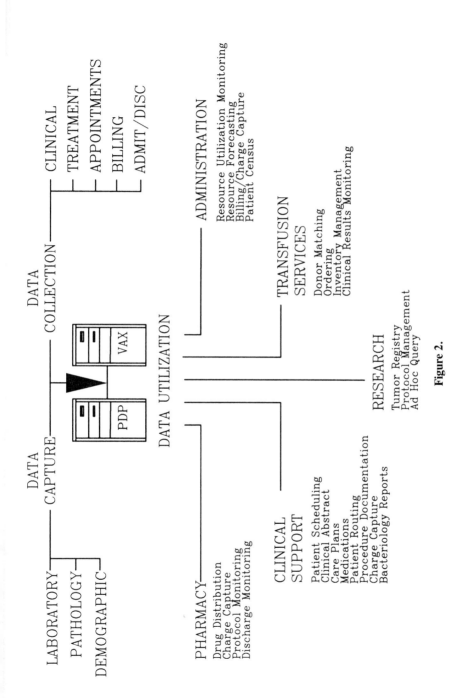

Figure 2.

an abstract of key demographic data, and some essential administrative information. These data are included in most reports in various degrees of detail.
Data should be represented in time-oriented tabular form. Examples are test
results, vital signs, coded performance measures, and daily totals of drug
administration. These data can be displayed as plots or flow sheets.
Some clinical data cannot be represented as flow sheets or plots and require
specially formatted reports. Examples are microbacteriology reports, daily
drug administration profiles, and displays of blood product transfusions. The
format of the output will depend on the data structure and the orientation of the
user. To illustrate, the physician and the pharmacist require different displays
of the same drug administration data.
Treatment data should be organized using fixed sequences of therapies and tests
to monitor the patient response. Such data include both the patient-indepen-
dent plans and the daily treatment recommendations as modified for each
inpatient.

Because the OCIS may contain hundreds of therapy days for an individual
currently being treated, and because there may be over a hundred data items
collected during a single therapy day, the key function of OCIS is to collect the
patient information rapidly and accurately and make it available to the health
care team in appropriately focused displays. This implies that some data will be
plotted, other data listed in greater detail, and some data presented in formats
designed to facilitate the recognition of events and trends.

Table 2 is extracted from the *OCIS Users' Manual*. It lists alphabetically those
functions supported by the system that will be of the greatest interest to clinicians. Most of these functions produce outputs that are used in medical decision
making. How these outputs are used is discussed in Chapter 2. A description of
the displays and the tools used to manage the data entry and display is contained
in Chapter 4. The protocol-directed care system is presented in Chapter 5.

Ancillary Clinical Functions

There are two functions supported by OCIS that focus on both the patient and the
operational units. These are the pharmacy, which integrates its internal processing with the OCIS data collection and display functions, and the blood product
support system, which manages a broad range of functions from product collection to transfusion management. These two systems are described in Chapters 6
and 7.

Administrative Functions

Much of the data collected by OCIS can be used to support administrative activities. In fact, in an integrated environment it is difficult to separate administrative
from care-oriented activities. For example, The Tumor Registry manages an
abstract and summary of the diagnosis and treatments for all Oncology Center

Table 2. OCIS User's Manual Listing of Functions, 1988

Function Name	Description	Page Number
Abstract (A) Complete diagnostic history	Tumor registry coding, patient history and symptoms, diagnosis, morphology, protocol IDs/dates, and physician follow-up information	VO-4
Admissions scheduled (SA)	Displays a listing of patients who are currently scheduled to be admitted into the Oncology Center	OP-15
Appointments By patient (PT) By provider (PR) By clinic (CL)	Short or full listing of appointments scheduled with emphasis on either provider, patient, or clinic appointments; dates can be specified	OP-9
Bacteriology report (B) By date By specimen By organism	Up-to-date results of patient specimens, organisms found, and antibiotics with susceptibility factors	VO-7
BMT screen display (PLAN)	Shows the BMT date, the number of days following transplant, the primary and associate nurse(s)	IP-2
Blood and body fluid precautions list (BF)	Provides a list of all active patients positive for blood and body fluid precautions by serology	UT-6
Body surface area (BS)	Calculates a patient's BSA on the basis of a given height and weight; calculates the dose for drugs on the basis of a given dose per square meter	AN-5
CCPDS number conversion (CC)	Provides the actual HNO and name of a patient when it has been hidden or encrypted by OCIS	DM-11
Census (C)	Flexible format that includes patient information, inpatient admits, OPD visits, protocol activity, and specific patient treatment responses and comments with diagnosis information	VO-11
Chemistry screen (CHEM)	Displays routine chemistry values for any desired date on a per-unit basis and is time specific	IP-3
Chi-square (CS)	A calculation routine used for patient statistical analysis	AN-3
Clinical items Item Groups (IG) Item Names (IT)	Provides an alphabetical listing of the data item names (e.g., WBC, RBC, AMPH) used within OCIS	DM-7
Counts — outpatient (C)	Displays the routine hematology values of all outpatients being seen on the current day; values include the time results were collected and can be listed by provider, by medical oncology or radiology oncology	OP-8
Cumulative doses (CD)	A calculation routine that provides the total dosage given to a specific patient since first admission	AN-6

Table 2. (*Continued*)

Function Name	Description	Page Number
Data (D) Today's data Latest data Search data item	Includes daily clinical data for each patient seen in the Oncology Center for any given date. User selects data range and search data	VO-12
Date difference (DD)	A calculation routine that results in the total number of days between any two dates given	AN-4
Dictionaries (Y)	Several functions that are used for referencing interhospital physicians, protocol IDs, preformatted plot, and flow definitions and data items within OCIS	DM-2
Flow— horizontal (F) Preformatted Special order	A tabular representation of patient data showing any specified clinical values for seven days/dates in columns	VO-17
Flow— vertical (F)	A tabular representation of patient data showing up to seven data elements in columns for values collected over long periods of time	VO-19
Hematology counts (COUNTS) Individual All or print	Provides the most recent hematology values of the current day for each patient on an inpatient unit	IP-4
Hematology screen (HEM)	Provides time-specific routine hematology values of a unit for any given date	IP-3
Hospital names	See *Physicians, referring* in this list.	
Inpatient census screen display	Displays the HNO, name, age, race, sex, room number, admission dates, and estimated length of stay for patients who are currently admitted to one of the Oncology Center units	UT-5
Item ID (IT)	Provides the full name for a data element abbreviation that may be used in OCIS displays	VO-15
Message system (W)	Electronic mail with editing capabilities for OCIS users with a password	UT-2
Output definitions (OD)	Provides the data structures and data elements for the available preformatted plots and flows	DM-4
Pain table (PAIN)	Provides conversions of narcotic analgesic doses and routes of administration; also lists pain medications	UT-7
Personal data base (PD)	A menu of varied options that allow development and manipulation of a personal database	AN-8
Physicians (JHOC) (JP)	Given a last name and initial, provides an alphabetical listing of JHOC physicians with the full name and ID number	DM-9

Table 2. (*Continued*)

Function Name	Description	Page Number
Physicians, refer-ring (RP)	Given a physician's last name and initial or a begin-ning hospital name, provides an alphabetical list for access to full names, addresses, ID/phone numbers for a specified physician or hospital	DM-10
Plots (P) Preformatted Special order	A graphic/linear representation of related data items showing changes and patterns on a plotted grid	VO-23
Protocol ID (PR)	Provides a protocol list for selection of full protocol name, description, status, and overview	DM-3
Provider schedule (VP)	Provides a current day display of the baseline schedule and times of availability for a provider or nurse	OP-5
Provider summary (PS)	Using a specified date, displays a schedule of appointments with patient names for a specified provider or nurse	OP-6
Registration (R)	Displays a patient's name, address, insurance infor-mation, and pro fee comment	OP-4
Schedule (S) CH	Shows all scheduled appointments, tests, and proce-dures for a requested radiology or medical oncol-ogy patient; user specifies the date	VO-27
Search (S)	Provides the last 10 values of any selected data ele-ment for any patient	VO-16
Transfusions (TR) NS Transfusion plan Transfusion history Transfusion reactions Platelet match-ing data Lymphocytoxic-ity Glossary of blood products	Provides an extensive reference for an individual patient's blood transfusion information	VO-32
Treatment sequence plan (T) X PLAN	Shows a patient's current treatment with start day and number of days on treatment; shows standing orders, daily care plans, clinical findings, and protocol definitions	VO-28
Unlisted functions	See inpatient census section	IP-1

Table 2. (*Continued*)

Function Name	Description	Page Number
View listings		
Patient's by		
protocol		0P-12
Protocol		
descriptions		OP-14
Scheduled		
admits		OP-15
Projected census		OP-16
View option line (V)	A command line that offers a selected patient's abstract, bacti reports, census, scheduling, data, flows, plots and other information	VO-2

patients. This information can be used in patient care, research, or Center management. By first addressing the clinical needs, the data that exist can be applied in other contexts. Chapter 8 discusses these uses of the database.

Research Functions

The Oncology Center conducts both laboratory and clinical research, and participates in four multi-institutional cooperative clinical protocol groups: the Eastern Cooperative Oncology Group, the Pediatric Oncology Group, the Radiation Therapy Oncology Group, and the Gynecology Oncology Group. The OCIS database serves as a central resource to support these activities. Clinical data routinely are copied over into research databases, and the OCIS database has been expanded to record items of interest in a clinical study, for example, outcome measures. In some cases, research laboratory data are also entered into OCIS for use in patient care or integration into clinical research protocols. At any point in time there are well over 150 clinical studies being conducted at the Center— approximately one-half are of a cooperative group nature and one-half are internal. OCIS provides tools to manage the administration of the research and to organize the data to be analyzed.

Users requiring large data extractions from the OCIS system file a request with appropriate OCIS staff and receive clearance. Data requests are scrutinized with regard to the resulting use of data and are cleared through the internal Clinical Research Committee. All requests are accompanied by a formal commitment to maintain patient confidentiality. Additional restrictions are placed on requests for research data coming from outside the Oncology Center.

Within the Center, there also is an increasing trend toward the electronic transfer of data between systems. Because OCIS was designed for clinical patient management, the structure of the OCIS database may require reformatting to manage some aspects of clinical research. As a result, there are plans at the

Center for integrating the hierarchical OCIS database with a relational database. In this model the OCIS database will be used to collect essential clinical data, and the relational database will be used to monitor clinical research activity and provide a natural interface for ad hoc queries or statistical analysis of data. Details are discussed in Chapter 9.

Administration of OCIS

Operation of OCIS is the responsibility of Oncology Information Systems (OIS). This organization has a clinical and research orientation and does not have a primary role in the financial and administrative functions. However, its director is charged with the coordination of the procurement and integration of all Oncology Center computer resources. Some of the facilities located in the Oncology Center are controlled by other Hospital organizations. The satellite pharmacy is the principle example. In what follows, the organization of the Information Center and its computer resources are described.

Oncology Information Systems

The OIS has a full-time staff of 28 that includes a director, a senior manager, a development leader, a maintenance leader, 4 maintenance programmers, 2 development programmers, a systems supervisor, a network supervisor, 5 operators, 8 data collection personnel, a PC technician, and several administrative staff. The great majority of these individuals support the development and maintenance of OCIS. All OIS staff have cross-coverage responsibilities for OCIS.

Figure 3 displays the general information flow, organizational structure, and administrative responsibilities from an Oncology Center perspective. OIS is responsible for the 24-hour-a-day operation of oncology computer and communications equipment, developing communications capabilities with other facilities in the Hospital, the centralization collection of clinical information, and the development and maintenance of the necessary clinical management applications.

A unique position within OIS is that of the clinical data coordinator. The coordinators are assigned to specific clinical units within the Oncology Center and become closely integrated with the units' medical staffs. They are responsible for a variety of routine and specialized data collection and entry tasks. They also serve as the primary physician interface with the system for specialized reports and queries. Thus, although all physicians and medical staff have on-line access to a multitude of generalized data query functions and reports, the OIS staff also provides routine access to the database without requiring special provider action. This is a very helpful feature in an environment in which interns, residents, postgraduate fellows, and attending physicians all change assignments frequently.

The OIS staff also provides clinical data interfaces and technical guidance for other computer-based activities within the Center and throughout the Hospital. The development of specialized applications that are not direct patient care func-

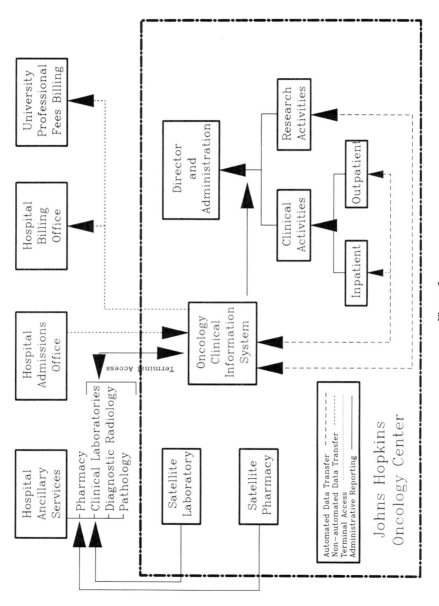

Figure 3.

tions is handled in a decentralized manner. For example, although the centralized collection and management of general clinical research data is the responsibility of the biostatistics component of the Oncology Center, close ties with the OCIS database are essential. The management of the Hospital's Tumor Registry is performed by a hospital-funded component of the Center which is supported by OIS computing resources and staff. Data processing in support of administration is performed by a separate group in OIS that has high-level access to the OCIS database. In most instances, the OIS staff is responsible for recommending automation solutions for other areas of the Center. In many instances OIS both develops and maintains these applications.

OCIS Computer Resources

The OCIS is presently composed of over 5000 TEDIUM programs (9000 MUMPS routines), 1300 relations, and 2500 data elements. The database contains information on over 55,000 individual cancer patients seen throughout The Johns Hopkins Hospital, of which over 20,000 were seen at the Oncology Center. There is on-line information on approximately 500,000 Center patient days. These include over 25,000,000 separate data points. Complete microbacteriology data are available for all Center patients seen after 1984 (approximately 35% of the Center's total patient population).

Data are collected in two ways. The majority of the data is collected electronically from analytic laboratory instruments both within the Center and throughout the Medical Institutions. For laboratories in the Center, data are collected and displayed in real time. Externally recorded data are collected in batches and added to the patient records every two hours. All data are subjected to an extensive validation process before they are added to an active data set.

Where electronic data capture is not possible, as in the case of the recording of vital signs (temperature, pulse, blood pressure), the data are recorded by nurses or doctors in a hard-copy form and later entered by data coordinators and other data entry personnel. (Because the computer requires very little operational support, computer operators perform most of the manual data entry.) Very few individuals have authority to enter data into the system. This limited access to data entry and electronic data capture provides a controlled mechanism for ensuring the completeness and accuracy of data within the system.

Presently, the Oncology Center computing hardware consists of two PDP-11/84[6] computers, one MicroVAX II,[6] and three MicroVAX 3600[6] series computers, and over 140 IBM PCs[7]. These computers are linked over an Ethernet[8] architecture network using distributed database software, namely, InterSystems' M/net[9] and DECnet[6] (See Figure 1). Approximately 170 terminals and 120 personal computers can be connected through a Gandalf StarMaster[10] data switch to

---

[6]PDP-11/84, MicroVAX 360 & MicroVAX II are tradenames of the Digital Equipment Corp. [7]IBM Corp. [8]Xerox Corp. [9]Intersystems Corp. [10]Gandalf Corp.

any of the Oncology computing and peripheral resources. Peripheral resources include a 40-page-per-minute network laser printer that has PostScript capabilities, two 800-line-per-minute line printers, several smaller special-function character printers, and a large-bed plotter. The switch also can serve as a means of low-level communication between PCs within the Oncology Center and for on-line communication with other institutional computing resources. OCIS operates on the two PDP-11/84 computers and two MicroVAX 3600s. It has access to all the other peripherals as well.

The critical role that OCIS plays in the Center requires that it be in operation 7 days a week, 24 hours a day. Although two PDP computers are the minimum required for normal system operation, the system is structured to provide a form of fault tolerance. If one of the computers and/or its associated peripherals fails, all critical functions can be moved to a backup processor until appropriate repair is made. Critical users are virtually remapped through the data switch to be connected with the operational computer should one of the systems fail. The Micro-VAX systems can also serve as backups for each other and the PDP systems. Several very critical applications are maintained concurrently in both the PDP and VAX environments to provide an extremely low probability of extended down time. This backup strategy will be expanded in the future to cover the majority of OCIS functions. Any future functional expansion of OCIS, such as bedside data entry and a user query system, will be placed on the MicroVAX computers. Operators are available 24 hours a day and perform routine maintenance and backup functions for the PDP, VAX, and switching systems.

The Oncology Center network is connected with The Johns Hopkins Hospital Ethernet network through a filtering LAN bridge (See Figure 1). Individual devices can communicate with the Hospital network and associated devices through a Bridge CS-1 interface. The majority of computing facilities within The Johns Hopkins Medical Institutions are connected to this network. Thus, individuals within the Center that have either terminal or PC access to OCIS also have access to a variety of other services within the institution. Such services include medical literature searching, radiology, pathology and laboratory reporting systems, a centralized patient demographic database, and a variety of electronic mail systems. Conversely, with proper authorization, individuals throughout the Medical Institutions have full access to the OCIS database and associated functions. Thus, the information systems within the Oncology Center are integrated with other systems throughout the Hospital.

Future Directions

Luck is a major ingredient in any successful venture. The OCIS is not an exception. When development began in 1976, we had a vision and the courage of the naive. We tried to build a system to help manage a complex process. As described in the chapters that follow, some of our initial goals proved unrealistic. But we adopted a philosophy and structure that demonstrated itself to be remarkably resilient. The OCIS grew and prospered. Technology changed, and networks obscured the boundary between the original OCIS and the automated tools used in the clinical, research, education, and administrative functions of the Oncology Center.

As the basic design philosophy in building the system was one of iteration and evolution, it is likely that there will continue to be ongoing phases of development. These developmental phases will probably include the integration of elements such as parallel processing, enhanced decision support and expert systems, some form of artificial intelligence, and on-line access to image data. However, in each new phase of development the iterative and interactive design philosophy that has made the overall system successful will be repeated and built upon.

The initial developers of OCIS are no longer associated with it; in fact, all have left the Oncology Center. A new generation of managers and developers is presently adding to the system and integrating it with other Johns Hopkins systems. Versions of the OCIS have been exported to two other cancer centers. We hope that readers will learn from what follows and that portions of OCIS will appear in other settings and systems.

2
Data Management in Clinical Decision Making

Raymond E. Lenhard, Jr., M.D.

Introduction

The Oncology Clinical Information System (OCIS) is a comprehensive computing system that provides organized and complete medical information to physicians, nurses, medical students, and other health care providers at logical times in the patient's management. Although implemented in a cancer center, the principles that have been used in its development and many of the applications that are in daily use are equally applicable to general medicine. Physicians caring for patients with cancer face common medical problems that are not specific to patients with cancer. Conversely, physicians in other medical specialties are concerned with the same data management and decision-making issues that confront oncologists.

Decisions in medicine should be based on information that is not only reliable, complete, and timely, but also presented in a way that leads to the correct decision. Many models of computer-assisted decision support have been explored over the last several decades. The differences in these systems seem primarily to be how the responsibility for processing data are distributed between man and machine.

In designing an information system that supports medical decision making, there are several philosophical issues that must be decided. First, one must determine the primary unit of concern. For example, one can design a system around admissions, outpatient visits, billing sequences, or patients. In the episodic care of nonreturning patients, there is no loss of information when each treatment sequence is independent. However, for long-term follow-up and continuing care, as one typically finds in a cancer center setting, any distinction between events and data resulting from admissions and outpatient encounters is artificial. Therefore, the OCIS was designed to manage the information about a patient in an integrated unit so that it could report on findings and therapy regardless of episode, location, or source of care.

The next philosophic issue to be resolved involves the kinds of knowledge to be used by the system. In an artificial intelligence paradigm, the goal is to have the necessary knowledge stored in the computer to guide the diagnostic or patient management decision making. Heuristics provide satisfactory (as opposed to optimal) advice, and much of the effort in developing a knowledge-based system goes into the process of collecting and formalizing that knowledge base (an activity called knowledge engineering). For complex medical domains, however, these artificial intelligence applications are still research programs.

If one recognizes, therefore, that it is premature to organize most of the medical knowledge used to diagnose and manage patient care in a knowledge base, then alternative forms of knowledge organization are required. In the design of the OCIS we have divided the responsibility of knowledge management between the physician and the system. All knowledge organization activities that can be described with some precision (i.e., are routine or can be stated algorithmically) are relegated to the system. Examples include the organization of clinical data in medically meaningful ways, the capture of routine therapy clusters and formal protocol sequences, and the association of data displays with clinical situations. Clearly, these system data organization tasks represent functions that should be both natural and designed to assist the provider in applying his or her knowledge. In this case the OCIS exhibits its intelligence by reducing the information overload and presenting the data in forms that help in rapidly finding the best solutions to the current medical problems.

The third philosophical issue to be decided relates to system closure. That is, how closely linked should the system be to the operational process. For example, a laboratory system is closed with respect to orders, result reporting, and charge determination; every order that comes in must produce a result and some charge action. However, the laboratory system is not closed in the care process; its reports may be unread, and there may be no response to abnormal results. Of course, systems with alerts attempt to close this processing loop by demanding a response when certain events are recognized. In the case of OCIS, the goal is for the system to behave in an intelligent manner and complement the physician's knowledge. This implies that the system must be integrated into the care process so that it can respond appropriately. Thus, it must know something about the patient's status to produce the most effective reports.

In summary, then, we see that the OCIS was designed to store and organize all patient data in an integrated fashion. It also manages well-understood knowledge to assist a broad range of medical providers in the various aspects of patient care. To be effective, it is necessary that the OCIS be integrated into the care process. Where recommendations are made, it is essential that the OCIS be informed of the resulting action. However, it is equally important that the OCIS not intrude on the process. It should be perceived to be a useful tool. For some providers, there may not even be an awareness of its presence — only a recognition that the Oncology Center always manages its medical records in this way. In these situations the OCIS is a clear success; it invisibly supplies an intelligent data management facility that naturally supports the physician's decision making.

The remainder of this chapter illustrates how clinical data are related to patient management and how OCIS, designed to meet the preceding philosophical objectives, supports the process. The organization of the automated medical record is described first. It is presented as a layered structure in which the patient's name and identifier are at the top; below it are the census data that record major events, and below that is the abstract that contains an overview of the medical record narrative. The clinical data provide additional information, and a variety of formats and reports is available to complement the physician's knowledge. Several clinical examples are given; these illustrate how this intelligent display of data improves patient care. More detailed descriptions of the OCIS tools are contained in the chapters of Part II.

Patient Identification and Census

In a hospital or group practice there is considerable cross-coverage of patients by physicians and office nurses. Patients who come to the outpatient clinic or emergency room, or telephone a general number for the practice need to be identified as belonging to the practice group. They can be served best if the person responding to the patient has rapid access to information about their diagnosis and current treatment.

First, the patient must be identified as a participant in that care system. The OCIS census provides the correct name, history number, age, and diagnosis. In addition, the date on which the patient was first seen and the last outpatient visit are immediately available. All hospital stays with admission and discharge data and reason for admission are also displayed. This information is available on line, 24 hours a day, for 56,000 patients. It is an example of administrative information that is collected as a by-product of each encounter and not specifically entered into the system for this purpose. Figure 1 shows a typical encounter screen as it might be used by a registrar, primary nurse, or physician to identify the patient.

The Abstract

The abstract is, as the name implies, a collection of pertinent information presented in abstracted form for rapid reference during the course of diagnosis and treatment (Figure 2). An OCIS abstract is completed on all patients at The Johns Hopkins Oncology Center and is available on line, as is all other information, 24 hours a day, 7 days a week.

Based on the data collected on all patients by The Johns Hopkins Hospital Tumor Registry, the abstract contains medical information presented in chronological order in a sequence similar to that used by physicians to describe a patient to a colleague. The demographics are commonly used by care providers to contact the patient or their relatives. The diagnosis section provides ICD-9 coded

```
7779992   PATIENT,THREE                 36 W F  LUNG, ADENOCARCINOMA

     2N PRIMARY NURSE: CATHY    2N ASSOCIATE NURSE: MARTHA

 OUTPATIENT VISITS
  FIRST MED/550 VISIT: 11/03/87
  LAST MED/550 VISIT: 04/20/88
  FIRST RAD ONC VISIT: 10/30/87
  LAST RAD ONC VISIT: 04/08/88
 ADMISSIONS
  2N      11/03/87  11/09/87 DISCHARGED 6   R/O CORD COMPRESSION
  2N      11/15/87  11/18/87 DISCHARGED 3   5FU
                                            CHEMOTHERAPY
  2N      03/14/88  03/18/88 DISCHARGED 4   MYELOGRAM,PAIN CONTROL
  2N      03/21/88  03/24/88 DISCHARGED 3
                                            OTHER COMPLICATIONS
  2N      03/30/88  04/01/88 DISCHARGED 2   MRI/CORD COMPRESSION
                                            OTHER COMPLICATIONS
 PROTOCOL ACTIVITY
  INDIV   2N        11/07/87
                      COMMENT: CYT-ADRIA-MTX-5-FU-LEUCOVORIN

 REFFERING PHYSICIAN/HOSPITAL
       PHYSICIAN,TEST    REFERRING/FOLLOWING PHYSICIAN
                   413 TULIP LANE
                   ANYWHERE, MI 49043      1-555-1212
```

Figure 1. A typical encounter screen.

diagnoses and other Tumor Registry information. In addition, the free text report of the pathology or cytopathology diagnosis is collected on each patient as part of the Tumor Registry data entry function.

Following the diagnostic information, a table of chronological events is presented. These data are entered by data coordinators and summarize each hospitalization and each change in treatment. Each entry is a single line of text showing pertinent diagnostic tests, procedures, and treatments. Surgical procedures, such as biopsies and their results, are included, as are major surgical therapeutic procedures. In addition, tests, such as estrogen receptors in breast cancer and the presence of hormone or tumor markers such as CEA, AFP, or myeloma protein, are shown with their numerical results.

Treatments also are shown in the abstract. Radiation therapy is described by site, total dose, and the duration of treatment, but not in such detail as specific field size, dose fractions, or treatment machine source. A typical radiation therapy statement is shown in Figure 2, recording that 5000 rads were given to the right chest wall and 4500 rads to the right supraclavicular area and showing the associated dates of treatment. Chemotherapy and hormone administration are similarly collected, showing what drug was given, the dose fraction, and duration, but not cumulative dose. Figure 2 shows that Tamoxifen was administered beginning in June 1987.

The next section in the abstract is a short history and physical examination section with information about the patient's occupations, toxic exposures, and cancer-related personal lifestyle factors, such as smoking history.

Finally, the abstract provides updated information on which physicians and nurses are responsible for the care of the patient. Both the doctor following the patient at Johns Hopkins and the personal physician and referring physician in the community are listed. This information provides an important link to the patient's primary physician and shows where follow-up care will be given and follow-up information should be sent.

JOHNS HOPKINS HOSPITAL
ONCOLOGY CENTER

HISTORY NO: 777 99 91
NAME: PATIENT,TWO
DATE: 04/26/88

PATIENT,TWO
1234 ADDRESS ROAD
ANYWHERE, MI 48043

PHONE 999-9999   CLASS ONCOLOGY
SPOUSE   SEER 021/21093
BIRTH DATE 01/01/27   POB 999
        MAR. STATUS SINGLE

SEX FEMALE   RACE CAUCASIAN
MOTHER/FATHER PATIENT,MOTHER - PATIENT,FATHER
FOLLOW UP STATUS: 02/88 NO EVIDENCE OF DISEASE

```
: DIAGNOSIS PRIMARY - 1
:--------------------------------------------------------------------
:SURVIVAL TIME:  0 YEAR(S)  11 MONTH(S)      AGE AT DX: 60
:--------------------------------------------------------------------
:   JHH DIAGNOSIS     03/13/87  CARCINOMA OF RIGHT BREAST
:
:SITE:                174.2    UPPER-INNER QUADRANT OF BREAST
:MORPHOLOGY:          8500/39  INFILTRATING DUCT CARCINOMA
:GRADE:               NOT DETERMINED, N/S, N/A
:LATERALITY:          RIGHT ORIGIN OF PRIMARY
:EXTENT:              LOCALIZED
:    METASTATIC SITES:    NONE
:    STAGE IDENTIFIER:    STAGE I T2 N0 M0 PER RAD ONC
:TUMOR SIZE:          3.5 X 3 X 3 CM
:BASIS OF DIAGNOSIS:  HISTOLOGY, CYTOLOGY, X-RAY (CT SCAN OF CHEST AND
:                     ABD)
:
:REPORT SECTION
:
:   NM4329 - CYTOLOGY - BREAST ASPIRATION: CONSISTENT WITH ADENOCARCINOMA.
:
:   87-4670 - 1,2,3,4. RIGHT BREAST AND AXILLA (SIMPLE MASTECTOMY AND
:AXILLARY LYMPH NODE DISSECTION): INFILTRATING DUCT CARCINOMA OF BREAST. THE
:SKIN, NIPPLE AND TWENTY-SIX (26) AXILLARY LYMPH NODES ARE NEGATIVE FOR
:TUMOR. 5. INTERPECTORAL REGION (BX): ONE (1) LYMPH NODE NEGATIVE FOR TUMOR.
:SPECIAL NOTES:
:
:   BONE SCAN AND CT SCAN OF THE CHEST WERE NEGATIVE FOR TUMOR. CT SCAN OF
:THE CHEST AND ABDOMEN (03/03/87) 3 CM MASS MEDIAL ASPECT OF RIGHT BREAST
:MOST CONSISTENT WITH A CARCINOMA. TUMOR MARKER: CEA 2.0
:
:--------------------------------------------------------------------
: TREATMENT PRIMARY - 1
:--------------------------------------------------------------------
: FROM      TO    : LOC : TYPE : PURP : DESCRIPTION
:03/03/87:        : JHH : D    :      : CT SCAN OF CHEST AND ABD
:03/13/87:        : JHH : B    :      : NEEDLE BIOPSY RIGHT BREAST MASS
:                 :     :      :      : (NM4329)
:03/18/87:        : JHH : S    :      : SIMPLE MASTECTOMY AND AXILLARY
:                 :     :      :      : LYMPH NODE DISSECTION (87-4670)
:03/18/87:        : JHH : E    :      : 200 (ER), 11 (PR)
:05/14/87:06/19/87: JHH : R    :      : RIGHT CHEST WALL, 5000R X 36 DAYS
:05/15/87:06/22/87: JHH : R    :      : RIGHT SUPRACLAVICULAR REGION, 4500R
:                 :     :      :      : X 32 DAYS
:06/09/87:        : JHH : C    :      : TAMOXIFEN
:--------------------------------------------------------------------
: PROTOCOL ACTIVITY
:--------------------------------------------------------------------
:                    NO PROTOCOL ACTIVITY
:--------------------------------------------------------------------
: HISTORY
:--------------------------------------------------------------------
:ONSET OF SYMPTOMS:   MASS NOTED IN RIGHT BREAST 2/87.
:FAMILY HISTORY:      MOTHER AND SISTER WITH BREAST CARCINOMA - MOTHER
:                     DIED  WITH CARCINOMA.
:MEDICAL HISTORY:     HYPERTENSION
:CONGENITAL DEFECTS:  NEG
:ALLERGY:             NEG
:OCCUPATION:          SECRETARY
:EXPOSURE:            N/S
:COMMENTS:
:--------------------------------------------------------------------
: FOLLOW UP
:--------------------------------------------------------------------
: DATE  : LST SN : COND : QUAL : SOURCE COMMENTS
:       : 09/87  : NED  : SU   : PER MED ONC
:       : 11/87  : NED  : SU   : PER ONC OPD NOTE
:       : 02/88  : NED  : SU   : PER RAD ONC CLINIC NOTE
:--------------------------------------------------------------------
:PHYSICIAN/HOSPITAL REFERENCE
:    PHYSICIAN,TEST   REFERRING/FOLLOWING PHYSICIAN
:                 413 TULIP LANE
:                 ANYWHERE, MI 49043   1-555-1212
:
:MED ONC   CLINIC LAST VISITED
:--------------------------------------------------------------------
            END OF ABSTRACT
```

Inpatient Data Management

OCIS was primarily intended to help support information management of complex patients with chronic medical problems who have repeated admissions to the hospital and frequent outpatient visits.

Patients on the acute inpatient nursing unit present a special problem in data management. This is because of the large volume of information that is returned and the way in which that information is collected and reported. Requests for laboratory services are sent in chronological order, but each laboratory test has a different time required for completion and return of results to the requesting physician. In a high-data-volume environment, the physician finds it difficult to recall which tests have been reported and which are still pending. In addition, when the tests results return, they are not delivered in the same chronological order in which they were sent. Physicians spend considerable time organizing this information either on paper or in their memory. Frequently, they are required to telephone several laboratories to get recent information that may not have been reported to them. This manual time-consuming effort is driven by the level of illness of the patient and the urgency for getting information as quickly as possible. As physicians have only a limited amount of time to allocate to each patient, time spent correcting errors of omission and processing data must compete for time spent in direct patient care and family interactions and in making decisions based on available information. OCIS is designed to substitute for this manual effort and to free the physician's time for patient care and decision making.

At Johns Hopkins and many other hospitals, a common organizational plan is the clustering of patients with similar medical problems on a single inpatient unit. This is done as a logical extension of medical specialization to provide optimal medical care. In the Oncology Center, acute leukemia, bone marrow transplantation, and other specialized diseases are clustered on a single nursing unit. Of course, this is not unique to oncology as renal dialysis units, coronary care units, and other facilities are also designed around specific illnesses. Although this makes the management of patients more effective, using nurse specialists and specially trained medical support personnel who will respond to a medical emergency in a reliable and consistent way, it makes data management more difficult. Not only do these patients have large amounts of information returning to the physician for evaluation, but the problem of assessing the importance of each individual value is accentuated because of the similarity of the patients housed on that unit. Patients in kidney failure clustered on a dialysis unit all have very similar problems, and each has a similar limited set of laboratory results that define his or her disease and treatment status. Gathering a full set of laboratory values, ensuring that there are no missing data, and then weighing this information against other related data and against itself as it changes over time constitute a major source of information overload for physicians.

◄ **Figure 2.** An OCIS abstract.

An Example

A good example of how OCIS was designed to manage the problem of information processing can be illustrated by a clinical inpatient unit containing ten patients with acute leukemia. We shall follow this scenario of acute leukemia management throughout the next several sections. In these illustrative cases dates have been artificially compressed and several weeks of hospitalization are truncated for ease of discussion.

Patients with leukemia have indicators of their primary illness that can be quantified in the laboratory and reported as a numerical value. These markers are the white blood cell count and the white blood cell differential. These cells, which both define the presence of the disease and quantify its extent, are both enumerated and examined for morphological characteristics. Enumeration generally is done by an automated particle counter linked to a computer. The results are expressed as particles (cells) per cubic millimeter (mm^3) of fluid (blood). For example, the white blood cell count (wbc) may be reported as $7000/mm^3$.

Leukemia is characterized by both increased numbers of cells circulating in the blood and the abnormal morphology of these cells, determined by examining stained fixed blood smears under a microscope. Treatment strategy is based on the administration of medications or groups of medications from different chemical classes to destroy the leukemic cells and their precursors, but leave the normal cell precursors relatively intact. Successful treatment outcome is assessed by a return of normal white blood cells to normal numbers and the absence of all abnormal leukemic cells. To reach this successful outcome (commonly referred to as a complete remission), patients must be supported through at least three major medical complications of the disease and its treatment. These are:

Infection. There is an increase in the risk of infection because of the disease. This risk is made worse by chemotherapy, which further lowers the remaining normal white blood cells, making the patient highly susceptible to infection and at high risk of dying, unless the presence of infection is detected and treated in a timely and appropriate fashion.

Hemorrhage. Because there is a lowering of the patient's platelet count by both the disease and the chemotherapy, patients are at risk of bleeding because of their inability to carry out normal blood clotting. The support strategy for this complication is the administration of transfusions of platelets derived from normal donors, to provide the necessary numbers of platelets needed for normal clotting. Platelet transfusions are administered daily until the patient's normal platelets recover.

Complex medical problems. Fluid and electrolyte balance is an example of the difficult medical problems requiring attention to detail and repetitive calculations. A balance must be maintained between the amount of salt and fluids taken in by mouth or by intravenous drip and the amount of fluid that is put out through urine, perspiration, and bowel movements.

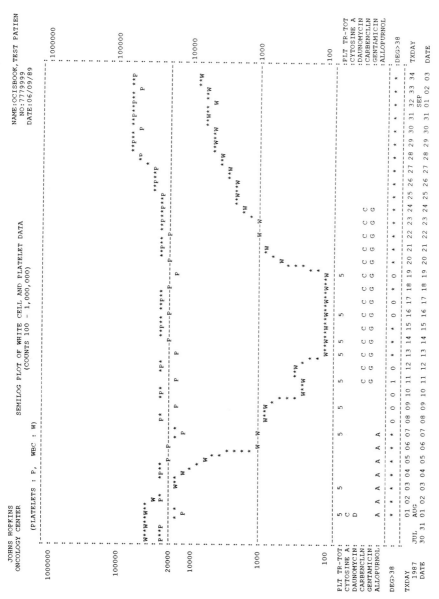

Figure 3. Semilog plot of white cell and platelet data.

```
JOHNS HOPKINS ONCOLOGY CENTER                 HISTORY NO: 777 99 99
                                              NAME: OCISBOOK,TEST PATIENT
                                              DATE: 06/13/89
COMP FLOW                                                FILE COPY      1
                                                         PAGE  1
:----------------:-------:-------:-------:-------:-------:-------:-------:
:                :30JUL87:31JUL87:01AUG87:02AUG87:03AUG87:04AUG87:05AUG87:
:    TXDAY       :       :       :DAY  1:DAY  2:DAY  3:DAY  4:DAY  5:
:PAT STATUS------:-------:-------:-------:-------:-------:-------:-------:
:TEMP-MAX   DEG C:       :       :  37.0:  37.2:  37.0:  37.3:  37.3:
:BODY WT AM KG   :       :       :    54:    54:    54:    56:  56.5:
:TOTL INTAK ML   :       :       :   2.5:   3.5:   3.0:   4.0:   3.5:
:TOTL OUT   ML   :       :       :   1.5:   2.0:   1.5:   2.0:   1.5:
:IN/OUT DIF ML   :       :       :   1.0:   1.5:   1.5:   2.0:   2.0:
:BLD PROD  ------:-------:-------:-------:-------:-------:-------:-------:
:PLT TR-TOT      :       :       :     5:       :     5:       :       :
:HEMATOLOGY------:-------:-------:-------:-------:-------:-------:-------:
:WBC       #/CU :  40000* 42000* 39000* 30000* 15000*  12000:   5000:
:PLATELETS /MM3 :  24000* 26000* 12000* 22000* 16000* 25000* 20000*
:SGGT      MIU/L:       :       :       :       :       :       :       :
:OUT CTS   ------:-------:-------:-------:-------:-------:-------:-------:
:MEDICATION------:-------:-------:-------:-------:-------:-------:-------:
:CYTOSINE A MG   :       :       :    50:       :       :       :       :
:DAUNOMYCIN MG   :       :       :    20:       :       :       :       :
:ALLOPURNOL MG   :       :       :   100:   100:   100:   100:   100:
:----------------:-------:-------:-------:-------:-------:-------:-------:
```

Figure 4. Comp flow screen.

Each of the above demonstrates a need for rapid, accurate, and well-correlated data presented in formats that show related information from tests done in several laboratories displayed relative to each other. Figure 3 shows a typical, relatively uncomplicated, clinical course of a single patient and is described in some detail.

Infection. Just before treatment on August 1, the white blood cell count (w) is elevated to 40,000/mm.[3] This is significantly higher than normal (between 4500 and 11,000/mm.[3]) In addition, the platelet count (p) is depressed to fewer than 20,000 because of the leukemia (normal platelet count 150-350,000/mm^3). Two treatments (chemotherapy and platelet transfusion) are therefore shown along the bottom of the plot. The first is chemotherapy for the primary disease to destroy the leukemic cells. This is administered on August 1 (treatment day 1) and is shown at the bottom of the figure as days that Daunomycin (daunorubicin) and Cytosine A (cytosine arabinoside) are given. Neither dose nor schedule is shown on the graph, but only the fact that on that day treatment was administered. This same information is shown in detail in Figure 4, where the actual doses and blood counts are displayed.

Chemotherapy drug doses are frequently calculated on the basis of milligrams per square meter of the patient's body surface area. OCIS assists in chemotherapy administration by providing a facility for doctors, nurses, and other staff to calculate the patient's body surface as a function of height and weight. This calculation can be used by the physician to plan the original dose, by the nurse as a verification before administering the medication, and by the pharmacist in preparing the medication for administration. These internal checks lessen the risk of dose miscalculation for medications that are used at the high levels of tolerance at which overdose can be a risk to the patient's life.

As the administration of chemotherapy is a major event, it is often used as the starting point for measuring the time to the occurrence of many other events. OCIS provides a chronological "event counter," which can be started at the time of a treatment or other specified event. This is seen at the bottom of Figure 3. It shows that the day on which the two chemotherapy treatments were administered is day "one" (August 1, 1987).

The toxic results of chemotherapy on the white blood cell count can be recognized in Figures 3 and 4. The disease responds as expected with the white blood cell count falling from 40,000/mm³ to 800/mm³ by the eighth day following chemotherapy. This is a graphic representation of a successful response to treatment and shows that the appropriate medication was selected.

As noted above, successful treatment requires major support for infectious disease, bleeding, and fluid balance. On day 11 after chemotherapy, the anticipated infection emerges. This can be seen in the OCIS displays in two ways. First, on the standard white blood cell and platelet count graph, an asterisk is displayed along the bottom line to indicate that the patient has a normal temperature on that date. When the asterisk is replaced by a number, it indicates the number of degrees above 38.3°C, a threshold that requires that the patient be started on antibiotics. Actual temperature values are displayed in Figure 4, and graphically (T) in Figure 5. In this figure another important feature of OCIS is shown, the use of threshold lines. A horizontal line has been drawn across the entire graph at the level of a temperature of 38.3°C. In the medical setting described here, all numbers below this temperature are normal, and all above are abnormal and require immediate antibiotic administration following a predetermined treatment plan. These guides to treatment decisions have high visual impact and help the physician, nurse, and other care providers to separate at a glance patients who are normal from those who have abnormal findings.

Medical response to common clinical problems have been reduced to a standard regimen to help doctors, nurses, and other technical personnel respond rapidly in a preplanned fashion. It is known that all patients with low white blood counts have a risk of infection. Therefore, it is the physician's job to detect the problem promptly, to weigh successfully the importance of fever in the clinical setting, and to react appropriately. This commonly happens late at night when a full staff of senior physicians is not immediately available for consultation. The algorithm for infection states that when a patient's white blood cell count is less than 1000/mm³, and the temperature is greater than 38.3°C, then antibiotics must be started, as the patient is presumed to have a life-threatening infection that must be treated immediately. This protocol-driven medical approach has been shown to prevent sudden death from acute overwhelming bacterial infection in this class of patients. Rapid initiation of treatment with antibiotics that are lethal to bacteria is credited as one of the most important support strategies in this disease. This has allowed patients to be entered safely into high-risk chemotherapy treatment protocols that are designed to be curative, but require meticulous attention to detail.

In a clinical setting where there are multiple patients with leukemia in an inpatient unit, each is at a different point in time in his or her treatment course. The sorting and weighting of information are time-consuming manual tasks that are not easily done by the least senior member of the medical staff in an emergency situation. OCIS displays link medical treatment to specific indicators. In this way

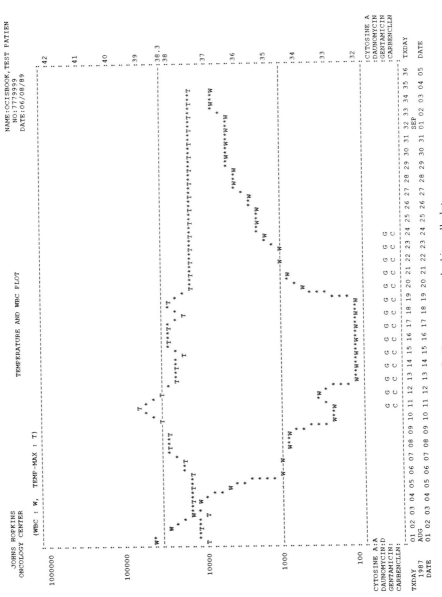

Figure 5. Temperature and white cell plot.

OCIS applies the experience and knowledge of senior staff to influencing decisions that are made in a defined clinical setting without requiring senior staff members to be physically present. This use of routine support plans is part of the goal of OCIS and has proved to be one of its most successful features.

In this illustrative case antibiotics were begun on day 11 when the patient's temperature rose to 39.0°C. The correctness of the selection of antibiotics and the timeliness of the decision were verified by a prompt return of the temperature to below the fever threshold level. Antibiotics were then continued until both the patient remained free of fever and his white blood cell count (composed of normal rather than leukemic cells) returned to safe levels above 1000/mm³. Then, antibiotics were carefully withdrawn. The patient's temperature remained normal and the risk of acute sepsis was judged to be over.

Hemorrhage. Platelets are the necessary normal blood component for allowing blood to clot to prevent or stop bleeding. Returning to Figure 3, one can see that the patient had a platelet count on admission of 24,000/mm³. Our experience has taught us that the risk of hemorrhage rises above an acceptable level when the platelet count is less than 20,000. Therefore, on this graph, a second limit line is drawn at 20,000 using the scale on the right of the graph to assist in blood product support. Blood Bank transfusion specialists monitor the status of all patients being treated for any cancer in the Oncology Center and, by following the slope and direction of the plot, they can anticipate the need for transfusion and have preplanned blood products ready for transfusion of patients. Using OCIS, the Blood Bank has developed a creative prospective inventory and donor management program to provide high-quality and timely platelet transfusion services, while minimizing operating overhead and the need to respond to unexpected emergency demands. As shown on the graph, on August 1 the patient's platelets were below 20,000 and platelet transfusions were correctly administered, resulting in a rise of the platelets above 20,000 on the following day.

The administration of life-saving human-derived platelet products that are in short supply (as well as the quality control review of our support system) can be monitored by senior staff members using this tool. Each transfusion is shown as a number showing how many units of platelets were given. This also is presented in tabular form in Figure 4. As the patient's leukemia improves, the platelet counts advance toward normal. The fact that the counts are maintained spontaneously, without the need for additional platelet transfusions, is evidence for the success of the treatment.

Management of Fluid Balance. The third support problem to be discussed is the management of fluid balance. This problem is common to the management of heart, liver, and kidney disease, and it serves as a good example of the generalization of OCIS applications to the management of a broad range of medical problems.

The related data in the management of this problem are patient body weight, amount of fluid taken in as oral and intravenous fluids, fluid lost in urine, bowel movements and from the skin, and proportions of salts taken in and lost. These relations change with activity and temperature, and both foods and medications may contain large amounts of salt. In the ill patient, the normal mechanisms for regulating this complicated equilibrium are frequently dysfunctional. The physician needs to help manage these factors and relies heavily on measurement of the daily weight and the input and loss of fluids. Graphic representation of these relations are helpful. On such a plot, a line can be drawn from the baseline weight and used to show change up or down from that number. Fluid and salt equilibrium should correlate with body weight. The persistence of an input/output imbalance, with more fluid taken in than is lost, can place a strain on the heart and lead to accumulation of fluid in the lungs and resultant respiratory distress, an emergency that requires prompt action.

Sodium salt is closely linked with fluid balance in this medical problem. Salt intake contributes to fluid retention and its balance must also be calculated, adding further to the complexity of this management problem. With the amount of sodium salt administered to the patient coming from a variety of sources, such as food, medications, and intravenous fluids, the calculation of sodium input may be difficult to obtain. The most important measure may be a global evaluation of the dynamic relationship between the patient's weight and fluid input/output balance. Further sophistication of this measurement, to provide a more accurate clinical management plot, can be built into the system in models that account for insensible loss of fluid through the skin relative to patient temperature and loss of sodium via other body fluids.

Assessment of Clinical Data—Implied Intelligence

Laboratory and clinical data are usually not assessed as abstract numbers in the practice of medicine. Most data must be clustered with related data items to be clinically relevant. The magnitude of difference between sequential values and the rate of change between these values are both critical for medical decisions. A scenario using a kidney function test, such as serum creatinine, illustrates this point.

The chemistry laboratory has reported an abnormal value of 4 mg/dl. This value is well above the normal range (<1.2 mg/dl) and should be reported immediately to the physician as emergency intervention may be needed.

The physician's responsibility is to respond appropriately to this value. There are several possible clinical settings that would lead to completely different interpretations of this abnormal value.

Two weeks ago the patient was seen as an outpatient and the serum creatinine was 1.2 mg/dl. A rapid increase to 4.0 mg/dl represents a serious emergency. The patient needs to be seen immediately and admitted to the hospital for acute medical management.

Two weeks ago the patient's creatinine was 4 mg/dl. The patient has chronic kidney failure and nothing has changed over the last two weeks. The result of 4 mg, although abnormal, is stable and represents a chronic condition calling for no new medical treatment. The patient does not need emergency care.

Two weeks ago the serum creatinine was 7.5 mg/dl. Over the last two weeks medical management has succeeded in decreasing the creatinine to 4.0. This represents not an emergency, but a sign of improvement and successful therapeutic response to current management. In this instance the result viewed by the laboratory as an emergency is actually an indication that the current treatments are successful.

A laboratory value, therefore, cannot be considered an absolute number and cannot be evaluated without knowing the last value and the rate and direction of change between these numbers. Clinical information systems should take these simple principles into consideration. Modern automated systems should include this level of "implied intelligence."

The OCIS organizes the patient data so that they may be viewed in medically meaningful presentations. Examples of groupings that present data from more than one database include:

Serum calcium displayed with the serum albumin so that bound and unbound serum calcium can be considered.

Cerebral spinal fluid glucose, simultaneous serum glucose, and CSF white blood cell count displayed together. This example is also an educational comment from the system for, if one or more of these values is not present in the system, the physician can be made aware that evaluation of the CSF glucose, in the absence of the other two values, may be unreliable.

The use of tabular and graphic information and meaningful groupings are two examples of implied intelligence that appear throughout the OCIS system. Many of the tables and graphs are prepared by specialists on the senior faculty and help to give less experienced doctors and nurses displays of data that not only show the results, but also suggest an appropriate action that might be taken in response to those results. The OCIS developers believe strongly that information systems have a responsibility for displaying data in a way that increases the likelihood of the physician's arriving at the correct decision in the most timely fashion. Therefore, the expansion of this function is a key goal in all subsequent phases of development.

Outpatients

Medicine is increasingly being practiced in an outpatient setting. Although many of the data items are the same, the information-processing environment is entirely different from the acute inpatient setting described above. Patient visits to the outpatient clinic are episodic, with irregular intervals of time between encounters. The physician sees many other patients in the time between outpatient visits, and it is often difficult to recall pertinent facts for any given patient and to assess accurately which laboratory results are changing and how rapidly change is occurring. In addition, many laboratory tests are either carried out at the completion of a visit or requested to be done at the next visit. Consequently,

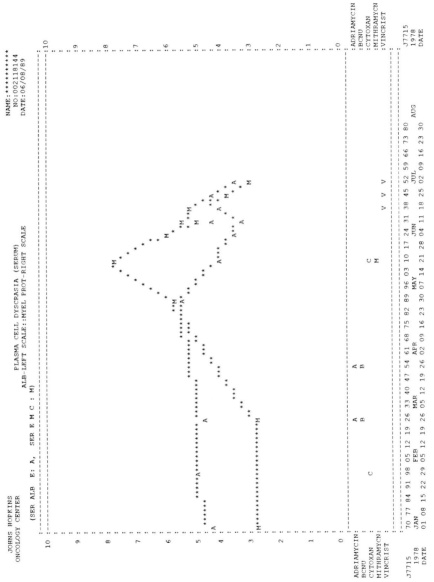

Figure 6. Plasma cell dyscrasia.

there are long delays between the time an action is initiated and the results of the action are reported.

When the laboratory or radiographic results are reported, correlation with previous values necessitates the retrieval of a chart that has been returned to the file. This process of outpatient results reporting and the frequency of delays in retrieving the paper chart lead to a dependence on the physician's memory for recall of previous laboratory values and tend to focus the physician on those results that are significantly abnormal. Subtle, slowing changing trends are easily overlooked until the absolute value becomes sufficiently abnormal to call attention to itself. Slowly progressive anemia, weight loss, or an increasing laboratory marker of extent of disease, such as the CEA test, are all examples of this clinical problem.

A good example of the worth of an information system in monitoring long-term trends in chronic disease is illustrated by the protein marker of multiple myeloma. Figure 6 shows the M-protein measured over a six-month period and demonstrates a gradual worsening of the disease that takes place in weekly or monthly intervals rather than the hourly or daily dramatic changes illustrated previously in the inpatient setting. If early intervention is important in reversing a disease process before symptoms appear or serious organ dysfunction occurs, then long-term trend analysis by either graphic or mathematical means requires an information system that takes into consideration outpatient events and integrates inpatient and outpatient data. It also emphasizes the need for prospective reminders for collection of information at appropriate intervals, such as routine follow-up "pap" smears, chest x-rays, or measurement of a blood test marker of disease. Modern information systems need to support the practice of anticipatory medicine by showing early trends that can be modified by outpatient care, thus avoiding emergencies that could have been anticipated by the careful analysis of trends of multiple variables. This approach is medically important but difficult to achieve in an outpatient setting that relies exclusively on a paper record. As outpatient medicine becomes the standard of care, outpatient information systems are becoming a necessity.

Research Support

A by-product of the OCIS system is the support of clinical research. All information collected for medical management can be used both for prospective as well as retrospective analysis. The data are easily accessed and organized into treatment groups. The use of this information for research also emphasizes the need for careful control of the quality of data collection and enhances the credibility of the system for clinical care. The system has been invaluable for detecting unexpected toxicities by collecting individual data and grouping them into research clusters. Such a grouping can help the investigator to recognize an abnormality that occurs in several patients at a specific period of time after a new treatment is given, instead of interpreting it as an unusual event in an individual patient.

To support this level of analysis, OCIS allows down-loading of information into a clinical research database for further statistical analysis using other computers and statistical tools. It also assists the Cancer Center Research Office, which collects and enters into the general system dates of entry for a study, completion of the study for a particular patient, and assessment of results of treatment. By using electronic mail, notification and updating of information between the clinical areas and the research office are facilitated. Investigators are able to search the database and derive lists of patients who are in their studies and to monitor centrally the collection of information and its quality. The database can be searched periodically by the study chairman to monitor the progress of patients in the study and to determine whether appropriate testing was done by the staff collaborating on the study.

Research reminders can be linked to the appointment system. Much clinical research is directed by prospective protocols. In this environment a group of patients to be studied is defined, treatments to be studied are described, and a set of parameters to be measured to assess the effects of the treatment are selected. These need to be collected at predefined intervals to allow analysis of similar values collected at similar intervals from a time of intervention. The data collection system can be supported by a simple scheduling system, and compliance with the plan can be monitored by a patient query shortly after the scheduled visit to ensure correct and complete collection and to detect errors in a timely enough way to allow for corrective action to take place. If a well-directed medical information system is in place, the additional costs of clinical research can be minimized and the power of the entire system augmented by incremental additions of special research information to the basic medical data set, providing additional benefit to the clinician while serving the needs of clinical research.

Summary

OCIS was originally designed as a medical support system functioning in the environment of a cancer center, but our experience with it is generalizable to the management of medical problems seen in a community hospital. The system's success is due in large part to the accuracy, timeliness, and relevance of the information contained. It is important that clinicians perceive that it provides valuable information and that by using OCIS, the quality of medical care is improved. With the focus of medical care moving from the inpatient to the outpatient setting, OCIS becomes an increasingly powerful tool for integrating medical management of inpatients and outpatients. This patient-oriented approach can limit the cost of medical care by supporting planned collection of information before a patient is admitted to the hospital and carrying inpatient information forward into the outpatient clinic for continuity of care. OCIS is a good model for hospital systems of the 1990s.

3
Development History
Bruce I. Blum

Introduction

This chapter presents a historical overview of the OCIS. Because the OCIS is a software system, this history is necessarily one of software development. There are two basic themes in this chapter. The first, which is consistent with the central focus of this book, concentrates on what the OCIS does and how it is used. The second is that of software implementation—especially in the context of clinical information systems. In this view the OCIS is considered a case study.

The development of the OCIS did not occur in a vacuum; there were many interacting and overlapping events that affected its design and application. For example, a new development environment TEDIUM[1] was used in the second phase of OCIS implementation. This impacted the development process and also provided new insights into the process. Also, experience with the OCIS was carried over to the implementation of clinical information systems elsewhere in the hospital.

As one of the lead designers, I clearly left my mark on the OCIS. At the same time, the development of the OCIS taught me much about medical informatics and software engineering. I would like to capture some of that exchange in this chapter. Therefore, I shall use the first person singular to indicate my recollections and opinions, and I shall present the history from a very personal (as opposed to institutional) perspective.

The remainder of the chapter is divided into four sections. The first contains an overview of the software development process (or software process as it is now called). The goal is to establish a common understanding of how systems are implemented. The next section presents a summary of the OCIS development history. This is described from a functional perspective, that is, what did the OCIS do and when did it do it? The third section contains an overview of the tools

---

[1]TEDIUM is a trademark of Tedious Enterprises, Inc.

that the development team used: MUMPS and TEDIUM. The final section evaluates OCIS with a special emphasis on the development activity.

For persons with a limited computer background, reading the first two sections may be sufficient. The section on the software tools is oriented to technical readers and is not necessary for an understanding of the project history. The final evaluation section reports on data collected to help us calibrate the development effort. It is technically oriented, and we believe that it will be of interest to many of the readers; most of the clinical evaluations, however, are included in the chapters in Part II.

The Software Process

Software engineering is the discipline concerned with the process of implementing and maintaining large computer applications. The goals of software engineering are to deliver and maintain the necessary functionality and quality in the required time period within the budgeted costs. There are several "life cycle models" that have been designed to facilitate the management of the process. The first subsection describes the most commonly used development approach, the "waterfall model." The next subsection examines the software process from a different "essential" perspective, and the final subsection concludes with some observations about software development and the OCIS.

The Waterfall Software Life Cycle Model

This model gets its name from the "waterfall diagram" presented in Figure 1. As shown there, the model organizes the development process into a series of steps or phases. The output of one phase becomes the input to the next. In this way the phases are managed serially; one cannot begin a new phase until all the issues in the previous one have been resolved. Naturally, as development progresses, changes to earlier assumptions are made, and feedback is required. This feedback is shown as the dotted lines in the figure. The phases in the model include all activities from the initial analysis through the product's retirement. Hence it is called a life cycle model.

The labels in the boxes (i.e., the names of the phases) vary from diagram to diagram. However, they always follow the flow used in any intellectual or construction process: Decide what is to be done, decide how to do it, do it, and evaluate the results. This is how we build bridges and airplanes, conduct scientific research, and implement computer applications.

Using the terms of Figure 1, the process begins with an analysis step in which it is determined what the software product should support. The result of this step is a requirements document that describes what the system should do; it does not indicate how the system should achieve these goals. That is, it tells "what," but not "how."

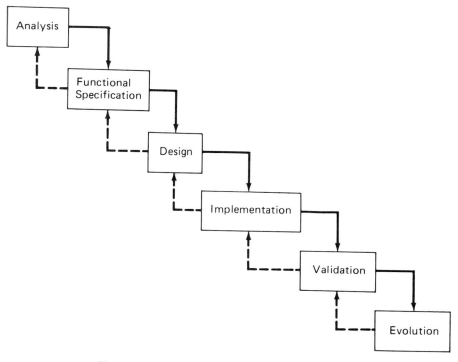

Figure 1. The traditional software life cycle model.

The design describes how the software product should be implemented. At the highest level it defines how the functions are to be distributed among the modules (the *functional specification*). Once this has been determined, a detailed design follows. (It is documented as *design specifications*.) As the designs are refined, implementation (i.e., coding and debugging) follows. Naturally, some portions of the system are implemented before others; that is, implementation begins before the entire design phase is completed. However, in this model one cannot begin the implementation of a module until its design is complete.

After products are implemented, they are tested. First the programs are tested as individual entities (unit testing); then the tested products are integrated and retested in larger components. Finally, the entire system is tested to see if it conforms to the initial requirements statement. In effect, the design process is one of decomposing the whole into smaller and smaller parts, while the testing is the inverse of this process. Design begins with a single requirements document and ends with a large collection of computer programs; testing begins with these programs and ends with a single tested system.

This waterfall model was adapted from the hardware development life cycle model. It has been used with software for almost two decades. It is particularly effective for large projects in which it is necessary to coordinate the implementation of hardware and software components; similar management tools can be applied to all components. The model is also interesting because we have a great deal of empirical data that describe the process.

In planning for a software project, one typically uses a 40–20–40 rule that states that

40% of the effort should be allocated for analysis of the requirements and design;
20% of the effort should be allocated to the programming process, that is, coding and debugging;
40% of the effort should be allocated to testing of the finished product.

Notice that the process of writing code is a very small portion of the entire project.

As the result of studying many large projects we also have found that:

Most errors are design errors; relatively few errors are made in translating a design into code.
The later in the life cycle that an error is identified, the more expensive it will be to correct it. The cost ratio can be as high as 1 : 100.
The more persons working on a project, the lower the productivity of each individual. That is, a programmer working alone may be able to produce ten times more product in a given time than when working as a member of a very large team. Communication among team members and the management of large development efforts both reduce individual performance.
There is evidence to suggest that the productivity of an individual is the same regardless of the programming language used. That is, the same number of lines of output will be produced per effort day for assembly language, COBOL, or MUMPS. An industry average of two delivered lines of code per effort hour is common; this effort includes all analysis, design, testing, and documentation.

Again, these results indicate that the writing of programs is a very small part of the process.

The discussion so far has been limited to the development phases of the life cycle. Once the product has been accepted, it is placed in operational use. Any changes to the product that follow are considered maintenance – or as indicated in the figure, evolution. Evolution may represent anywhere from half to three-quarters of the total life cycle cost. That is, an organization will spend, on the average, twice as much to maintain a software product as it did to implement it.

A naive view of maintenance is that it is an activity devoted to the correction of errors. However, studies of project histories have shown that

20% of the maintenance effort is to correct errors, that is, corrective maintenance;
25% of the maintenance effort is to adapt the software to meet changed requirements, that is, adaptive maintenance;
55% of the maintenance effort is to enhance existing features or to add new functions, that is, perfective maintenance.

Thus, maintenance (or evolution) is a positive sign that the software product is used and is evolving with the organization's needs.

Most of the results just reported are based on experience with the waterfall process model. One of the major advantages of that model is that we have experience in its application. However, it should be recognized that this process model assumes the writing of a requirements document that can serve as a contract for the development stages. In effect, once the requirements are defined, they will be fixed until the finished system is available to be tested against these requirements.

When the hardware and software development are conducted in parallel, this is a reasonable approach. Clearly, one cannot start to fabricate hardware until the design drawings are complete. But software is not hardware. It can be changed easily; the cost of fabrication is negligible. Thus, although it may be convenient to manage software in this waterfall model style, there are practical, alternative process models. This is especially true for applications in which the requirements are understood poorly or are subject to change. To see how the software process can be modified to accommodate such applications, the next subsection reexamines the software process from another perspective.

An Essential Software Process Model

One of the major concerns of the waterfall model is the management of the process. It allocates what has to be done into well-defined tasks that can be monitored and controlled. One danger of this model is that one may lose sight of the essential steps of the process by concentrating on the objects being managed. In this subsection I present what I call an essential process model. I view the software process as an intellectual activity in which one identifies needs and builds programs to produce a software system that meets those needs.

In this essential model the emphasis is on the process of determining what the software is to do. The process of building the programs is not considered very important. Recall, that most errors are design—and not programming—errors. Thus, if we know what it is we want to do, we should be able to implement a system that meets our needs. In this context implementation is not a problem-solving activity in the domain of application; it simply represents housekeeping, that is, a delay between the time that a solution has been postulated and the time that a realization of that solution is available for evaluation.

What I have written in the previous paragraphs reflects a personal view. That is why I use the first person singular; one may not find other computer scientists referring to this essential model. Having warned the reader of my personal biases, I now return to reporting on concepts that are accepted throughout the software engineering community. As a framework for the discussion, I use the model shown in Figure 2.

This essential model concentrates on the problem-solving activities of the software process. It follows the canonical problem-solving process of deciding what to do, deciding how to do it, doing it, and evaluating the results. In this case the software process is described as a sequence of transformations that go from a

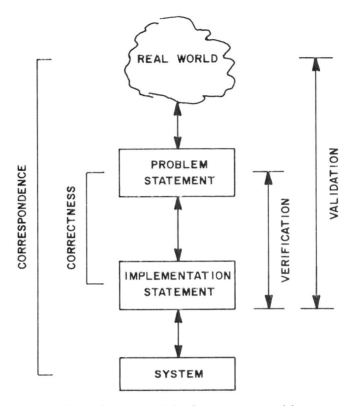

Figure 2. An essential software process model.

real-world need to a system that satisfies that need. The transformation from the real world to the problem statement is the decision of what to do, and the transformation into the implementation statement involves the next three steps. (The perspective of this model is the application domain; the aggregation of the implementation steps as a single transformation reflects my application view of program development as housekeeping.)

In this model the real world is viewed as a poorly understood dynamic object with operations that can be improved through the use of a software system. Naturally, this software system includes software plus hardware and people. Recognizing this need and identifying an appropriate set of responses to it are subjective processes. There are no "correct" requirements documents. Thus, this model starts with a transformation from the real world to a statement of the problem to be solved with a software system. This problem statement is what previously has been called the requirements specification.

Once the problem statement exists, it is used as the source document for the implementation. The transformation from the problem statement to the implementation statement (i.e., the code and documentation) represents the bulk of the development process: deciding how to do it, doing it, and evaluating the final result. The final transformation in this model is the creation of a system (as opposed to a collection of computer programs). This involves training, facility modifications, changes to operating procedures, and so on.

After the system is complete, it is embedded in the real world, thereby changing the real world, its needs, and the problem statement. Thus, this model is not a "life cycle" model; rather it is the description of a single iteration of the process. For real-world problems in which the problem is poorly understood, small problems are solved in early iterations, and the experience gained is used in defining subsequent problem statements. This is sometimes referred to as evolutionary development, and the preliminary implementations are often called prototypes.

The model in Figure 2 also indicates two quality measures with their associated evaluation processes:

Correctness. This is a logical property that describes how well a product meets its parent specification. Correctness is always with respect to some formal document. One can measure the correctness of the system with respect to the requirements specification; that is, does the system perform all the functions as they were described in the specification? In the same way, a computer program can be correct only with respect to its design specification; program correctness is never a property of the program alone. The process of determining correctness is called verification. (The root is the Latin *veritas* meaning truth.)

Correspondence. This is a subjective property of the final system that measures how well the product meets the needs of the environment. Correspondence can be determined only after the system is complete. The process of predicting correspondence is called validation. (The root is the Latin *validus* meaning strong or worth.)

Note that the two properties are independent of each other. One can have a system that is correct but does not correspond (e.g., the product was delivered as specified, but it does not do what is needed), or one can have a system that corresponds but is incorrect (e.g., the delivered system has some useful reports that were not included in the requirements specification.)

As shown in Figure 2, validation begins as the project starts. All validation activities are subjective (cognitive), and the validation techniques are built upon examinations of the design concepts in order to discover whether the right product is being implemented. Verification, on the other hand, can be objective, but it cannot begin until there are documents against which to test the correctness. Testing, by the way, simply implies the discovery of errors. A good test will identify errors; a bad test will not. Thus, the absence of errors during testing may give little insight into the quality of the software. One can only determine correctness by means of a proof with respect to some previous statement. And, of course, a correct system may not correspond.

The advantages of this essential model are that:

It presents a problem-solving perspective. The resultant system is viewed as a
tool that provides some useful function to its users. The fact that it is a software
product is obscured.

The implementation of the software is considered to be a simple transformation
from the application perspective; naturally, this may not be the case when considered from the perspective of the software development team.

It is not a life cycle model. The life cycle is viewed as a series of iterations of this
model. Some early iterations may produce prototypes that are discarded; later
iterations represent the maintenance activities.

The obvious shortcoming of this model is that it does not address any of the
management issues.

Developing Clinical Information Systems

The previous two subsections on the software process are valid for all application
domains. This subsection makes some observations that are specific to the
domain of clinical information systems (CIS). This class of system maintains
clinical data in a large, permanent database to support patient care and medical
decision making. The applications typically use off-the-shelf hardware and software systems, and they have few real-time or computational demands. Relative
to other application domains, the computer technology for the CIS is mature.
This implies that, once the requirements for a CIS have been established, it
should not be difficult to implement a product that meets these requirements.

Another way of considering the relative maturity of the CIS technology is to
view it in the context of risk. Figure 3 presents two dimensions of risk. The application risk is a measure of the certainty that a valid requirements specification
can be written, that is, one that will define a system that corresponds to the
environment's needs. Technical risk, on the other hand, measures the certainty
that it is possible to produce a product that will meet the requirements, that is,
that a correct implementation can be produced. Because the CIS uses a mature
technology, almost all applications have low technical risk.

One lowers application risk through experience in the specific domain. If the
users or developers have a clear understanding of their needs, the risk will be low.
If, on the other hand, there is no experience with this particular application, then
the risk can be lowered only by gaining experience. This may be done by reading
about the experience of others with similar applications (the justification for
writing this book) or by learning from hands-on experience with prototypes and
similar applications.

Note that two groups must learn about the application in order to lower the
risk. The developers must understand the organization's needs in order to specify
a useful product. The users also need to understand what the technology can do
and how it will alter their work. Thus, there is a dual problem-solving activity.
Each of the problem solvers begins with mental models of what the "ultimate system" will do. It is only after experience with using the CIS that these mental

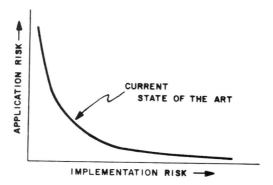

Figure 3. Two dimensions of risk.

models are refined. Recall that, in the essential model, the implemented system is embedded in the real world, thereby altering it and the problem statement; we seldom are farsighted enough to anticipate the changes introduced by the new system.

Thus, we may conclude that the development of a complex CIS in a relatively new domain will have high application risk. Implementation will require learning by trial and iteration. The developers will need to have experience in both computer systems and their applications in a medical setting. Because of the high cost of failure, evolutionary development is mandated. Small failures can be accepted as learning experiences, but a major failure would be recognized for what it is.

The OCIS, of course, is an example of a CIS. It is a complex system that charts new waters. Although its developers had a general understanding of what it was to do, there was much to learn. Therefore, the OCIS development history followed the guidelines outlined in the previous paragraphs. How it did this is the subject of the next section.

OCIS Development History

I begin this section with some personal observations. In 1974 the Applied Physics Laboratory (APL), that part of Johns Hopkins University for which I work, offered to help The Johns Hopkins Hospital design and implement a small clinical information system for their outpatient medical clinic. This system would manage a *mini*mal medical *record* (the minirecord) that would provide an on-line summary problem list and medication summary for use when the full chart was not available. APL provided a programmer plus dial-up computer support for this prototype Minirecord System.

Of course, I was that programmer. At the time, I had over a dozen years of experience with the development of moderately large information systems. But this was my first application in a medical environment, and I did not know this application domain. I was lucky, and I learned rapidly. Fortunately, the Minirecord System prototype was a success. Consequently, when Dr. Donald Simborg, then the director of the Clinical Information Systems Division of the Department of Biomedical Engineering, left the School of Medicine to move to California, I was invited by Dr. Richard Johns, the department chairman, to assume that position.

At the same time, work was proceeding on the construction of a new building for a comprehensive cancer center at Johns Hopkins. The Johns Hopkins Oncology Center (JHOC), as it came to be called, would contain 60 inpatient beds, large outpatient facilities, a major radiation therapy complex, and laboratory space for research. In 1975 a scaled-down version of the JHOC was operating out of a Johns Hopkins clinic for outpatients and a unit in the Baltimore City Hospitals for inpatients.

As a result of their experience in these units, the medical oncologists had a good model of the type of care they intended to provide. Most of the antitumor drugs were given in precisely timed sequences, toxicities and complications were anticipated and monitored, and there was experience in the use of plots and displays to suggest trends. The goal was to formalize the care of all medial oncology patients by (a) establishing protocols—some of which were for research and others specialized for individualized care—and (b) using modern data management techniques to monitor the patients' status.

It was immediately obvious that these goals could be met only if the care process was linked to an automated system. The manual preparation of graphs had demonstrated their utility; the use of a manual approach, however, would not scale up to a 60-bed center. Thus, the JHOC directorship had two choices: constrain the care to the level that could be supported by a manual system, or apply automation to the care process. Notice that, to a certain extent, this automation would eliminate the potential labor costs associated with the data technicians required to manage and plot all the clinical data. However, because it would not be practical to maintain this type of data management manually, automation was not really a labor-saving tool. Rather, it was an enabling device; it enabled the JHOC to provide the data management support that it considered necessary.

Because it was obvious that patient care in the JHOC would require automated support, Dr. Albert Owens, the director, planned for a computer room with cables to each patient room and clinical area. Dr. Raymond Lenhard, the chief of medical oncology, was given responsibility for the information management activities. And, in 1975, I was given an appointment in the Oncology Center and asked to guide in the development of what we came to call the Oncology Clinical Information System (OCIS).

Thus, in 1975, with no domain knowledge, I was responsible for a division in the School of Medicine plus the implementation of the OCIS. Fortunately, I had the assistance of two domain specialists—Drs. Johns and Lenhard—to guide me in the various development activities. I had two titles, no computer, no staff, and considerable optimism. The latter, of course, is a prerequisite for the computing profession.

Before continuing with the narrative, it will be helpful to present an organizational overview. As already stated, I worked for APL; I was given an interdivisional assignment with the School of Medicine that continued until 1983. Within the School of Medicine I was responsible for a division in the Department of Biomedical Engineering (BME). The division staff doubled in 1977 when Elizabeth McColligan joined us after completing a master's degree in medical computing. She also succeeded me as the division director when I decided to return to APL. In 1978, as work on the OCIS expanded, we began to add more computer professionals to the BME staff.

Most of the JHOC Information Center staff were Hospital employees. (The Johns Hopkins Hospital is administratively and legally distinct from the School of Medicine.) Therefore, most of the people hired to work in the information center were hospital employees. All jobs that were considered to be operational and/or long term were assigned to the JHOC staff (i.e., hospital employees). Short-term software development activities were assigned to the BME staff (i.e., university employees). The goal was to have the people who desired a long-term association with the JHOC remain with it by means of either their initial hire or a later transfer. In actual practice, work assignments were similar for the JHOC and BME development team members. However, few of the OCIS staff members had any prior computer experience when hired.

The reason that it is important to recognize that there were several organizations cooperating in the OCIS development is that this fact impacted on the development process. The OCIS implementation was only one of my responsibilities; my other assignments allowed me time to work out the TEDIUM concepts, participate in professional meetings, and consult in the development of other clinical systems. As time went on, the BME staff members were given new assignments: The Minirecord System became the Core Record System, and new systems were prototyped or implemented for the Department of Anesthesiology and Critical Care, the Department of Social Work, and the University Health Service. Each of these activities borrowed from the OCIS experience and, at the same time, contributed to it.

Finally, it is useful to recognize that the informality of this multiorganizational development also contributed to the OCIS success. There were no rigid contracts, and all staff members were peers independent of their home organization. Because I recognized that I would return to APL, operational responsibility for the OCIS was transferred to the JHOC during a three-year phaseover. Because the BME staff members perceived that new projects would always materialize, they were comfortable in doing the development and then providing consultation as they moved on to another assignment.

To conclude this introduction with an epilogue, the Clinical Information System Division of BME no longer exists. I left the School of Medicine because I chose to concentrate on software engineering. APL supported me in the culminating activity of writing *Clinical Information Systems*, and now I am active in computer science research. Elizabeth McColligan left BME to take a position with the Ohio State University. The rest of the division's BME staff has moved on to other positions; several staff members now have jobs within the Hospital. Thus, even though the division had great success, it no longer exists.

The Oncology Center was not affected by either the changes in the BME's or its own staff. The Center's director, Dr. Owens, became President of The Johns Hopkins Hospital in 1987. Dr. Lenhard left the Oncology Center in 1984 to head a hospital-wide clinical information system organization; he is now Vice President of Information Systems. Each brought to his present position an awareness of how the effective management of clinical information can improve the delivery of care. They all left behind a well-managed operational system.

John Enterline succeeded me as Technical Director of the Information Center. His background as a statistician brought a different perspective that added significantly to the growth of the OCIS and computer application within the JHOC. OCIS is now a permanent part of the JHOC, and the remainder of this section details its early history as summarized in Figure 4. The Phase III history and status, together with a discussion of the plans for further development, are presented in Chapter 9.

The Prototype System

Recall that work on the OCIS began in 1975 before the building was available or there was a computer. The first objective was to determine what the system was to do and how it could be implemented. It was decided that a prototype would be programmed on the APL computer. The goal was to gain some insight into how the OCIS should operate. Ideally, the prototype would also provide some useful functionality to the JHOC.

Dr. Lenhard, in addition to his responsibilities as the chief of Medical Oncology, was responsible for all clinical information management within the JHOC. One of the largest of these tasks was the maintenance of The Johns Hopkins Hospital (JHH) Tumor Registry. The Tumor Registry is a registry of all patients diagnosed at JHH as having cancer. It is a hospital-wide registry, required by the American College of Surgeons (ACS), and is not restricted to patients treated at The JHOC. (Only a small subset of the cancer patients treated at JHH are cared for in The JHOC; The JHOC, however, provides consultation services for all such patients. Patients treated in The JHOC generally are limited to those with diagnoses actively being studied by the Center's faculty.)

The JHH Tumor Registry was managed by Anne Kammer. In 1975 the registry was maintained as paper records with an automated summary stored on magnetic tape. This automated file contained the information required by the ACS, along with some additional data. It was organized in the form of 80 character unit records. Each record contained the patient identifier, the history (dates and status), topography (location of the tumor), and morphology (cell type and stage) for each primary tumor site. (In a tumor registry each primary site is independent, and a patient may have more than one primary tumor.)

The first task was to define a format for an extended tumor registry that would meet all the ACS requirements and also satisfy the anticipated reporting needs

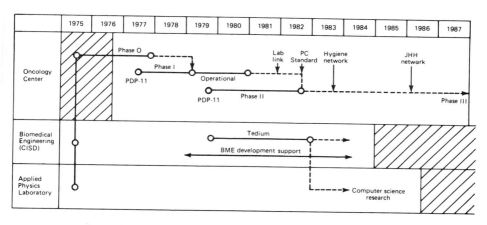

Figure 4. Overview of OCIS development history.

for both JHH and the JHOC researchers. A compact coded system would meet the needs of the first two groups, but it was doubtful that it could satisfy the needs of the faculty. Thus, after several iterations, a tumor registry abstract—essentially the same as the OCIS abstract shown in Chapter 2—was designed. The next step was to write the programs for entering and updating these abstracts and to convert the existing tumor registry tape to the new format.

The prototype tumor registry program was written in PL/1 and run on an IBM mainframe located in Laurel, Maryland, some 25 miles away from the JHOC. Since this was 1975, punch cards were used as the input medium. An APL/JHU/JHH courier picked up the punch cards from the Tumor Registry each day, delivered them to the APL computing center for a run, and returned a listing of update errors to the Tumor Registry to be corrected in time for the next day's processing. Routine reports were printed, and occasional searches were run.

From today's perspective this was a very primitive system. However, it did several things. First, it did something useful. Before the prototype, the tumor registry was on a single magnetic tape. There were no reports or error-checking tools. The only output was a tape listing. The new prototype replaced a manual system with an automated system that offered some reporting facilities. It also verified the old data and provided a limited search facility for data going back to 1964. Although there was a small user community for the tumor registry, that small group was satisfied that a computer system would be of value.

The second thing that the prototype did was to establish the format for the patient identification node of the OCIS. The format chosen for this prototype defined what information—coded and textual—was considered necessary for all patients treated at the JHOC. For these patients, the complete abstract would be filled out; for the other JHH Tumor Registry patients, only the basic (i.e., readily available or ACS required) fields needed to be entered.

Work on the OCIS started in July 1975; by the end of the year the tumor registry system was operational. A perception of progress had been planted. Once the abstract was in production, work began on the design of the formats for the flow sheets and plots. Several iterations were tried, and we gradually converged on the formats shown in Chapter 2. Clearly, the processing cycle was so slow that none of these displays could be of any value in a clinical setting.

But we did learn from our prototype. Even though the JHOC did not get its computer until August 1977, we nevertheless felt that we had enough understanding of the problem to present three papers on the OCIS in 1977. Of course, these publications reflect the then state of the art in refereeing papers on the subject; there were not too many reports with evaluated results to choose from.

The Phase I System

Once we felt that we had learned as much as we could from the prototype system, we began to work on the Phase I system that would operate from a dedicated computer located in the JHOC. The new facilities for the Center were opened mid-1976, and by October of that year all units were in operation.

An Information Center was established to manage the data processing within the JHOC. Hospital systems were used for billing and administrative purposes; the Information Center was concerned only with clinical applications and the Tumor Registry. It was located on the main floor of the new building and had a small computer room, cables from that room to 250 locations throughout the JHOC, but no computer.

Financial support for the Information Center operations came out of the patient care income. Some research funds were available to support special applications, but—as one might expect—after moving into the new building there was little money available for a computer. Fortunately, a gift from the Educational Foundation of America freed the funds to purchase the Phase I computer.

A PDP-11/70 was ordered with 256K words of memory, support for 32 terminals, and 44 million bytes of mass storage. The cost was on the order of a quarter of a million dollars, a fact that helps explain why there were so few clinical information systems in the 1970s. In any event, a computer was on order, a programming language was chosen, and implementation of the Phase I system began.

It was decided to develop the OCIS in MUMPS. There were several reasons for this choice. First, an examination of the language suggested that it would be easy to learn and use. Second, the Clinical Laboratory was developing its system using MUMPS, and the director of that activity, Dr. Robert Miller, offered us computer time and consulting assistance.

The commitment to MUMPS proved to be a good choice. The OCIS computer was installed in August 1977, the data from the prototype system were converted to the new system by December, and in April 1978, the terminals at the clinical stations provided on-line access to the patient data. The Phase I system continued to grow in functionality until 1979, when it was decided to freeze the system so that everyone could concentrate on a Phase II system. However, it was not until June 1980 that work stopped on Phase I.

The Phase I system relied on the insights gained from working with the prototype. In theory, we knew what we wanted to do. Briefly, we expected to capture all tabularly represented data—test results, drug doses, tumor measurements—and list them in flow sheets or plots. Textual information would be printed as abstracts, and special types of data, such as the microbiology reports, would require custom programs.

The goal was to present all this information to the clinical staff in formats that were appropriate for the patient's disease, therapy, and status. In addition, because most patients were treated using a preestablished therapy plan (protocol), we wanted to have the patient database interact with the plans in printing out daily care plans that listed the tests, recommended therapies, and follow-up for each patient.

We designed the system to operate in a "cafeteria" style. That is, the staff could use whatever features of the system found helpful. The Information Center staff would be available to insulate the clinical users from the system details. Not that the system was hard to use; it was just a question of familiarity with computer applications.

The Phase I system in 1979 was almost the same, functionally, as the later Phase II system. The following features were available on line from any inpatient unit or outpatient clinic:

Abstracts and the Tumor Registry. A database of 25,000 patients was available on line; queries generally were managed by modifying report programs.

Clinical Data Display. The data were available at CRTs in three formats: horizontal and vertical flow sheets and listings of the day's data. (The printed output included the flow sheets plus plots.) There also were special programs for microbacteriology reporting.

Patient Census. Summary patient data for each admission, protocol start, and outpatient treatment were recorded.

Daily Care Plans. Starting in April 1979, two units used protocol-directed care for the ordering of all morning tests, as well as for the printing of therapy reminders.

Transfusion Summary. This was the first increment in the hemopheresis system. A summary of each patient's transfusion history was available.

The outpatient units also had access to scheduling programs. Other management and administrative applications were implemented, and—on paper—the Phase I OCIS was indeed a very powerful system. However, what was installed was really a set of programs and not yet a system. It would take years to transform the OCIS into an effective clinical system. This last observation requires some explanation.

For a clinical information system to be effective, it must provide timely access to the data and it must be available without fail. Obviously, no one-computer system can meet the availability requirement. The timeliness condition, however, depends on more than equipment; it relies on people and procedures.

When the Information Center was in its planning stages, Dr. Lenhard recognized that the clinical staff would need the assistance of clinically oriented data technicians who could serve as the links between the users and the OCIS. The title of "clinical data coordinator" was descriptive, but it represented a concept that required several years of experimentation to refine.

In addition to deciding what was reasonable to expect of the clinical data coordinators, we also had to establish procedures for the operational flow. Because the MUMPS system required little operator maintenance, the computer operators doubled as the data entry staff. The system was up six days a week, two shifts a day. Within its equipment constraints, it was reliable. It could process up to 20 concurrent tasks, but as the number of tasks approached 20, the response time degraded. In effect, the Phase I system was a victim of its success. It did many things well, showed great promise, but still fell short of the performance required.

Therefore, a second computer was ordered in 1978. This two-computer system would add reliability to the functionality of the Phase I system. Naturally, it would be called the Phase II system.

The Phase II System

The goal of the Phase II system was to provide the same functionality as the earlier system in a two-computer configuration. In preparing the prototype, we had gone from nothing to a demonstration. We did this quickly, and the potential users were impressed. When we prepared the Phase I system, we went from nothing to an operational system, and this too we did quickly. As work began, the users felt that this would be a very good system once the equipment limitations were overcome. They looked forward to having a Phase II system that would meet their needs.

However, in implementing a Phase II system, we would be going from something that existed to something that worked even better. Surprisingly, this turned out to be a much more difficult task than I had expected. When we started, I told the users that development would take one year and that, when we were done, the new system would look just like the old one. I was wrong. It took three years from the time the second computer was installed (August 1979) until the Phase I system was retired and the new two-computer system was operational (August 1982). What was installed had greater functionality, but its lateness was its key attribute.

This was a hard lesson to learn. The new system consisted of 3500 programs with a data model of 850 relations. A data-processing group would be impressed to know that this was done in three years by a staff of under eight full-time equivalents, who also had to maintain the Phase I system, convert a database with 37,000 patients to a new format, and provide almost uninterrupted service to the clinical staff. But the users went through two years of wondering when the system would be finished, and—no matter how heroic our EDP efforts were—the users were right to complain.

What made the problem so difficult was that the language used for the Phase I system (MUMPS-11) was no longer being supported. It was replaced by the new Standard MUMPS. There were three choices: translate from MUMPS-11 to Standard MUMPS and thereby lose some of the benefits of the new standard, reprogram the entire system in Standard MUMPS, or do something else. We chose the last option.

At the time the decision was made, we were involved in the maintenance of the Phase I system. MUMPS was designed to operate in very small computers, and it therefore used a compact notation to save space. This notation made programs difficult to read, allowed the use of clever tricks, and was a barrier to the maintenance of any code not authored by the maintaining programmer. We have seen from an earlier section that the long-term cost of maintenance is much greater than that of the initial development. By the age of only two years, the Phase I OCIS already had become very difficult to maintain.

Another problem was that the system seemed to have been built as a collection of individual clusters with various levels of completeness. In an information system, one expects that every input will be validated, that user prompts will be based on common conventions, and that help messages will be available. However, such were not always the case with the Phase I system. One could guess from the interface who wrote the code. Moreover, the temptation to introduce 95% complete code into production often led to the acceptance of invalid inputs and a resulting degradation of the database.

In parallel with this conversion decision, some work that offered new insights was underway in BME. Through a generous contract with IBM, BME was lent a Series/1 computer so that we could experiment with it for a patient management application. Recognizing the repetition involved in developing such an application, we began to build a specialized tool called SIMPLE. (The "we" here were Ken Bakalar, Martin Trocki, and myself.) It turned out that what was simple to do was not very interesting. Nevertheless, the result was a different approach to software development that I later came to call TEDIUM.

Thus, in 1979, as we began to plan for the Phase II system, I was convinced that reprogramming the system in MUMPS would be difficult to control and would result in a system that would be hard to maintain. I also had the germ of an idea — TEDIUM — that would make everything much easier (someday). And so, in 1979 we set out to maintain a large system (Phase I), develop a new programming environment (TEDIUM) for a new language (Standard MUMPS), and implement a two-computer version of that system (Phase II). All in one year. No wonder I was wrong.

Fortunately, we knew what we wanted to do; we had our Phase I experience. Among the programming staff, Alan Sacker served as the system manager and kept the systems going. Liz McColligan led the effort on the daily care plans, and Ken Bakalar designed the scheduling language. (Incidently, we received a great deal of help from Dr. Robert Friedman and Jacki Horowitz of Boston University in the design of the protocol system.) Ping Chang and Sue Powell worked on the plots and flows, Martin Trocki did the microbacteriology reports, Chris Brunn designed the outpatient system, and Jean Causey developed the pharmacy system.

In 1982, as the Phase II went into operation and the BME staff was phased out, new people were added: Farideh Momeni (who is now the lead OCIS designer) contributed a variety of new features, Mark Borinski helped develop the blood product system, and Jerry Rouch maintained and augmented the abstract and tumor registry system.

This list includes only the development staff. Of equal importance were the contributions of the OCIS users, who made us understand the problems that we had to solve, and of the Information Center staff—clinical data coordinators, computer operators, and administrative support—who made OCIS work. However, in the interest of not making a long chapter even longer, I shall simply acknowledge their collective help.

What are the lessons from the Phase II history? First, the programming profession is always optimistic. An often cited rule of thumb for estimating is to get the best estimate and then double it. (Of course, if the best estimate already has been doubled. . . .) Second, there are two things that we must understand before we undertake a development effort: what we are to do, and how we will implement it. In this case we understood only the former, and the cost of developing TEDIUM and learning to use it impacted the schedule considerably. If we did not have a solid understanding of the first, then I am sure that we would have failed completely.

Finally, one should never underestimate the cost of maintaining and converting an ongoing system. Even though we nominally began work on Phase II in 1979, it was not until mid-1980 that most of the staff was freed from the maintenance activities and available to work on the new system. Also, because the Phase I system was new, it could be installed incrementally. Although some new Phase II features were operational in early 1982, its final installation required the complete replacement of the Phase I system.

Beyond Phase II

Obviously, the Phase II system was completed, and it is successful. It is the topic of the remainder of this book. To conclude the historical narrative, in 1982 we began to interface the OCIS with the clinical laboratory so that results could be batched and transmitted electronically. Later, computer interfaces were developed between the JHOC laboratories and the OCIS. Once this was done, clinicians used the OCIS as the primary mechanism for viewing results; it was the most complete and timely source.

The pharmacy system was developed using the unit dose model first designed by Dr. Simborg. (Its implementation history is contained in Chapter 6.) Links were installed between the OCIS and the associated hospital systems. The OCIS computers were upgraded, new and more powerful Standard MUMPS versions were installed, and both mass memory and the number of on-line terminals grew. A listing of the current configuration is shown in Figure 1 of Chapter 1. In parallel with this, personal computers proliferated throughout the Oncology Center, and small networks were installed in the laboratories and the administrative areas. The Phase III system, which integrates these resources with the Hospital network and the School of Hygiene computer, is described in Chapter 9, along with a brief overview of the future plans for the OCIS and computing in the Oncology Center.

The Software Tools

The history of the OCIS development is closely associated with the tools used in its implementation. The speed with which the early versions were produced and the ease with which the current system is maintained cannot be understood without some introduction to the tools used in its development.

The OCIS is implemented as a set of Standard MUMPS programs. These programs run under a MUMPS operating system. These same programs run under a variety of other operating systems, such as DEC VMS, IBM VM, UNIX,[2] and MS-DOS. The OCIS was designed using TEDIUM. TEDIUM is a program generator, written in Standard MUMPS, that generates Standard MUMPS code. The generated code does not require TEDIUM to operate.

In the following two subsections, I present a brief introduction to MUMPS and TEDIUM. The discussion contains some technical detail, and readers who do not have an interest in computing and system development may wish to move directly to the section on evaluation.

An Introduction to MUMPS

The Massachusetts General Hospital Utility Multi-Programming System (MUMPS) was developed in the late 1960s when computers were expensive and resources were limited. Targeted for the new breed of minicomputers, MUMPS was intended to provide interactive support and data management facilities for the kinds of complex file structures that are common in medical applications.

In the 1970s most MUMPS systems used the DEC PDP 11 computers, and there were a variety of proprietary MUMPS and MUMPS-like systems. (The DEC version for the PDP 11 was called MUMPS-11.) In the mid-1970s the MUMPS Users' Group (MUG) organized a standardization activity, and the new Standard MUMPS was available in time for the Phase II conversion. In what follows, we consider only that standarrd version and describe only those features that contribute to an understanding of the OCIS.

MUMPS is an interpretative language. With this type of language there is a program called the interpreter, that reads the program as data and executes its commands. An interpretive language can be contrasted with a compiled language, in which the program is transformed into a machine-processible form by a program called a compiler. This object code is loaded into the computer, and it directly executes each instruction.

---

[2]UNIX is a trademark of AT&T Bell Laboratories.

With an interpretative language one is essentially a level away from the machine instructions. The program interacts with the interpreter, and the interpreter interacts with the computer. Thus it is possible to stop a program, examine the values being processed (i.e., the machine state), alter the program, and continue execution. In fact, because the interpreter treats the program as data, one even can pass data to the interpreter for execution. In MUMPS this is called indirection.

The advantage of a compiled language is that all processes are converted to efficient machine code. Thus, performance with a compiled language should be better. An interpreter must parse, verify, and execute each line of code every time it is processed. In general, one uses an interpretative language when testing or debugging a program or when one wants to delay a decision about what a program is to do (or how it is to do it). The latter is called delayed, or run-time, binding. Compiled programs always rely on early, or compile-time, binding. That is, all control paths are determined when the programs are compiled, and no changes can be made to take advantage of run-time knowledge.

Except for situations in which delayed binding is necessary, as is the case with some artificial intelligence applications, the efficiency of compilation is preferred. Therefore, some languages offer an interpretative debugger, along with a compiler for the operational system. Most MUMPS systems now use a form of compilation. The system converts each program into a parsed and verified intermediate form called pseudocode or p-code. This code can be processed rapidly by the interpreter, which is also available to support the user's interactive needs, such as debugging support.

The command structure of MUMPS is organized around the line. Each command can be abbreviated as a single letter. For example,

    WRITE "Hello world"

could be written

    W "Hello world"

Both will write the message, "Hello world." Assignment uses a SET command (similar to the BASIC LET), and many variable/expression pairs may be supplied. For example,

    SX=1,Y=2*X,Z=(X+Y)/Y

MUMPS commands allow the user to append a conditional to a command. That command will be executed only if the condition has been met. Each line has an optional label separated by a tab character (<tab>) from the command string. The GO command transfers control to another line (or program). For example,

    <tab>S I=0
    LINE<tab>S I=I+1 D^PROGRAM G:I<10 LINE

will cause D^PROGRAM to be executed 10 times. The DO command is similar to a call command, and ^PROGRAM is a program, stored on disk, to be called. The same loop can be more succinctly written with the FOR instruction:

F I=1:1:10 D^PROGRAM

The syntax of the FOR reads, for I going from 1 by 1 to 10, do what follows through the end of this line.

The circumflex (which is referred to as an up arrow by MUMPS programmers) indicates that the object referenced is on the disk. The above statements without the circumflex, that is, D PROGRAM, would transfer control to the label PROGRAM (assumed to be already in working memory). In either case control returns to the next command when the called section of code encounters a QUIT command or reaches the end of the program text.

The same convention is used to differentiate between data in working memory (X(1)) and data stored on disk (^X(1)). The latter is called a global. Thus, one can read or write from disk using the same commands that one uses when dealing with data in working memory. For example,

S X=1,Y=^Z(1)*X,^Z(Y)=X

sets the local variable X to 1, sets the local variable Y to the global Z value with the index 1, and stores in the global Z with the index Y the value of X. Notice that the line includes one read from disk and one write to disk.

Although the syntax and commands are interesting, the real power of MUMPS is in its data manager. Data (in both working memory and permanent storage) are organized as a sparse array. In a sparse array, storage is allocated only when an array value exists. For example, in a traditional language, a 3 by 4 matrix, say M(3,4), will be allocated 12 storage locations. In the sparse array of MUMPS, however, storage is allocated only when a value is assigned through either a SET or READ command. Thus,

S M(1,1)=1,M(3,2)=2

will set only two locations in the matrix M. The remaining 10 matrix elements are undefined, unless, of course, they had been set prior to this line.

The sparse array concept allocates storage only for those array elements to be stored. Because MUMPS is a nondeclarative language, the programmer need not declare how much storage is to be allocated for an array (or global). The statement

S M(1)=1,M(1,1)=2,M(1,2,3)=3

establishes M as a hierarchy with entries at three levels. This statement is similar to the previous statement in which M was viewed as a matrix. The difference is in how the programmer will use M. (Note that in the second case M(1,1) has a value associated with it, whereas M(1,2) points to the node M(1,2,3) but may not have a value associated with it.)

As we have seen, the sparse array is a very powerful and flexible structure. Its greatest strength, however, lies in the fact that index terms may be character strings. In this way, one can extend the sparse array to implement a hierarchical patient file:

^PAT("1234567")="Jones,Mary#WF35"
^PAT("1234567","ADR",1)="10 Main Street"
^PAT("1234567","ADR",2)="Anytown, MW 12345"
^PAT("1234567", "PROB, "87/01/12") = "Head cold"

In the first node, the # is used as a separator; the patient name field is of arbitrary length, and the # indicates the end of the name and the start of the race/sex/age field. (There are many MUMPS commands and functions that facilitate operating on character strings like this.)

The circumflex indicates that the data will be stored on disk. All entries (records) will be stored in lexical or numerical order. For that reason, the date is shown in the form of year/month/day. Given this ordering of the globals, one can construct a name index as follows:

^PATNAME("Jones,Mary","1234567")=""

In this case there are two index terms; the second is required to allow for two different Mary Jones entries. Because one is interested only in the index terms, the value assigned to this sparse array node is the null string, that is, a character string with zero length. (Because all globals are stored in lexical key order, MUMPS does not need a sort routine. Sorting is done by writing a global with the desired index.)

The global notation can be extended to identify which partition in the MUMPS system stores a global. In the OCIS case, development is done in a partition called DEV, and the production system is maintained in a partition called PRD. To test programs in DEV, one can read production globals with the notation

^["PRD"]GLOBAL(. . . .

This notation can be extended to multiple machines as well. In the OCIS, some globals are stored on the OLD machine and some on the NEW machine. Thus, the OCIS tends to use the general form for a MUMPS distributed system of

^["OLD"]["PRD"]GLOBAL(. . . .

From this very brief introduction to MUMPS it is clear that it is a very powerful and flexible language. What are its shortcomings? First, the ability to do so much so easily is an invitation to create programs that are difficult to maintain. For example, in the previous illustrations, what does the sparse array M stand for? It would be almost impossible to understand its structure without documentation. Yet the dynamic, friendly MUMPS development environment does not encourage the creation *and maintenance* of good documentation. Of course, this is a human problem that is not limited to the MUMPS programming language.

The problem is compounded, however, by the terse MUMPS style; it is difficult to manage a large system and understand the code of other programmers.

Because of the limitations of MUMPS, the difficulty in maintaining a consistent system style, and the need to provide tools that would facilitate the evolution of the OCIS, I chose to implement the Phase II system using a development environment called TEDIUM. Before describing TEDIUM, let me observe that this was a very bold, perhaps even foolish, high-risk decision that turned out to be a good one.

One objective of this chapter is to offer lessons learned. Consequently, I conclude this subsection with the following observation. MUMPS, by itself or with some of the available productivity tools, offers an excellent environment for some types of system development. As with most languages and environments, there are deficiencies. Yet one should not rush to design new environments that correct those deficiencies. As the stunt driver tells the enraptured teenagers in his audience, please don't go home and try this with the family sedan. With that word of warning, let me now tell you how I "solved" the problem of developing software.

An Introduction to TEDIUM

The Environment for Developing Information Utility Machines (TEDIUM) was first implemented in 1979. It was written in TEDIUM and MUMPS, and it went through several iterations. The version of the system that I report on here was frozen in 1982. I shall not try to describe the history of TEDIUM or how I envisioned its use in the Phase II development activity. Rather, I shall concentrate on how I understand TEDIUM today. The goal is to provide a background for understanding the OCIS evaluation of the next section.

In several places I have made the point that, in software development, there are two separate problems to be solved: what the application is to do, and how to detail its implementation. In theory, if one can specify fully what the application is to do and also define all the programming conventions to be followed, then one should be able to give these instructions to a programmer and, without further dialogue, receive a correct program. In this view, the designer decides what is to be done, and the programmer translates this decision into code.

TEDIUM follows this division of the problem domains. The designer works within the context of a system style. This defines all the standards and conventions to be used by the programmer; for example, every input procedure must perform validity checking, and every user interaction must offer a help message. Within this style, the designer specifies what is to be done. These specifications are very compact; the reuse information already specified and constructs already defined. They are called, therefore, minimal specifications.

The minimal specifications describe what the program is to do from the perspective of the application. That is, the designer is asked to visualize how the user will interact with the system. Implementation details are avoided unless (a) they are required for efficiency purposes or (b) the TEDIUM specification language has no effective way to describe the desired actions. Thus, the designer is not a programmer; he is an analyst who should describe the system as it is to be used.

Once the minimal specification and system style are available, there is little creative activity left. If, in theory, a programmer could take these documents and, without further instruction, create a correct program, then there is no reason why the programmer's actions should not be formalized and automated. This is what TEDIUM attempts to do. It views specification as a value-adding activity, but it considers programming to be only housekeeping. The latter does not add to our determination of what the application should do. Therefore, TEDIUM uses program generation to create programs from the specifications. That is, it automates the programming.

The ability of TEDIUM to limit the development process has several advantages. Referring back to the section on software engineering, we know that the number of "lines of code" produced per effort day is independent of language. Consequently, a higher level language will result in more functionality for a fixed effort. Second, because the greatest life cycle cost is associated with maintenance, a compact and application-oriented specification should be relatively easy to maintain.

The greatest advantage of the TEDIUM program generation approach, however, is derived from the fact that most TEDIUM products are of high application risk. That is, it is not clear that the designer knows what is required, and therefore the resultant specification may not correspond to the user's needs. With TEDIUM the designer may specify an application (or part of it), rapidly generate the code, and test the behavior of that specification.

The process of incrementally testing a prototype system is often called rapid prototyping. One develops a test system, experiments with it, and then uses the knowledge gained for the implementation of the next prototype or the final product. In most cases each prototype is discarded, and only the experience with its use is retained.

TEDIUM uses a different model for prototyping. In this case a sculpture metaphor is used. One begins with a model of what is desired. This model is shaped, perhaps recast, until the result is aesthetically pleasing, that is, it corresponds. At this point the final prototype becomes the delivered product. (The program generator ensures that all conventions defined by the system style are included in each prototype; thus, each prototype is functionally complete, i.e., it is never simply the shell of a target application.) The method is called system sculpture.

On the basis of this description, TEDIUM may be viewed as an application design language that generates programs. The reason it can generate programs is that the domain of information systems is relatively mature; we understand how to implement them. The TEDIUM version used for the OCIS generates MUMPS code. That code is perceived to be as efficient as custom-crafted code. Fortunately, there are enough good MUMPS implementations available so that slight losses in efficiency do not impact overall performance.

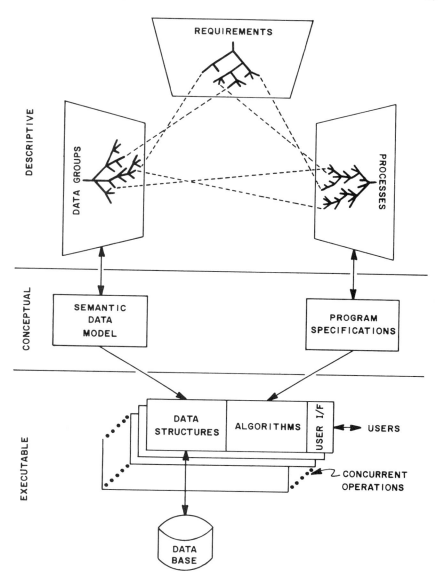

Figure 5. Three levels of application representation.

Even though the generated code is MUMPS, there is little in TEDIUM that depends on MUMPS. The objects that TEDIUM works on are called applications. All specifications are stored in an application database (ADB), and the contents of the ADB are shared by all specifications in that application. The ADB contains two levels of information. This is shown in Figure 5.

The top level, called the descriptive level, describes what the system should do. This is presented from three perspectives.

Requirements. What the application is expected to do. This often is a definition of the system's objectives and goals without any operational specifics.

Processes. Descriptions of the process that the application is to support. Frequently, these describe procedural flows.

Data Groups. Descriptions of the entities to be modeled in the database.

There are links among the three perspectives, and each is described in both outline and text form.

At the next, or conceptual level there are two types of specification. The semantic data model describes the database as a relational data model with additional constraints. For example, the patient data structure might be defined, in part, as

PAT(PATID)=NAME,RACE,SEX,AGE

This represents a symbolic specification for the MUMPS global example given above. With this definition, the TEDIUM commands can refer to NAME, RACE, or SEX by name without concern for how the variables are stored or accessed; that is, the housekeeping is eliminated.

In this illustration, the variable PATID is underlined. This is an example of a semantic constraint. It implies that the table (relation) PAT serves as a dictionary for all valid values of PATID. Every input of PATID, anywhere in the application, will be validated against the PAT table automatically. Again, we see how TEDIUM concisely captures the designers' intent and distributes it throughout all the programs in the application.

The second class of specification is for programs, which determine the functions to be implemented. There are two types of program specifications:

Generic Specifications. These specify often-used functions such as the creation of a menu or the implementation of a file management program for a table. These tend to be declarative, but procedural commands can be inserted.

Common Specifications. These are written using the TEDIUM command language; they are always procedural.

The TEDIUM command language permits the designer to specify the program flow with very little housekeeping overhead. For example, the command

Input PATID

will generate code that prompts for a value of PATID, checks the input for existence in the table PAT, performs any other input validation, and responds to a help request by listing out the definition of PATID from the data dictionary. Once a valid PATID exists, one could set the patient's name with the command

Get NAME in PAT

The conventions used for the interactive dialogue and data access are all established by the system style.

The ADB allows the designer to associate tables in the data model with data group descriptions and program specifications with the process descriptions. The program generator uses the program specifications and the associated data model definitions to produce MUMPS programs. These represent the lowest, or implementation, level. The generated programs are maintained by the MUMPS environment. Because they do not include any information that is not already in the ADB, they are not considered to be part of the ADB.

Notice that the ADB contains two categories of information. At the descriptive level there is subjective information. Text is used to convey concepts; decisions are made regarding what should be included and what level of detail should be supplied. Even the links between the descriptive and conceptual objects are based on a subjective determination of what will be helpful in the context of design, operations, or maintenance. At the conceptual level, on the other hand, the objects represent a complete specification of some aspect of the application design. They always describe exactly what is implemented; therefore, we consider them to be objective documentation.

During initial implementation the ADB can be considered the application design as created by the system sculpture process. It reduces redundancy, identifies inconsistencies, and provides the designer with limited local views of the application. The average program specification is 15 lines in length and normally can be displayed as one or two CRT pages. The text in the ADB is used for help messages, manual preparation, and application documentation.

From the maintenance perspective, the ADB may be viewed as a knowledge base that describes the application. The subjective information provides a road map to the system. It suppresses detail and assists the designer in identifying what conceptual objects relate to the problem being investigated. The objective information adds detail and describes the system completely. Cross-references are updated with each generation; they identify which programs call (are called by) which programs and access (read or write) which tables. Thus, the designer can sit down at a terminal, interactively identify a program or table, see how that object interacts with other objects, review all definitions, and then make and test changes. Because the objective documentation is the generator's input, this documentation is always complete and up-to-date.

On the basis of this brief introduction, one would expect TEDIUM applications to be more compact than the equivalent MUMPS code, always well documented, and described in application, rather than implementation, terms. The price that one pays in using TEDIUM is the loss of the convenience of interpretative debugging, the need to specify a program completely before it can be tested, and the occasional rough edges associated with a locally developed product. Clearly, it is more fun to write programs in MUMPS, but the production of an operational system entails considerable tedium. TEDIUM addresses the second issue; how well it does that is examined in the following section.

Table 1. OCIS Database Growth

Type of Database Entry	August		
	1982	1986	1987
Patients	37,000	50,000	56,000
Tumor Registry entries*	33,000	41,000	44,000
Patients admitted to JHOC	15,000	18,000	22,000
Patients with clinical data	8,800	18,000	22,000
Patient days	216,000	458,000	557,000
Unique data points	4,500K	14,000K	16,000K
Patients with microbacteriology data	3,000	7,000	9,000
Patient days	16,000	109,000	133,000
Reports	200,000	365,000	428,000

*Total hospital patients.

OCIS Development Evaluation

This chapter has considered the history of the OCIS with a special emphasis on the development of its software. An evaluation of the OCIS as a clinical tool is distributed throughout the following chapters, which describe its features. In reading those evaluations, however, one must keep in mind that the OCIS was designed for a cancer center for the purpose of delivering a level of care that could not be supported effectively with a manual system. Thus, the OCIS was intended to enable this type of care; it was not developed to justify its existence on the basis of cost savings.

Today, the staff cannot order morning laboratory tests, view in-house laboratory results, examine the Tumor Registry, schedule a visit, or review a local medical record without using the OCIS. Many clinicians are not aware that they are using OCIS; they think of it as a set of specialized applications used by others. Nevertheless, the JHOC could not operate without the OCIS. Moreover, the existence of the OCIS acts as a base for the addition of integrated features that could not be implemented independently. Table 1 illustrates the size, scope, and growth of the OCIS database; it suggests how the JHOC has come to rely upon the OCIS.

I suggest that it is best to evaluate the OCIS in the context of the visions of the JHOC founders, Dr. Owens and Dr. Lenhard in particular. The next chapters will provide anecdotal examples that justify the system's worth—clinically as

Table 2. OCIS Development Effort

Organization	75	76	77	78	79	80	81	82	83	84	85	86	87	Total
Oncology Center*			1	2	2	2	4	7	7	7	5	5	5	
Biomedical Engineering*	1	1	2	5	7	8	5	3	1					
Total FTE	0.5	0.5	2.5	6	6.5	8.5	7	6.5	6	6	4.5	4.5	4.5	63.5

*Counts individuals, not all full time.

well as financially. However, from a historical perspective, it would be improper to suggest that the OCIS had a set of well-defined, clearly stated (and therefore evaluatable) objectives, for example, to realize an economic benefit. The OCIS was not a research project when it was started a decade earlier, and it was never supported by research funds. The goal was to use the available technology (which was very expensive by today's standards) to implement a system that would aid in patient care. That it was successful (and incidently saved money) is the justification for this book.

Of course, the OCIS is also a software product, and I am now engaged in software engineering research. Therefore, it is fitting that I conclude this long and somewhat egocentric chapter with an evaluation of the OCIS development history. This discussion will be limited to the Phase II system. Table 2 summarizes the development and maintenance effort over the system's lifetime.

There are several ways of evaluating a software effort. The term "evaluate" usually implies an evaluation with respect to a standard or set of goals. In the section on software engineering, two quality goals were identified. Verification was concerned with the correctness of a system with respect to its specification. Inasmuch as the OCIS is generated from its specifications, it must be correct. The fact that it is used in life-endangering situations suggests that its users also perceive it to be defect free. The second quality measure, validation, considers how well the system meets the environment's needs. The following chapters provide ample evidence of its correspondence.

Another way of evaluating a software project is to compare its development history with that of other similar projects. But TEDIUM introduces a new development method (system sculpture), and it is not clear how the OCIS results relate to other projects. Thus, even though this is a section on evaluation, I will not evaluate the OCIS project. Rather I will present some characterizing metrics that describe both this project in particular and the software process in general.

To begin, I note that there is very little difference in this project between development and maintenance. Organizationally, the same staff members and users are involved. The OCIS is viewed as a resource to support the JHOC needs; it is not a product to be built, delivered, and frozen. Thus, one would expect the OCIS to grow continuously. Moreover, one would expect older programs to be replaced by newer programs. Tables 3 and 4 show that both these expectations are realized.

Table 3 presents the relative growth of the OCIS. Each program is about 15 lines long. Using a formula to include the data definitions, the OCIS application

Table 3. Growth of the OCIS Definition

Year	Programs	Tables	Elements
1982	2177	456	1251
1983	3662	848	2025
1984	5024	1045	2398
1986	5541	1375	2613

Table 4. New OCIS Programs by Year

Year	New Programs
1980	17
1981	625
1982	1388
1983	990
1984	1014
1985	737
1986	770

*In production use, December 1986.

consists of about 85,000 "lines of code." This code is, of course, its minimal specification. An earlier study showed that each TEDIUM specification line produced 4 lines of MUMPS code. Thus, the specification is the equivalent of 340,000 lines of MUMPS code. (Because a TEDIUM program may generate more than one MUMPS routine, there are over 9000 OCIS MUMPS routines.)

There was also a study that indicated that one line of TEDIUM would provide the functionality of 20 lines of COBOL. If that is true, then the OCIS would be a 1,700,000-line COBOL application. The point is, there is a difference between the size of the problem specification and the size of the implementation. The more compact the representation, the easier it will be to build and maintain the product. Bigger clearly is not better.

Table 4 shows the number of new programs that were written each year. The data are taken from a 1986 analysis of the programs then in production use, but the general pattern is clear. In 1980 very little was done. Most work involved maintenance of the Phase I system and learning about TEDIUM. The 1981 effort also was hampered by the TEDIUM training (and debugging) effort. Nevertheless, a staff of seven full-time equivalents produced 625 tested programs — about one program for every two effort days. By 1982, the staff was familiar with TEDIUM, and individual productivity doubled. Tested programs were being installed at the rate of one per effort day.

In the previous section it was stated that a goal of TEDIUM was to have the designer specify the programs from the perspective of the application. It has been shown already that this specification approach is compact, that is, minimal. The

Table 5. Measures of Program Generation by Year

	1981	1982	1983	1984	1985	1986*
Number of programs	625	1377	950	1014	731	430
Mean generations	25.14	18.08	13.48	12.78	10.32	7.03
Median generations	27	13	10	8	7	5
Mode of generations	18	8	4	5	3	2
90th percentile	44	37	29	27	25	15

*Through September.

Table 6. Distribution of Program Generations (1980–1984)

Percentile	Upper Bound (Number of Generations)
10	3
20	5
30	7
40	9
50	11
60	14
70	17
80	22
90	31

question now is: Does TEDIUM allow the designer to express himself effectively? To provide insight into this property of TEDIUM, I have recorded each time that a designer edits a specification. A small number of edits (or generations) indicates that the language is expressive. A large number of edits may have many meanings; for example, the problem is not well understood, the designer incrementally develops programs, or the environment is not expressive.

Table 5 summarizes some measures of generation (editing) activity by year. Notice that the numbers are higher in the earlier years. This reflects two facts. First, the early years involved more learning; thus more errors would be made in debugging. Second, older programs will be more subject to revision as changes are made to the system. The data do show, however, that TEDIUM is an expressive environment. On the basis of the 1986 data, an average of only six edits is required for a production program. Table 6 presents some data from a 1984 analysis. In this case only half of the 5000 OCIS programs had been edited more than ten times; this number included all debugging and maintenance changes.

The final two tables offer some insight into the OCIS maintenance activity. Since 1985 all maintenance has been performed by a staff of four programmers and a system manager who programs half of the time. This staff is responsible for maintaining 1600 programs that they did not write, plus maintaining and adding to a large, complex application. Only one member of this staff had professional programming experience prior to employment by the JHOC.

Table 7 displays the activities of the principal contributors to the OCIS. The BME staff members are identified by a B, and the JHOC members are denoted by an O. The table shows the number of programs in production use in 1986, by year and designer. Table 8 shows the average number of program generations (edits) for the data in Table 7. One can recognize the learning process. In the case of O4's 1982 and 1983 activity, the large number of programs produced are the result of copying and modifying existing programs. This reuse obscures true "productivity." Still, the data in Table 8 clearly show that, as the designers learn their job and how to use their tools, their profiles become almost identical; there are few individual differences.

Table 7. New Programs by Year and Designer

Designer	81	82	83	84	85	86*
B1	228	228	7			
B2	25	48	16			
B3	38					
B4	98	14				
B5	50	236	101	30		
B6	32	88				
B7	17					
O1	45	27	48	9		
B8/O2		226	258	214	159	97
O3	3	15	22	10	29	6
O4	38	256	292	390	174	161
O5	31	171	143	254	233	115
O6		23	57	94		
O7		33	5	3		
O8					135	49

*January through September only.

Not shown in all these tables is the fact that the OCIS staff is dedicated and stable. Few people have left the JHOC, and those who now make up the Information Center have a clear understanding of the OCIS, the JHOC, and its users' needs. The members of the staff have gone through a long apprenticeship, and they are very familiar with both the application domain and the OCIS implementation. This fact is a necessary condition for the system's development and maintenance success.

To conclude this evaluation, the OCIS was developed using TEDIUM, and now it is necessary to live with TEDIUM or reprogram the entire system. At one point, an objective analysis of the system was conducted and other development approaches considered. There were no feasible alternatives. There is anecdotal evidence that TEDIUM provides an effective environment for the OCIS. Some TEDIUM users, who were reluctant at first to work with the environment, have told me that they could not maintain the OCIS without it or that they would be pleased to act as a reference for other potential users. Someone who installed the OCIS in Australia said that he could not accomplish that task if it were not for TEDIUM.

Of course, I find the TEDIUM endorsements gratifying; I continue to use it as a tool in my current research. However, I find even more satisfying the fact that I could participate in the development of the OCIS, walk away from the JHOC in 1983, and come back to see the system in use, enhanced, and an integral part of the JHOC operations. In closing this section on evaluation, I am reminded of Dr. Octo Barnett's three criteria for evaluating a clinical system: Will people use it? Will people pay for it? Will people steal it? The first two questions were answered in the affirmative in the 1970s. Let us hope that this book will contribute to the theft of our concepts.

Table 8. Program Generations by Year and Designer

Designer	81	82	83	84	85	86*
B1	23.8	11.9	3.6			
B2	22.2	15.0	9.1			
B3	25.4					
B4	27.0	23.0				
B5	25.5	16.4	13.5	13.5		
B6	23.1	16.5				
B7	13.3					
O1	16.3	12.9	10.2	12.7		
B8/O2		23.1	14.0	13.0	9.2	6.0
O3	14.3	9.4	9.5	5.4	18.6	5.3
O4	42.4	19.6	12.5	12.6	10.1	5.8
O5	33.0	24.3	13.5	14.1	10.3	5.8
O6		16.0	22.0	10.9		
O7		12.6	27.2	12.0		
O8					10.3	7.5

*January through September only.

References

There clearly is no need for any OCIS references. However, for readers interested in the software process, there is a collection in this series called *Implementing Health Care Information Systems* (H.F. Orthner and B.I. Blum, Editors, Springer-Verlag, New York, 1989). It includes chapters on software development, MUMPS, and TEDIUM. For readers wishing additional information about MUMPS, the MUMPS Users' Group offers primers and reference manuals. Their address is MUG, 4321 Hartwick Road, College Park, MD 20740. A more complete discussion of TEDIUM is available in B.I. Blum, *TEDIUM and the Software Process*, MIT Press, Boston, MA, 1989.

II
Functional Description

This section contains a detailed description of the functional components of OCIS from the perspective of its use in the Oncology Center. Each chapter contains a general introduction followed by a presentation of the OCIS tools in the context of their use. In most cases, the chapters have been written by the principal users of the applications.

4
Clinical Data Management
Gloria J. Stuart[1], Bruce I. Blum,
and Raymond E. Lenhard, Jr.

Introduction

The primary objective of the OCIS, as described in Chapters 1 and 2, is to
manage patient data and to present clinical information in a manner that facilitates medical decision making. This means that the OCIS must be able to produce
reports in a variety of formats for each category of clinical data. To accomplish
this, the OCIS also requires tools to define the desired formats, to produce
the outputs at the appropriate times, and to collect the data in a timely and accurate fashion.

The OCIS clinical reports are patient oriented, and the system offers a variety
of mechanisms for viewing a report. When the patient is being treated as an inpatient, the patient record is linked to an Oncology Center nursing unit. Table 1 lists
the current inpatient units. Each unit has associated with it a home screen that
identifies the patients currently in the unit. Figure 1 illustrates a sample inpatient
screen. Access to the data for a patient is accomplished by entering the number
to the left of the name. Thus, to view the data for Patient C, one would enter "3."

When patients have been discharged, the clinical information is available by
entering either the patient name or identification number. For patients being
treated as outpatients, the appointment subsystem, which associates patients
with clinic (and physician) appointments, provides another means of accessing
patient information.

Clinical information is maintained on line for both active and deceased
patients. The inpatient and outpatient data are merged, and summary abstracts
are maintained. The primary goal of the OCIS is to display information that will
facilitate the treatment of patients at the Center. The following subsections

---

[1]Gloria J. Stuart is presently Manager of the OCIS system. She has been in the health care field
for over 20 years and has been affiliated with OCIS for the past 9 years. Prior to her position as
Manager of OCIS she worked for the Pediatric Oncology Division and held the position of supervisor
of data coordinators.

Table 1. JHOC Inpatient Units

Unit	Number of Beds	Primary Diseases Treated
2 North	14	Solid tumor
2 South	14	Leukemia
3 North	22	Solid tumor
3 South	20	Bone marrow transplant
Pediatrics	14	Pediatric malignancies

describe the kinds of data that OCIS maintains and some of the functions that are associated with the maintenance of the data and reports. Naturally, there are administrative and nonclinical uses for the same data; these are discussed in Chapter 8.

The Clinical Data

OCIS maintains clinical, support, and administrative data. All clinical data are patient oriented and keyed by The Johns Hopkins history number (HNO). This is a seven-digit number (with an optional eighth check digit) assigned to the patient and used for all inpatient stays and outpatient encounters. Assignment of the history number is the responsibility of the Johns Hopkins Hospital Medical Records Department, and the JHOC staff assumes the responsibility for seeing that the correct HNO is manually entered into the OCIS database.

Associated with the HNO are the patient's name, demographic information, and administrative data. The OCIS duplicates portions of the central hospital system, but there has been no attempt to link the two patient identification systems electronically. Relative to the rest of the hospital, the JHOC sees a small number of patients over an extended period of time and has the facilities to verify that the correct HNO is being used. The OCIS does not require all of the administrative information used by the central business office, and it collects information not

```
JOHNS HOPKINS ONCOLOGY CENTER    INPATIENT CENSUS    2S    07/15/86

NO   HIST NO   NAME         AGE R S   ROOM   ADM DATE   EST LOS
 1   7777777   PATIENT,A    41  W F   367    07/13/86     15
 2   6666666   PATIENT,B    24  B F   365    06/30/86     15
 3   7654321   PATIENT,C    41  B M   333    06/29/86     15
 4   1234567   PATIENT,D    15  W F   369    05/20/86      4
 5   1231234   PATIENT,E    19  W M   322    06/12/86     15

 ENTER SEQUENCE NUMBER:
```

Figure 1. Inpatient home screen with unit census.

used by the other systems. For example, there are provisions for both a home and local address, and the name can be of arbitrary length and written in both upper- and lowercase.

Below the level of the patient identifier, there is a record of all patient treatments administered at JHOC. This is maintained in a *census* file containing a summary of admissions, outpatient activities, diagnoses, and therapies. The census is augmented by an *abstract* of the patient's medical record, which includes both medical and administrative data.

Although the census and abstract both contain some clinical data, they are used primarily as a summary to identify the patient, the disease, and an overview of the treatment. The clinical data are reported in more detail. Several categories of data are retained.

Tabular Data. These data can be represented as a triple consisting of an identifer, a time or date, and a value. Examples are laboratory results, cumulative daily medication doses, and subjective scales for performance. These data are displayed in the form of *plots* and *flow sheets*. Special formats are also provided to display current laboratory results on line, that is, the data reports.

Bacteriology Data. These data follow a general pattern, but they require special report formats. There may be many organisms found in a single specimen and many antibiotic sensitivities for each organism. The bacteriology reports organize the data by time, specimen, and organism.

Treatment Plans. The protocol-directed care plans, described in Chapter 5, rely on treatment plans that are initiated, reviewed, and canceled by the Oncology Center physicians. Some of the *treatment sequence plan* displays that they use are presented here briefly.

Pharmacy Information. The OCIS tabular displays of medications summarize activity in the form of daily accumulations. Clearly, greater granularity is required for patient management. The pharmacy system, described in Chapter 6, provides tools for reviewing drug profiles and supporting medication administration. Most of the provider-oriented outputs are integrated into the other data displays and are not discussed in this chapter.

Transfusion Data. The presentation of this category of data must include the patient status before and after the transfusion, the kind of product used, and other information relevant to the planning of future transfusions. Although the display of these data are considered part of the blood product management subsystem described in Chapter 7, the *blood transfusion summary* report is an important tool in patient care.

Special Functions. There are a variety of special data management functions that can be managed easily when there is a comprehensive database available to support them. Examples include the computation of body surface area and the management of pain medications.

The OCIS philosophy is that all reports should be available on line from any terminal provided that the viewer has the appropriate authorization. (See Chapter 8 for a description of the authority system.) Because paper records can display more information and are more portable, all reports are available in hard-copy form as well. The OCIS has a task-scheduling system (see Chapter 8) that produces outputs whenever required, typically in time for morning rounds for inpatients and before visits for outpatients. Finally, we note that it is OCIS policy not to archive data. Thus, the provider has access to all information about a patient beginning with his or her initial treatment at the Oncology Center.

The equipment available for the initial implementation had a major impact on the appearance of the OCIS reports. In this era of microcomputers and bit-mapped displays, it sometimes is difficult to recall what the state of the art was in the mid-1970s. Because many of the clinical reports have an "old fashioned" feel, we close this introduction with some background on this artifact.

At the time that the OCIS equipment was procured, there were two choices regarding a high-speed printer. One could opt for upper- and lowercase, or one could have the uppercase character set repeated twice, thereby doubling the printer's throughput. We chose the latter option, a standard selection at that time. Unfortunately, the system treated the lowercase characters as nonprinting characters, and so the database was built in uppercase only. When we purchased the second computer, we added the ability to print upper- and lowercase, but the logistics of associating an output with a printer trapped us into continuing with uppercase abstracts, etc. It was only the introduction of the Phase III system that freed us from this limitation.

If printers were expensive in the mid-1970s, then plotters were even more expensive. In order to get the desired throughput, we elected to use character printing for our plots. When the 11×14 computer paper proved too cumbersome, we purchased an electrostatic printer and produced the plots in a landscape orientation on $8\frac{1}{2} \times 11$ paper. The clinicians became accustomed to our plot formats, and there has been no demand to convert to a new format as the appropriate equipment has become less costly.

Finally, we note that OCIS does not use full-screen cursor control for any of its functions. (This fact would not be apparent from the examples in this book.) This also goes back to the mid-1970s. Although today there are over 200 OCIS terminals, our original system had only 8. We added to this number as we could, buying a variety of terminals that relied on evolving standards. Because of this diversity, we elected to restrict the OCIS applications to the common functions supported by all terminals, that is, clear screen, home, and scroll. Such is the fate of those who are among the first to implement.

Administrative Data

Recall that most of the JHOC administrative functions are performed by other hospital or university systems, for example, inpatient billing, admissions, professional fees. Thus the OCIS administrative functions are limited to those activities that are integrated with the patient care functions. In some cases OCIS tools parallel those of the central hospital systems; this duplication is required because of the interactions between the administrative and clinical systems.

OCIS supports the following clinically oriented administrative functions. Each of these functions uses some of the clinical data for other purposes. More complete discussions of each function are contained in Chapter 8. They are catalogued here simply to remind the reader that, once a clinical database has been established, there are many uses for it.

Admission, Discharge, and Transfer (ADT). Although the central hospital system is responsible for the management of the ADT function, OCIS maintains schedules for both new and old patients; it provides an up-to-date locator for all patients in the Center, and it integrates discharge planning with the delivery of care. Projected admission and discharge dates are available on line or as printed reports.

Outpatient Scheduling. Preparation of reports and tests must be integrated with the patients' outpatient schedule. Therefore, OCIS must maintain a scheduling system. This system must provide access to information organized by patient, clinic unit, and provider.

Tumor Registry and Research Office. The Tumor Registry is a registry of all patients who are diagnosed as having cancer at The Johns Hopkins Hospital. The JHOC Research Office maintains records about all JHOC patients who have been treated on a protocol study. Both units must interact with the clinical operation of JHOC, but neither can be considered a clinical function.

Level-of-Care Reporting. A level-of-care nursing tool was developed at JHOC to record the intensity of care required by inpatients during their admission. This is recorded as a number from 1 to 5 and entered into the OCIS database. The number can be reported in the clinical displays; there also are special reports that are produced periodically.

Center Administration Reports. All of the data collected for patients can be organized by time or unit for use in Center management and planning. OCIS produces a large number of reports that describe Center activities in terms of occupancy rates, lengths of stay, diagnoses, protocols, etc.

Maintaining the Database

The emphasis in the previous subsections was on the use of the OCIS database. We now consider how the data are collected. This is done in one of two ways: automatically through electronic data transfer or by manual entry. The first has the obvious advantages of ease of use, timeliness, and a low error rate. In many situations, however, electronic transfer is not possible, and manual entry is required.

Electronic Data Entry. Data can be transmitted directly to OCIS from the Clinical Laboratory, the Hematology Laboratories located in JHOC, and from the pharmacy system. The link with the Clinical Laboratory is discussed in Chapter 8, and the interface with the pharmacy system is described in Chapter 6. The Clinical Laboratory and Pharmacy links manage an exchange of data between independent systems. There is a need for tools and procedures to coordinate dictionaries and identify mismatched history numbers. This extra processing results in a delay between the time data are available on the host system and the time that the data are in the OCIS database ready for reporting.

Communication with the hematology laboratories is managed in a more efficient fashion. Because of the Center's unique demands upon a hematology laboratory, the JHOC maintains two such laboratories. One is located in the inpatient facilities, where it is used by the inpatient units, the Medical Oncology Clinic, and the Radiation Oncology Department. A second laboratory is located off-site; it supports the Department of Hemapheresis and the Medical Oncology Consultation Service.

Three hematology analyzers in these laboratories provide the hematology results. The analyzers are linked directly to the OCIS computers. Results are generated via the Coulter counter, verified by the medical technologist, and sent directly to the OCIS database via electronic transfer. They are immediately reformatted for easy display on inpatient units. This has eliminated multiple calls to the Hematology Laboratory by physicians awaiting results on patients who potentially are in need of immediate blood product support. This is, perhaps, the most used facility offered by the OCIS.

Manual Data Entry. Operation of the OCIS data entry is divided into two categories. Routine, well-formatted data are entered by the computer operators. This fact implies that computer operations do not require much attending and that very little data remain to be entered manually. In fact, most of the data entered into the OCIS database require judgment regarding what should be entered and what the database contents should contain. As indicated in Chapter 1, the clinical data coordinator is responsible for this type of database maintenance.

The clinical data coordinator plays an important role with regard to the Oncology Information System. This position was developed specifically to serve as the interface between the health care providers and the programs and applications that reside in the OCIS. The clinical data coordinator has a comprehensive knowledge of the capabilities and limitations of the applications and is thus able to supply health care providers with the data in a format that best assists them in the daily clinical management of their patients.

Data coordinators are assigned to permanent locations within the Center and are regarded as members of the health care teams. The data coordinator assigned to the Bone Marrow Transplant (BMT) Unit, for example, has an office in that inpatient unit. Data coordinators attend daily rounds and provide updated computer reports on each patient. They attend routine meetings involving patient care; they are responsible for monitoring the data entered into the OCIS computer and serve as quality control mechanisms. In addition, they work with the health care providers to ensure that important data are captured and that new reports are developed to display that data in the best format.

Data coordinators serve each of the inpatient locations; Medical Oncology Clinic, Pediatric Oncology, and Hemapheresis. Although each area has specific duties unique to its location and program, data coordinators are cross-trained to provide coverage in other areas should the primary data coordinator be absent. This ensures continuous quality data support. Core coverage is provided on the weekends and holidays as well.

The data coordinator is the primary interface between the OCIS and the health care professional. To meet their obligations as clinical team members, data coordinators must possess sufficient knowledge of medicine to enable them to understand how to present the data in a manner that supports clinical care. Training is provided on the job, but all new employees have clinical work experience and college-level coursework in anatomy, physiology, and medical terminology. Although a programming background is not a necessity, a knowledge of data processing is helpful. Common data coordinator backgrounds include nursing, medical technology, and radiology.

To guarantee that the OCIS database contains correct and timely information, the data coordinator must assume responsibility for its validity. This implies that the data coordinators maintain appropriate internal dictionaries, schedule the listing of all periodic reports, enter the physicians' plans into the daily care plan system, verify that scheduled actions have been carried out, record clinical findings that must be extracted from the medical record (e.g., weights and temperatures), coordinate admission and discharge actions, and communicate with the Research Office regarding protocol starts. Clearly, this involves much more than manual data entry. By assuming these responsibilities, however, the clinical data coordinator eliminates the need for any other member of the clinical team to enter data into the OCIS. Thus the providers typically operate in a "read only" mode; they are users of the system.

Supporting Functions

We conclude this overview of the OCIS clinical data management functions by identifying briefly some of the support functions that are required to make the former operate effectively. The OCIS includes the following facilities.

Dictionaries of Terms. There are a variety of dictionaries used throughout the OCIS. Some identify the names of tests and findings. These provide short character identifiers, longer descriptive names, limits on the normal and allowable values, etc. Other dictionaries describe how to translate the data sent from the clinical laboratory and pharmacy system. There is a dictionary that describes all tests ordered in the hospital, what forms and containers should be used, where the specimen should be sent, etc. There are dictionaries for the units, the providers, the protocols, and so on.

Format Definition Output. The plots and flow sheets are considered to be reports produced by a report generator. The OCIS provides tools to define a format, edit or delete a report, and build a dictionary of available reports. Naturally, this dictionary of reports is integrated with the other dictionaries.

Routine Report Scheduling. Because the OCIS can produce so many different types of reports, it was essential that tools be provided to schedule the routine preparation of outputs for distribution to the clinical areas. Reports can be requested for delivery every day, on specific days of the week, when there is an outpatient visit, etc. A schedule may include several different reports, and many schedules may be active for a single patient.

Electronic Mail. The OCIS maintains an electronic mail facility that is used to send messages between the data coordinators and the Pharmacy, the Research Office, and other coordinators. The system can be used for communications among the staff or as a personal reminder system.

Data Sets for Analysis. Because the major orientation of the OCIS is patient care, little effort has been expended on the building of tools for retrospective data analysis. The system does have facilities for building data sets in formats that can be used directly by the standard statistical packages.

The Clinical Data Reports

This section presents an overview of the clinical data reports that the OCIS provides. In some cases the use of these reports has already been described, and the reference in this section is very brief. There are many other reports and system outputs beyond those that are described in this section. The criteria for selecting an output for presentation here include its importance to the JHOC staff and its potential interest to designers and users of other clinical systems.

As noted earlier, to view the clinical data, the provider first identifies the patient and then selects the desired report. Patient identification for inpatients is by selection from a display of the current unit census; selection for all other patients is by either name or history number. (The OCIS recognizes whether a number has been entered and, if so, does an HNO lookup. Otherwise, it displays all names that match the initial letters entered and allows the user to select from this list or reenter another name.) Once the patient has been identified, the OCIS responds with the "view" prompt shown in Figure 2.

The commands for selecting a report are given in parentheses. Most reports also have options; most can be displayed on line or printed. If a printed output is requested, the user indicates to whom the output should be delivered. In practice, however, most printed reports are scheduled for printing and delivery automatically. Terminal use normally is limited to the display of data.

Commands may be strung together without waiting for the prompt. For example, if the provider wants to see the follow-up information (F) in the abstract (A) for the third patient listed in the unit census (3), then it is possible to enter

    3, A, F

and get the display without having to respond to intermediate prompts. Conversely, if the provider is unfamiliar with the OCIS, it is possible to enter a question mark (?) at any prompt and get a help message. Finally, if the provider

```
(N)EXT  (A)BS  (B)ACT  (C)EN  (D)ATA  (F)LOW  (P)LOT  (S)CH  (T)X PLAN  (TR)NS
```

COMMAND	OPTION	FUNCTION
N	(N)EXT	DISPLAY PROMPT FOR NEXT PATIENT
A	(A)BS	DISPLAY ABSTRACT
B	(B)ACT	DISPLAY BACTERIOLOGY REPORT
C	(C)EN	DISPLAY CENSUS INFORMATION
D	(D)ATA	DISPLAY PATIENT CLINICAL DATA
F	(F)LOW	DISPLAY SPECIFIED FLOW SHEET
P	(P)LOT	DISPLAY SPECIFIED PLOT DIAGRAM
S	(S)CH	DISPLAY PATIENT SCHEDULE
T	(T)X PLAN	DISPLAY TREATMENT SEQUENCE PLAN
TR	(TR)NS	DISPLAY BLOOD TRANSFUSION SUMMARY

Figure 2. View options with description (page numbers refer to *Users' Manual*).

enters a return without previously entering any information, the first option in the list (usually considered to be the recommended default) is selected. Naturally, entering an invalid command results in the repeating of the prompt line.

The clinical data available to the providers can be divided into the higher level summaries of treatment, for example, the abstract and census, into displays of the clinical data, for example, the plots, flow sheets, and bacteriology data, or into other specialized reports. The following subsections examine some examples in each category.

Patient Summary Information

The OCIS patient summary information is relatively static. It is used for periodic reference, especially when the provider may not be familiar with the patient's history. For example, the admitting officer may review this information when making a priority decision regarding admission. Segments of the patient summary database also are included in other reports.

The Census Subsystem. The patient census is an extension of what one might normally think a census should contain. This subsystem began as historic record of all census activities and was gradually enlarged to its present form. Even though the name is misleading, it has been retained.

The OCIS patient identification consists of the patient's history number (HNO), name, and a demographic string consisting of age, race, and sex. (The

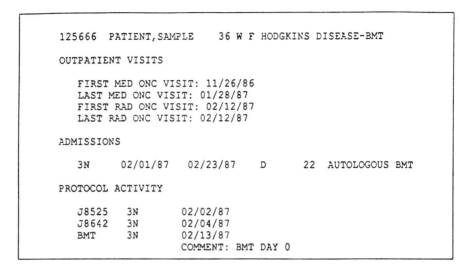

```
    125666  PATIENT,SAMPLE    36 W F HODGKINS DISEASE-BMT

 OUTPATIENT VISITS

     FIRST MED ONC VISIT: 11/26/86
     LAST MED ONC VISIT: 01/28/87
     FIRST RAD ONC VISIT: 02/12/87
     LAST RAD ONC VISIT: 02/12/87

 ADMISSIONS

     3N       02/01/87  02/23/87   D      22  AUTOLOGOUS BMT

 PROTOCOL ACTIVITY

     J8525   3N        02/02/87
     J8642   3N        02/04/87
     BMT     3N        02/13/87
                       COMMENT: BMT DAY 0
```

Figure 3. Sample census report with description.

age is updated each year automatically.) The census data consists of this identification information plus:

An optional text field. This text can be broken into strings with each string identified by a date. There are no Center standards regarding the use of this text field; its application varies from provider to provider.

A log of all hospital admissions, including the dates, length of stay (computed automatically), and final action, for example, discharged, transferred. There is an optional field for a brief comment.

A summary of the first and most recent outpatient visit for each clinic visited and/or radiation oncology treatment.

Patient diagnosis. A special Center disease dictionary is used so that patients may be grouped by disease in categories that are meaningful to JHOC. A more complete ICD categorization is available in the abstract, and there is also a field for the provider to write a clinical description of the diagnosis.

Protocol activity including the protocol, start and stop dates, where treated, outcome, and optional text field.

Figure 3 displays a sample census report. Other report formats may restrict some of the information displayed or order the information by diagnosis or protocol. (For a different census example, see Chapter 2, Figure 1.)

The Abstract. The abstract is an extension of the Tumor Registry record. It contains all the information necessary to satisfy the requirements of the American College of Surgeons and adds summary information of value to the OCIS clinicians. The use of the abstract in patient care was discussed in Chapter 2, and a

```
(C)OMPLETE  (I)D  (A)DM  (D)X  (R)ECR  (T)X  (P)R   (H)X   (F)U  PRI(N)T  (Q)UIT
```

NOTE: **TYPE: C <RET> (To view the entire Abstract of a chosen patient)

```
   (I)D  - Gives the IDENTIFICATION of patient, spouse, mother/father;
           Includes Marital Status, Birthday, Patient Address and
           Follow-up Status.

  (A)DM  - Tumor Registry Administration information; Access is limited
           to Tumor Registry Personnel.

   (D)X  - Gives specific DIAGNOSTIC/Tumor Registry information such as
           Morphology, Grade, Laterality, Metastatic Sites and Extent.

  (R)ECR - Provides Disease RECURRENCE data for patient.

   (T)X  - Summary of TREATMENT with dates and type (e.g. Surgery (S)
           or Chemotherapy (C).

   (P)R  - Gives Patient's Protocol Activity, Start and End Dates
           with Protocol Outcome.

   (H)X  - Gives HISTORY of patient to include initial Symptoms, Known
           Medical Abnormalities, Occupation, Exposure and Allergies.

   (F)U  - Gives Date of FOLLOW-UP, when the patient was last seen by
           a physician, his condition and any significant comments.

   (E)R  - Gives END RESULTS showing Date, Cause, and Source of
           patient's Death.

PRI(N)T  - Allows you to order a paper copy PRINT-OUT from OCIS.
```

Figure 4. Abstract display options.

sample abstract was shown in Figure 2 of that chapter. A discussion of the abstract from the perspective of the Tumor Registry is contained in Chapter 8. The on-line display of the abstract allows the user to page through the entire abstract or jump to any section of it. Figure 4 lists the abstract display options.

Tabular Clinical Data

In the OCIS, the data are divided into two categories: tabular data and special data. As the name implies, tabular data can be organized in a table (i.e., relation). The OCIS maintains the data in two tables. The Patient Data (PDATA) is indexed by HNO, date of the data, and name of the data item; each entry contains the value for that item, a normal/abnormal flag, and an optional (and seldom used) comment field. For data that may have more than one value reported each day, there is a Patient Data Time (PDATAT) file that adds the time of the value to the index.

The OCIS does not archive any data, and there are some 16 million data items on line. The MUMPS data access method facilitates immediate access to any value by date for a given patient. As discussed below, several of the standard reports can be built from data stored in this format. However, as discussed in Chapter 2, the key goal of the system is to display data in formats that are meaningful to the providers in the context of their current activity. Thus, there can be clashes between storage efficiency and display efficacy.

In the OCIS this clash is managed by replicating the tabular data in preformatted files so that the various displays can be produced rapidly. This is done periodically, usually at night just after the pharmacy data have been updated. The printed plots and flow sheets (which are generated from the tabular data) use this early morning state of the database. During the day, as the tabular data entries are updated, the updates are not reflected in the preformatted files. There are two reasons for this. First, the printed tabular displays satisfy most of the clinical needs; requests to view the most current data can be satisfied by listing from the Patient Data files or the unformatted flow format. Second, the processing demand to retain current preformatted files is heavy, and the high system load prevents more frequent updating during peak periods. (Compare this with the Ohio State University experience discussed in Chapter 10.)

The tabular data are displayed in the form of plots, flow sheets, and simple lists. For inpatient units, some summary data may also be displayed by unit. Examples of the most frequent displays are shown below; the use of these displays in a clinical situation was presented in Chapter 2.

Flow Sheets. The flow sheet is a tabular display of clinical data. Two formats are provided. The horizontal flow lists the dates as columns and the items as rows. The advantage of this format is that it can display all the appropriate clinical data for a limited number of days. (The narrow flow lists 7 columns on 8½ × 11 paper; the wide flow, which is very seldom used, lists 15 columns on 11 × 14 paper.) The disadvantage of the horizontal flow is that it cannot present long-term trends. For this reason, there also is a vertical flow that lists the data in columns and the dates (or times) in rows.

There are many flow-sheet formats; each is considered to be a special report for a particular need. Once the F command is entered, the user is asked to enter the name of the desired flow. A null return produces the default comprehensive flow that is shown in Figure 5. This horizontal flow sheet displays all the tabular clinical information for the patient for the period covered. The default is the most recent seven days of treatment as either an inpatient or outpatient. When browsing on line, there are options for starting with the earliest date or a selected date and paging forward and back.

At the top of the flow the patient identification, date of listing, unit, and flow name are printed. Below these are the dates of the data. For inpatients, the convention is to start listing with a Sunday in column one, except when the most current data are presented. If the patient is on protocol, then the protocol identification and day on protocol are shown. In Figure 5 the patient was started on two protocols on the same date. For BMT patients, the day of transplant is day 0, and negative protocol days can be listed.

```
JOHNS HOPKINS ONCOLOGY CENTER    2S          HISTORY NO: 777 77 77
                                             NAME: PATIENT,SAMPLE
    COMP FLOW                                DATE: 07/15/86
----------------:-------:-------:-------:-------:-------:-------:-------
                :08JUL86:09JUL86:10JUL86:11JUL86:12JUL86:13JUL86:14JUL86
      J8410     :DAY  19:DAY  20:DAY  21:DAY  22:DAY  23:DAY  24:DAY  25
      J8530     :DAY  19:DAY  20:DAY  21:DAY  22:DAY  23:DAY  24:DAY  25
PAT STATUS -----:-------:-------:-------:-------:-------:-------:-------
TEMP-MAX   DEG C:     38:  39.4:  37.8:  38.1:  38.0:  38.0:  37.8
TEMPERATUR DEG C:  37.9*:  38.5*  37.8:  37.4:  38.0*  38.0*  37.2
MAX BP     MM HG: 130/62: 150/70: 140/90: 168/70: 150/70: 154/78: 150/60
MAX PULSE       :    122:   110:   120:   100:   110:   120:   120
MAX RESPIR      :     28:    24:    32:    30:    26:    28:    28
BODY WT AM KG   :       :  85.4:  86.1:  84.0:  84.8:  84.5:  84.3
BD SUR AR  M SQ :       :     2:  2.01:  1.99:     2:     2:  1.99
FVC             :       :       :       :       :       :   1.8:   2.0
CARE LEVEL      :      4:     4:     4:     4:     4:     4:     4
FLUID (IV) ML   :   4120:  3410:  2990:       :  4130:  3595:  3965
FLUID (PO) ML   :    120:     0:   567:       :  2075:  1130:  1310
TOTL INTAK ML   :   4240:  3410:  3557:       :  6205:  4725:  5275
URINE OUT  ML   :   4425:  2000:  4050:       :  6795:  4620:  3300
LIQ STOOL  ML   :      0:     0:     0:       :     0:     0:    30
EMES OUT   ML   :      0:     0:   325:       :     0:   520:   100
TOTL OUT   ML   :   4425:  2000:  4375:       :  6795:  5140:  3430
IN/OUT DIF ML   :   -185:  1410:  -818:       :  -590:  -415:  1845
BLD PROD   ------:-------:-------:-------:-------:-------:-------:-------
PLT TR-TOT      :     13:       :       :    11:       :       :
PLT TRN-PH      :     13:       :       :    11:       :       :
HEMATOLOGY ----:-------:-------:-------:-------:-------:-------:-------
WBC        #/CU :   044*  099*   300*   300*   300*   300*    200
RBC        M/CU :  2.89*  3.55:  3.51:  3.11*  3.48:  3.79:   3.00
HGB        G/DL :   8.5*  10.4*  10.2*   9.1*  10.6*  11.6*    9.1
HCT        %    :  25.5*  32.1*  30.6*  26.8*  32.0*  34.4*   26.5
RETICLCYTE %    :       :   0.1*       :       :       :       :
PLATELETS  /MM3 :  76000* 56000* 41000* 78000* 54000* 39000*  32000
ABS NEUT        :       :       :    22:     6:       :       :     28
CHEMISTRY  -----:-------:-------:-------:-------:-------:-------:-------
SER NA     MEQ/L:   134*   142:   144:   145:   145:   147:    146
SER K      MEQ/L:   4.8:   4.5:   4.1:   3.6:   3.6:   3.8:    3.7
DIR BILI   MG/DL:   0.6*       :       :   1.1*       :       :
DIAGNOSTIC TESTS:-------:-------:-------:-------:-------:-------:-------
URINE K    NEQ/L:       :       :       :       :    53:       :
URINE CL   NEQ/L:       :       :       :       :    97:       :
MEDICATION ----:-------:-------:-------:-------:-------:-------:-------
HYDRCRTSNE MG   :       :    50:    50:    50:    50:    50:     50
FLUCYTOSIN GN   :       :       :     2:     2:     2:     2:      2
ACYCLOVIR  MG   :   1500:  2000:  3000:  3000:  3000:  3000:   3000
```

Figure 5. Portion of a sample comprehensive flow.

```
JOHNS HOPKINS ONCOLOGY CENTER 2S        HISTORY NO: 123  45  67
                                              NAME: SAMPLE,PATIENT
  HEMATOLOGY CTS                               DATE: 08/01/86
     1986      TEMP     WBC      PLTS    HCT  NEUT    BAND     ANEU
    MANAN      DEG C    #/CU     /MM3     %     %      %
  07/17  30    38.8:    066:    37000:   31.5:----:--------:------- :
  07/18  31    37.9:    154:    19000:   31.0:----:--------:------- :
  07/19  32    37.9:    187:    57000:   22.3:----:--------:------- :
  07/20  33    38.2:    231:    53000:   31.3:----:--------:------- :
  07/21  34    38.8:    200:    52000:   33.6:----:--------:
  07/22  35    39.3:    300:    48000:   30.9:----:--------:
  07/23  36    38.4:    300:    31000:   30.8:----:--------:
  07/24  37    38.4:    200:    57000:   26.1:----:--------:        1 :
  07/27  40    37.8:    330:    58000:   37.8:----:--------:------- :

  (C)URRENT   (E)ARLIEST   (D)ATE   (P)RINT   (Q)UIT
```

Figure 6. Sample vertical flow, unaligned format, terminal display.

The clinical data in the flow are grouped and ordered in clinically useful ways. A typical comprehensive flow may be three pages long. In Figure 5, the patient status data are given in the first block, blood product transfusions in the next block, hematology in the next, and so on. The medications exclude chemotherapy drugs; these are listed as a separate category. In each block, items are identified and data are listed only if values were reported during the period covered by the flow sheet. Abnormal values are indicated by an asterisk to the right of the value.

If the provider wants some other flow sheet, the initial characters are entered using the OCIS standard prompting convention. For example, entering "A" might return

```
1   ABIOT    (H, N)    ANTIBIOTIC FLOW
2   ACH      (V, N)    CHEM FLOW
3   ACPH     (V, N)    ACID PHOSPHATASE
4   . . . .
```

where the letters in parentheses indicate the type of flow, for example, horizontal, vertical, narrow. As described below, the provider may define new formats as necessary.

If a vertical flow is selected, the user must then select the format option. Unaligned is the default; other options include listing a line for each date even if no data are available (aligned), compressing the date field to preserve space (compressed), and including all data with a time (time). Because space is limited in the vertical flow, on-line users may select only one protocol to be listed. Figures 6 and 7 show two formats for the hematology counts flow sheet for patients during a period in July 1986. Each patient was on the MANAN protocol; day 30 was 7/17/86.

```
┌─────────────────────────────────────────────────────────────────┐
│                                                                   │
│  JOHNS HOPKINS ONCOLOGY CENTER              HISTORY NO: 123 45 67  │
│                                                 NAME: PATIENT,B    │
│  HEMATOLOGY CTS                                 DATE: 08/07/86     │
│                                                                   │
│      1986      TEMP   WBC    PLTS    HCT     NEUT  BAND  ANEU       │
│      MANAN    DEG C  #/CU   /MM3     %        %     %             │
│                                                                   │
│  07/24   37                                                       │
│            38.4:-----:---------:---------:-----:-----:-----:      │
│     6:30 AM ----:  200:  57000:     26.1:-----:-----:    14:      │
│  07/25   38      :     :         :         :     :     :     :    │
│            39.6:-----:---------:---------:-----:-----:-----:      │
│     6:30 AM ----:  066:  27000:     31.6:-----:-----:-----:      │
│     1:15 PM ----:-----:  54000:---------:-----:-----:-----:      │
│  07/26   39      :     :         :         :     :     :     :    │
│            38.5:-----:---------:---------:-----:-----:-----:      │
│     9:40 AM ----:  209:  73000:     29.3:-----:-----:-----:      │
│     5:00 PM ----:-----:  91000:---------:-----:-----:-----:      │
│                                                                   │
└─────────────────────────────────────────────────────────────────┘
```

Figure 7. Sample vertical flow, time format.

Plots. One of the most useful clinical displays for identifying trends is the plot. Several examples of their use were presented in Chapter 2, and an explanation for their character orientation was given above. Plots are available both on line and in printed form. The on-line plots are seldom used because of the limitations of the video screen: 80 × 24 characters as compared with 132 × 60 characters in the listing.

A sample plot is shown in Figure 8. It consists of two plotted items, platelet counts (P), and white blood cell counts (W). Both are plotted on a log scale from 100 to 1,000,000. (It is possible to plot up to four items with different scales on the same plot, but the resulting clutter makes this feature undesirable.) In this example, lines are drawn at 20,000 and 1000 to suggest decision boundaries.

Below the plot events are shown. In this case the first group of events is the administration of chemotherapy. There is no space to indicate the dosage; only the fact is indicated. A line separates the antibiotic medications, and the final group of events contains the temperature and the number of units of platelets and white blood cells transfused. (The asterisk in the temperature line indicates that the patient is afebrile; the number is degrees above 39° C.) From this plot one can see the effect of the chemotherapy upon the white blood cell count, the success of the therapies that respond to infection, and the use of platelet transfusions to prevent hemorrhage. (This plot was produced in 1981 with the Phase I OCIS; by comparing this sample with the plots in Chapter 2 it can be seen that the plot function has remained essentially unchanged since the late 1970s.)

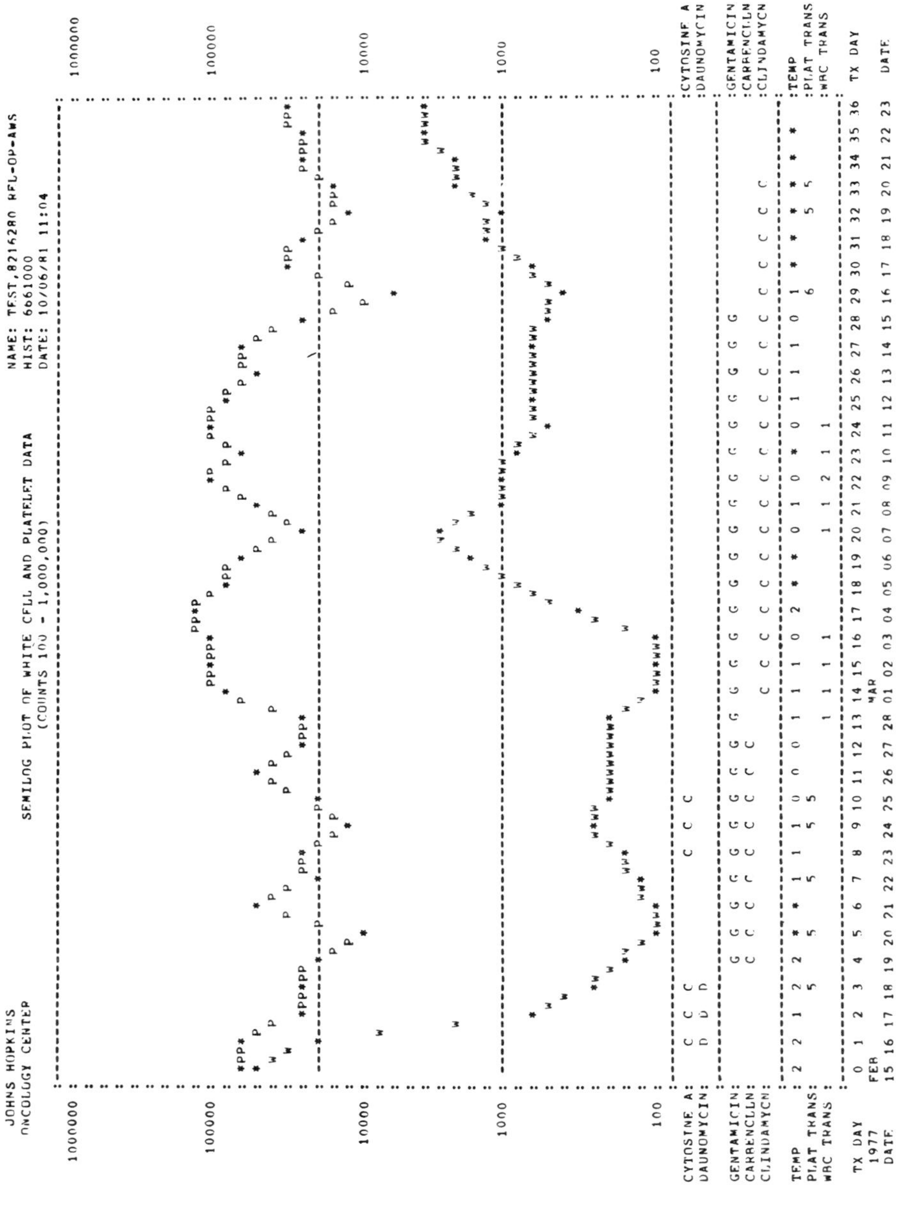

Figure 8. Sample plot.

On-line Displays. Although the flow-sheet and plot formats are available for on-line review, they were intended to provide access to more data than can be assimilated comfortably at a small video display. Consequently, they tend to be used in their printed form throughout JHOC. The database is constantly being updated, however, and the paper reports soon lose their timeliness. Therefore, the OCIS provides a variety of on-line data displays designed to report the most recent clinical values.

The standard format is called the Data format, and it is selected by using the "D" command of the view prompt string. This results in the listing of the option prompt line shown in Figure 9. The default is the data for the current day, and a sample listing is shown in Figure 10. In this case all clinical data reported for patient SAMPLE, PATIENT on 7/20/88 are grouped and listed. Where there is a time associated with a result, it is listed.

All data items are identified by a 6-character item code. The selection of this short code was based on the amount of space available in the listing. There is also a 10-character code that is used in the horizontal flows and a 20-character description. These codes are maintained in an Item Dictionary, which also includes an internal sort code (used to group the items and order them within a group), the format of the value (e.g., numerical or alphabetical code, pattern match), and the ranges of normal and unreasonable values (the latter suggesting a data entry error). The "I" option of the Data prompt allows the user to review the codes in the Item Dictionary. Figure 11 shows the sample response to

    I,TMP

as an input following the "D" command.

There are several other data display options. The Data Search (S) lists the most recent 10 values for the selected item. Figure 12 contains a sample output. There are also data display options available that allow the user to view data values for an entire inpatient unit. CHEM shows chemistry results for the patients on the 2S inpatient unit (Figure 13), HEM displays all hematology values for the 2S inpatient unit (Figure 14), and COUNTS displays a summary of critical hematology counts for the current day for the entire inpatient unit (Figure 15).

Bacteriology Reports

The reports from the tabular data are relatively simple to implement because there is a common format for most data, and the data of most interest are those of the current day. In the case of microbacteriology data reporting, there are many different formats, the data may not be reported until weeks after the specimen was submitted, and the amount and kind of data reported will vary with the test results. For these reasons, a separate reporting (and data entry) subsystem was created.

(T)ODAY (N)EXT (B)ACK (E)ARLY (L)ATE (D)ATE (P)RINT (I)TEM ID (S)EARCH

(Select one of these options to specify the time of patient data needed.)

DESCRIPTION OF DATA PROMPT OPTIONS

(T)ODAY – Gives all of the data values for the current day.

(N)EXT – Gives the data values for the next day.

(B)ACK – Depending on the current screen display date, this option
display the data collected from the previous day.

(E)ARLY – Provides the earliest data collected on any patient.

(L)ATE – Provides the most current data available on any patient.

(D)ATE – Allows you to specify patient data from any date using the
format MM/DD/YY.

(P)RINT – Orders a computer print-out of patient data for a date range

(I)TEM ID – Used to receive the full name of the data item
abbreviations that are used within the patient Data Display,
Flows, and/or Plots.

(S)EARCH – Gives the 10 most recent values for a specified Data Item.

Figure 9. Data display options with description.

```
1111111    SAMPLE,PATIENT  CLINICAL DATA      07/20/88

ITEMS FOR DATE - 07/07/88

PATIENT STATUS

      TMP    37.6  12:00A    TMP   37.1   4:00A    TMP    37.2   8:00A
      TMP    37.1  12:00P    TMP   37.4   4:00P    TMP    37.3   8:00P
      BP    130/80           PULS  92              RESP   20
      WT     81.5   4:00A    WT    82.9   4:00P    LVLC    3
      FLIV  6235             FLPO  120             UROT   7375
      URST     0             STLQ  2200            EMOT    0

BLOOD PRODUCT

      RBCTI    1   4:00P    RBCTI    1   5:00P    RBCT    2

LABORATORY

      WBC   3500*   7:40A    RBC    2.76*  7:40A   HGB      8.8*  7:40A
      HCT   26.9*   7:40A    MCV   97.3*   7:40A   MCH     31.9   7:40A
      MCHC  32.8    7:40A    RDW   14.6    7:40A   PLTS  129000*  7:40A
      SNA   136              SPOT   4.5            SCL    106
      SCO2   27             -GAP    8             SUN      6*
      SUN    7*              SCR    0.8            SCR     0.7    8:00A

MEDICATION

      ACYV  1000            NORFS   800           ALPRA   1.5
      CAF      2            KCL      30           PHEN    300
      SOBI    50

OTHER

      STOM     0            INF      1            SKN      0
      HCAT     0
```

(T)ODAY (B)ACK (E)ARLY (L)ATE (D)ATE (P)RINT (I)TEM ID (S)EARCH (Q)UIT

Figure 10. Sample standard data display.

The provider enters the Bact reporting system with the "B" command and is requested to supply a sort order and a date or range of dates. There are three orderings available.

Report by Date. This is the standard format. It lists all results by date. If antibiotic sensitivities are reported, these also are listed and documented. Figure 16 shows part of a date-ordered report.

Report by Specimen. In this case the user is prompted to select a specimen. OCIS lists out all sites from which a specimen was taken for this patient, and the user selects a site. The system then produces a report of the results of all cultures for this site within the given date range. Figure 17 contains a sample report on blood cultures.

Report by Organism. As in the case of the report by specimen, OCIS prompts with a list of all organisms reported for this patient, and the user selects an organism from that list. Figure 18 contains a report for cultures containing Candida Albicans.

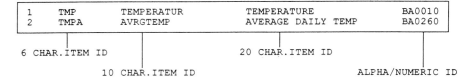

```
  1    TMP         TEMPERATUR          TEMPERATURE            BA0010
  2    TMPA        AVRGTEMP            AVERAGE DAILY TEMP      BA0260
```

```
6 CHAR.ITEM ID                     20 CHAR.ITEM ID

            10 CHAR.ITEM ID                          ALPHA/NUMERIC ID
```

Figure 11. Sample listing for Item Dictionary.

```
MOST  RECENT  VALUES  FOR  -  TMP

          09/25/88      37.6
          09/24/88      36.5
          09/23/88      36.5
          09/20/88      35.8
          09/18/88      34.6
          09/17/88      37.7
          09/16/88      36.4
          09/15/88      34.5
          09/12/88      36.6
          09/11/88      35.5
```

Figure 12. Sample Data Search listing.

```
JOHNS HOPKINS OCIS    CHEMISTRY RESULTS         3S     07/15/86

DATE: 07/15/86
=================================================================
7777777    PATIENT,A
--------------------         8:30 AM  --------------------------
GL    147         SNA   136                SPOT 4.2       SCL   106
CO2   14          SUN   63                 SCR   4.9
---------------------       11:00 AM      ----------------------
SCAL 8.5          SGL   262
---------------------        5:30 PM      ----------------------
SGL   260         SNA   135                SPOT 4.2       SCL  105
SCO2  14          SUN   66                 SCR   5.0
=================================================================
1111111    PATIENT,B
--------------------         6:15 AM      --------------------
STPR 5.1*         SALB 2.8*                TBLI 2.0*      DBLI 1.2*
SGOT 20           SGPT 43*                 SALK 81        SCAL 8.7*
SURC 1.5*         SGL  123*                SCHL 12        SPO4  3.7
SNA  136          SPOT 3.7                 SCL   10       SCO2 27
SUN  32*          SCR  0.9
--------------------         6:47 AM      --------------------
SNA   135         SPOT 3.4*
--------------------         8:00 AM      --------------------
SGL  122*         SNA  135                 SPOT 4.1       SUN  30*
```

Figure 13. Sample chemistry report.

```
JOHNS HOPKINS OCIS      HEMATOLOGY COUNTS     2S     07/15/86
DATE: 07/15/86
=============================================================
1212121    PATIENT,A
----------------------------- 7:00 AM -----------------------------
WBC     2800      PLTS 10000           HGB   11.0       HCT   32.4
RBC     3.69      RET   0.9            NEUT  48         BAND  2
LYMP    36        MONO  12             EOS   2
----------------------------- 9:35 PM -----------------------------
WBC     2500      PLTS  9770           HGB   12.1
=============================================================
3434343    PATIENT,B
----------------------------- 7:00 AM -----------------------------
WBC     3000      PLTS 18000           HGB   11.0       HCT   31.8
RBC     2.81      RET   0.77           NEUT  44         BAND  2
----------------------------- 9:35 PM -----------------------------
WBC     2850      PLTS  9000           HGB   11..1
```

Figure 14. Sample patient hematology report.

```
Inpatient Counts as of 10:04 A.M.      2N           6/25/86

HIST NO    NAME        HCT    WBC     PLTS      NEU   LYMP   TIME

1111111    Patient A   32     1500    150000    15    20     8:00am.
2222222    Patient B   37.2   3200    120000    81    2      7:15am.
3333333    Patient C   31.3   5400    40000*    14    4      6:57am.
```

Figure 15. Sample unit hematology report.

```
JOHNS HOPKINS ONCOLOGY CENTER            HISTORY NO: 1212121
                                         NAME: PATIENT,SAMPLE
MICROBIOLOGY DATA (BY DATE)              DATE: 08/26/86
--------------------------------------------------------------------
06/18/86  BLOOD   CLOSTRIDIUM RAMOSUM - BACT CULTURE; POSITIVE AT 2 DAYS;
                  IN ANAEROBIC BOTTLE (D525)
                  SUSCEPTIBILITY             A    B    C    D    E
                    PENICILLIN         (A)  0.1   1    4   16   16+
                    ERYTHROMYCIN       (A)  0.5   1    2    -    2+
                    CLINDAMYCIN        (C)  0.5   1    2    8    8+
                    TETRACYCLINE       (D)   1    2    4   16   16+
                    CHLORAMPHENICOL    (A)   2    4    8   16   16+
                    CARBENICILLIN      (A)   8   32  128  256  256
                    CEFOXITIN          (C)  0.5   4   16   32   32+
06/19/86  BLOOD   BACT CULTURE; NEGATIVE AT 7 DAYS (D639)
          THROAT  BACT CULTURE; HEAVY NORMAL RESPIRATORY FLORA AT 1 DAY
                  (R683)
                  FUNGAL CULTURE; NEGATIVE AS OF 06/30/86 (R683)
          URINE (CLEAN CATCH)      BACT CULTURE; URINE - LESS THAN 10,000
                  COLONIES PER ML--INSIGNIFICANT AT 1 DAY (V991)
```

Figure 16. Sample bacteriology report by date.

```
JOHNS HOPKINS ONCOLOGY CENTER              HISTORY NO: 1212121
                                              NAME: PATIENT,SAMPLE
MICROBIOLOGY DATA (BY SPECIMEN)               DATE: 08/26/86
-------------------------------------------------------------------
BLOOD
    06/18/86   CLOSTRIDIUM RAMOSUM - BACT CULTURE; POSITIVE AT 2 DAYS;
               IN ANAEROBIC BOTTLE (D525)
               SUSCEPTIBILITY            A     B     C     D     E
                  PENICILLIN      (A)   0.1    1     4    16    16+
                  ERYTHROMYCIN    (A)   0.5    1     2     -     2+
                  CLINDAMYCIN     (C)   0.5    1     2     8     8+
                  TETRACYCLINE    (D)    1     2     4    16    16+
                  CHLORAMPHENICOL (A)    2     4     8    16    16+
                  CARBENICILLIN   (A)    8    32   128   256   256
                  CEFOXITIN       (C)   0.5    4    16    32    32+

    06/19/86   BACT CULTURE; NEGATIVE AT 7 DAYS (D639)
    06/20/86   BACT CULTURE; NEGATIVE AT 7 DAYS (D761)
    06/21/86   BACT CULTURE; NEGATIVE AT 7 DAYS (D863)
```

Figure 17. Sample bacteriology report by specimen.

Schedules

Although the scheduling function is considered an administrative activity, providers require access to patient schedules. There are a variety of schedule reports available from the inpatient and outpatient scheduling systems. The "S" command of the view prompt line produces a summary schedule, as shown in Figure 19.

Treatment Plan Reports

Chapter 5 describes the OCIS daily care plan system. In this system we briefly describe some of the reports that this system makes available to the providers. The purpose of the treatment plans is to generate therapy recommendations

```
JOHNS HOPKINS ONCOLOGY CENTER              HISTORY NO: 1212121
                                              NAME: PATIENT,SAMPLE
MICROBIOLOGY DATA (BY ORGANISM)               DATE: 08/26/86
-------------------------------------------------------------------
CANDIDA ALBICANS

   06/23/86   THROAT    POSITIVE AT 2 DAYS (R734)
   06/30/86             FUNGAL CULTURE; POSITIVE AT 2 DAYS (R798)
              STOOL     FUNGAL CULTURE; POSITIVE AT 2 DAYS; LIGHT (T516)
              URINE     (CLEAN CATCH) FUNGAL CULTURE; POSITIVE AT
                        2 DAYS  (G822)
```

Figure 18. Sample bacteriology report by organism.

```
JOHNS HOPKINS OCIS        UNIVERSAL TERMINAL            08/09/88
APPOINTMENTS SCHEDULED FOR TEST,PATIENT    (7777777)
BEGINNING: 03/09/83 (WED)

DATE        TIME        TYPE      CLINIC    PROVIDER      COMMENT

03/09/83    10:00 AM    PRIMARY   ONC       TEST,DOC
             9:45 AM    LAB

03/13/83    10:00 AM    LAB

03/30/83     3:00 PM    PRIMARY   ONC       TEST,DOC      PER DR TEST
             1:45 PM    LAB
             2:00 PM    XRAY

04/01/83    10:00 AM    PRIMARY   OPD       NURSE
            10:00 AM    LAB

04/04/83    10:00 AM    LAB

05/11/83     1:00 PM    PRIMARY   ONC       TEST,DOC      PER DR TEST
            11:15 AM    LAB
```

Figure 19. Sample schedule report.

based on therapy plans and research protocols that define the general rules for care. The care rules are described as "treatment sequences," and a protocol may be defined by many different treatment sequences, for example, what to do at the start of a cycle of therapy and what the routine follow-up actions are.

Patients are managed by assigning them treatment sequences to create "standing orders." Figure 20 contains a patient's standing order list. Under blood procedures, the report indicates that a hematocrit (HCT) is required on day 1 according to the leukemia admission (LEUK ADM) treatment sequence and every day (Q1D) according to the leukemia follow-up (LEUK FOL) sequence. Under radiology procedures, the report indicates that a chest x-ray (CXR) is to be done beginning on day 7, every 3 days, until day 21 (B7/Q3D/C21) in accordance with the 8410 induction (8410 IND) sequence. The report also indicates when the test was done last, how many times it was done, and the day on the protocol. In this example it is day 53 in treatment sequence 8410 IND, and therefore no chest x-ray will be ordered.

Each day, plans are generated from the standing orders that indicate what therapies, procedures, and tests are recommended for the current day. The reports are produced in several formats. Figure 21 shows the form used by the providers. At the top is the standard OCIS patient heading. In this case it is augmented to include the patient's height and body surface area (BSA); these are used to compute drug doses. Below this are the text messages from the census system. Because these messages are optional, not all plans include this descriptive text. Next the protocols on which the patient has been entered are listed. Finally, the recommendations for tests and procedures to be ordered that day are presented.

```
                        ONCOLOGY INFORMATION SYSTEMS

              VIEW TX PLAN                        08/02/88

       121212: SAMPLE,PATIENT

       ORDER           SCHEDULE      CNT  LAST DONE  DAY #    T.SQ. ID
       ------------------------------------------------------------------
       BLOOD PROCEDURES:
       HCT             1             35   08/01/86   35       LEUK ADM
                       Q1D           35   08/01/86   35       LEUK FOL
       WBC             1             25   08/01/86   35       LEUK ADM
       HEM8            Q1D           35   08/01/88   35       LEUK FOL

       NURSING PROCEDURES:
       ECG             1             1    06/09/88   35       LEUK ADM

       RADIOLOGY PROCEDURES:
       CXR             B7/Q3D/C21    11   08/06/86   53       8410 IND

       P.A. PROCEDURES
       CSFC            3             1    06/30/86   53       8410

       PHYSICIAN PROCEDURES...
       THERAPY...
```

Figure 20. Extract from a standing order report.

Transfusion Reports

Chapter 7 describes the OCIS blood management system. In this section we briefly describe some of the features of that system that are available to the providers for their use in patient management. Figure 22 shows the transfusion option menu that is listed when the "TX" command is entered. Because the OCIS is used by the rotating house staff, as well as by the permanent staff and faculty, this menu provides access to both patient specific data and general introductory material.

For each patient, the menu provides access to plans and histories for both red blood cells and platelets. Figure 23 displays a red blood cell transfusion plan and Figure 24 a transfusion history starting on 9/12/86. For each date the history shows the protocol date (PD), the time at which the blood was drawn from the patient or the time at which it was transfused (if there is an RBC in the TR column), the hematocrit level (HCT), the normalized RBC increment (see below), a bleeding indicator (BLD where 0 is no bleeding and 4 is massive bleeding), the patient's weight (WT) and reticulocyte count (RET), and the average number of RBC units used per week (R PER WK).

There are similar reports for platelets. Figure 25 contains a platelet transfusion history. This is slightly more complex in that the donor platelets must be matched to the patient by HLA type. (This is discussed in further detail in Chapter 7.) In this report, the patient's HLA antigens are listed in the heading (A2,11 B13,46 BW4,6) and those of each transfused product in the HLA column. The MATCH column codes the degree of match between the patient's HLA type and that of the

```
JOHNS HOPKINS                       HISTORY NO: 2233333
ONCOLOGY CENTER                           NAME: PATIENT,SAMPLE
                                    PLAN DATE: 02/23/87
DAILY CARE PLAN                           MONDAY     PAGE 1


52 Y.O.  W F  M-1/ACUTE MYEL LEUK
                                       HT: 155.5 CM  BSA: 1.67 M2
SPECIAL NOTES:

    11/85 PAS POSITIVE. (OUTSIDE REPORT)

    11/11/85 ESTERASE NEGATIVE,MYELOPEROXIDASE NEGATIVE,PAS STAIN POSITIVE

    01/09/86 SKIN GRAFT

    11/11/85 MARROW CHROMOSOMES-ONLY 3 SLIDES COULD BE PREPARED FROM THE
    SAMPLE, AND NO METAPHASE CELLS WERE FOUND.

    02/04/87 PERIPHERAL BLOOD MARKERS - 8% BLASTS - MARKERS ARE THOSE OF
    THE MAJORITY POPULATION, T-LYMPHOCYTES. *NONDIAGNOSTIC* C.CIVIN


WEIGHTS:  ADMIN 64.1 KG    IDEAL 66.7 KG    CURRENT (02/19/87)  63.4 KG

PROTOCOLS:
                                       STARTED      DAY
  MANAN       MANNAN IMMUNOASSY        02/04/87     20
              MANNAN ASSAY
  INDIV       INDIVIDUAL THERAPY       02/06/87     18
              AC-D-VP16      ()

TEST AND PROCEDURES:

BLOOD AND SERUM TESTS
          HEMATOCRIT                   WBC
          PLT CNT                      WBC DIFF
URINE TESTS:
          24UR CR,PR
NURSING PROCEDURES
          FVC
          MYCOL-URINE                  SV CLT BCT
```

Figure 21. Sample physician's daily care plan.

product, and the final column is the product identifier. (The prefix SS indicates that the platelets were collected at JHOC.) The INCREM/HR is the number of transfused platelets (normalized for patient weight) that were retained over a given period. It can be seen from this report that the transfusion of the first product (with a match of 10100) was highly effective compared with the subsequent poor transfusion increment of only 57%.

In addition to the transfusion histories, there is a transfusion reaction history that is used to record any adverse reaction the patient has had to platelet transfusion and any premedications given to prevent such reactions. Figure 26 contains a sample report. There also are reports that cross match available products with patients and detail lymphocytotoxity cross matches. Finally,

TRANSFUSION OPTION MENU

```
+-------------------------------------------------------+
|         BLOOD TRANSFUSION INFORMATION                 |
|                                                       |
|         --------------------------------              |
|                                                       |
|   TRANSFUSION PLAN     : RED CELL          R          |
|                        : PLATELET          P          |
|                                                       |
|   TRANSFUSION HISTORY: RED CELL            RC         |
|                      : PLATELET            PL         |
|                                                       |
|   TRANSFUSION REACTION HISTORY             TR         |
|                                                       |
|   PLATELET CROSS MATCH DATA (RGT)          CM         |
|                                                       |
|   LYMPHOCYTOTOXICITY -                                |
|   CROSS MATCH DATA (QS)                    L          |
|                                                       |
|   HELP: GLOSSARY OF BLOOD                             |
|   PRODUCT TERMS & DEFINITIONS              G          |
|                                                       |
|   NEXT PATIENT                             N          |
|                                                       |
|   ENTER:                                              |
+-------------------------------------------------------+
```

Figure 22. Transfusion option menu.

```
            TRANSFUSION PLAN INFORMATION: RED CELL

========================================================================
   SAMPLE, PATIENT      1212123          APLASTIC ANEMIA - BMT

                 ** PREFERRED RED CELLS **

1.   IRRADIATED (TO PREVENT GVHD)
2.   LEUKOCYTE POOR (TO REDUCE RISK OF FEBRILE TRANSFUSION  (REACTION)
     WARNING: THIS TRANSFUSION PLAN MAY BE 72 HOURS OLD.  IF THERE HAS BEEN
     A CHANGE IN CLINICAL STATUS OR A TRANSFUSION REACTION, THIS PLAN MAY
     HAVE BEEN VERBALLY ALTERED.  IF THERE ARE ANY QUESTIONS, CALL BLOOD
     BANK (6580) OR DR. PLATELET (5020).


-------------------------------------------------------------------------
                      ** COMMENT **

     SUGGEST PREMED WITH DIPHENHYDRAMINE (092686) AND ACETAMINOPHEN
     (103086);SUGGEST LEUKO.POOR PLTS.(110686);PT. HAS MULTIPLE RED BLOOD
     CELL ANTIBODIES (110786)
========================================================================
```

Figure 23. Sample red blood cell transfusion plan.

TRANSFUSION HISTORY FOR RBC

```
JOHNS HOPKINS OCIS          UNIVERSAL TERMINAL        11/13/86

RBC TRANSFUSION DATA
STARTING 09/12/86 FOR 1212122  SAMPLE,PATIENT

DATE      PD  TIME  HCT  INCR/HR TR BLD WT  C IC RET  R PER WK

09/12/86  2   710A  33.9          0  59.2     0.6
09/13/86  3   752A  33.3          0  58.7
09/14/86  4   920A  33.6          1  57.8
09/15/86  5   832A  32.7          1  57.0     0.4
              900P  25.2
             1159P           RBC
09/16/86  6   415A           RBC 1  58.8
             1000A  33.5 6.5/06                       2/1.3
```

Figure 24. Sample red blood cell transfusion history.

```
JOHNS HOPKINS OCIS        TRANSFUSION SUMMARY        11/13/86

SAMPLE,PATIENT    1212122      B+    A2,11 B13,46 BW4,6

DATE      TIME   PL  INCREM/HR #UNITS      HLA       MATCH   PRODUCT

09/09/86 1220A   47  10725/1
          805A   45  10129/9
09/10/86  810A   34
         1030A            P11.1  A2,3 B7,14 BW6,6   10100  SS11709PX

         1130A   38  577/1
09/11/86  715A   23  -1587/21
         1115P            P10.4  A2,28 B44, BW4,4   10111  SS11732PX
```

Figure 25. Sample platelet transfusion history.

```
** TRANSFUSION REACTIONS (SINCE MARCH, 1985) --

   SAMPLE,PATIENT  2212122

                        APLASTIC ANEMIA - BMT
                    **   RED CELLS -- REACTIONS **
                                                      PREMEDI-
   PRODUCT      DATE      MODIFICATION      REACTION   CATION
   ----------------------------------------------------------------
   RED CELLS   11/06/86  LEUKOCYTE POOR  ALLERGY: URTICARIA  ACETAMIN

                        APLASTIC ANEMIA - BMT
                    **   PLATELETS -- REACTIONS **
                                                      PREMEDI-
   PRODUCT      DATE      MODIFICATION      REACTION   CATION
   ----------------------------------------------------------------
   PPC (AGE:3) 09/25/86  NONE            ALLERGIC: DYSPNEA   NONE
   -SUGGEST PREMED WITH DIPHENHYDRAMINE (092686)

   PPC (AGE:4) 10/28/86  SALINE RESUSPENDED  FEBRILE: CHILLS  ACETAMIN
                                                             DIPHENHY
   -SUGGEST PREMED WITH ACETAMINOPHEN (103086)
   PPC (AGE:5) 11/05/86  NONE              FEBRILE: CHILLS   ACETAMIN
                                          FEBRILE: FEVER    DIPHENHY
   -SUGGEST LEUKO.POOR PLTS.(110686)
```

Figure 26. Sample transfusion reaction history.

the transfusion menu provides a dictionary and some tutorial instruction (see Figure 27).

Special Reports

OCIS offers several other reports that are helpful to the providers. Some list data from special files. The blood and body fluid precautions report shown in Figure 28 identifies those active patients who are positive for blood and body fluid precautions by serology. There is also a PAIN function, described more fully in Chapter 6, that assists in converting one narcotic analgesic dose and route of administration to another dose and/or route of administration. This is especially helpful when preparing medications for patients about to be discharged. Figure 29 shows a sample of the narcotic information listing.

Providers also have access to the statistics and analysis menu shown in Figure 30. This provides access to sample-size calculation routines and quick calculation functions for computing chi-squares, date differences, body surface area, and cumulative doses. The PAIN function is available from this menu, as well as from other menus. Finally, the menu provides access to a personal database system; the demand for this feature has diminished as the number of personal computers in the JHOC has increased. (A separate "study" menu can be used to

```
                    TRANSFUSION GLOSSARY OF TERMS

        1.    WHOLE BLOOD
        2.    RED BLOOD CELLS
                 MODIFICATIONS:
        3.              LEUKOCYTE POOR RED CELLS
        4.              WASHED RED CELLS
        5.              FROZEN DEGLYCEROLIZED
        6.              CMV NEGATIVE RED CELLS
        7.              AUTOLOGOUS BLOOD
        8.              IRRADIATED
        9.    POOLED PLATELET CONCENTRATE
       10.    PLATELET CONCENTRATE, PHERESIS
                 MODIFICATIONS:
       11.              CONCENTRATED
       12.              CMV NEGATIVE
       13.              IRRADIATION
       14.              WASHED
       15.              LEUKOCYTE POOR PLATELETS
       16.              ABO COMPATIBLE
       17.    FRESH FROZEN PLASMA
       18.    GRANULOCYTES


   NUMBER OF DEFINITION REQUESTED ("RETURN" TO QUIT):
```

TERM	DEFINITION	INDICATIONS
LEUKOCYTE POOR RED CELLS	UNIT OF RED CELLS PROCESSED SUCH THAT 70% OF LEUKOCYTES HAVE BEEN REMOVED AND >70% OF RED CELLS RETAINED. CURRENTLY DONE BY A HARD SPIN & ADMINISTRATION WITH PALL FILTER; MAY ALSO BE DONE BY 1 LITER SALINE WASH.	*TO PREVENT FEBRILE TRANS-FUSION REACTIONS (GREATER THAN 1 DEGREE C UNEXPLAINED RISE IN TEMPERATURE DURING OR SHORTLY AFTER TRANSFUSION).

Figure 27. Transfusion dictionary display.

extract data sets for electronic transfer to other computers. Most clinical researchers prefer to work in their own environment, usually a networked PC.)

Clinical Support Functions

The previous section described the clinical outputs produced by the OCIS. From the providers' perspective, this represents what the system does for them. Yet, the production of those reports requires considerable OCIS infrastructure. We close this chapter with a brief summary of some of the hidden system features that are essential for the effective operation of a clinical information.

BLOOD AND BODY FLUID PRECAUTION LIST

ONCOLOGY   INFORMATION SYSTEM   07/20/88

```
+-----------------------------------------------------------------+
|                                                                 |
|  HEPATITIS BLOOD & BODY FLUID PRECAUTION PATIENTS               |
|                                                                 |
|  (LAST UPDATED: 07/18/88)                                       |
|                                                                 |
|  NAME            HNO        FIRST POSITIVE      LAST POSITIVE    |
|  -------------------------------------------------------------  |
|  PATIENT, A.    2238193        10/23/86           10/23/86       |
|  PATIENT, B.    2152021        03/14/85           03/14/85       |
|  PATIENT, C.    2020580        09/30/87           01/21/88       |
|  PATIENT, D.    1622570        02/05/88           02/05/88       |
|  PATIENT, E.    2319724        05/12/88           05/12/88       |
|  PATIENT, F.    2318449        04/20/88           04/20/88       |
|  PATIENT, G.    2256068        03/04/87           03/31/87       |
|                                                                 |
+-----------------------------------------------------------------+
```

Figure 28. Sample blood and body fluid precautions report.

```
+-----------------------------------------------------------------+
|                    NARCOTIC INFORMATION                         |
+-----------------------------------------------------------------+
|                           EQUI-ANALG.TO                         |
|  DRUG              FORM    10 MG MORPH.     RETAILED DOSE        |
|  -------------------------------------------------------------  |
|  CODEINE           SOLUTION      200    3 MG/ML*,  6 MG/ML       |
|                    SOLUTION                                     |
|                    (W/ACETAMNPHN)  200   12 MG/ML               |
|                                                                 |
|                    SYRINGE       130    15*, 30, 60             |
|                    TABLETS       200    15,30,60                |
|                                                                 |
|  DEMEROL           SOLUTION      300    10 MG/ML                |
|  (MEPERIDINE)      SYRINGE        75    25,50,75,100            |
|                    TABLETS       300    50,100*                 |
|                                                                 |
|  DILAUDID          SUPPOSITORY    ??    3                       |
|  (HYDROMORPHONE)   SYRINGE        1.5   1*,2,4,10*              |
|                    TABLET         7.5   1*,2,3*,4               |
|                                                                 |
|  METHADONE         SOLUTION       20    2 MG/ML,  5 MG/ML*      |
|  (DOLOPHINE)       SYRINGE        10    8*, 10                  |
|                    TABLETS        20    5,10,40 (DISKETTS)      |
|                                                                 |
|  MORPHINE          SOLUTION       60    2 MG/ML,4 MG/ML,20 MG/ML|
|                    SUPPOSITORY    ??    10 MG*                  |
|                    SYRINGE        10    1,2*,4*,8,10,15         |
|                    TABLET         60    10*, 15*, 30*           |
+-----------------------------------------------------------------+
```

Figure 29. Sample narcotic information display.

```
JOHNS HOPKINS OCIS STATISTICS AND ANALYSIS MENU  8/01/86

            FUNCTION                        ENTER

     SAMPLE SIZE CALCULATION
            PHASE II A                        SA
            PHASE II B                        SB
            PHASE III                         SC

     QUICK CALCULATION ROUTINES
            CHI-SQUARE                        CS
            DATE DIFFERENCE                   DD
            BODY SURFACE AREA                 BS
            CUMULATIVE DOSE (PAT BY MED)      CP
            CUMULATIVE DOSE (MED BY PAT)      CM

     PERSONAL DATA BASE                       PD

     OCCUPANCY STATISTICS                      O

     PAIN TABLE                              PAIN

     MEDICAL RECORD LABELS                     L

     ENTER:
```

Figure 30. Statistics and analysis menu.

System Dictionaries

Like any large information system, the OCIS relies upon dictionaries to provide generality. There are over 100 system dictionaries plus equal numbers for the daily care plan, pharmacy, and blood management systems. Many of the dictionaries are simple tables, for example, a table listing provider identification and name; others require a more complex structure, for example, a dictionary that associates the valid ZIP code ranges with a state.

For each dictionary, the OCIS requires programs to maintain the dictionary. Adding new terms is always easy to implement. However, editing and deleting existing entries can introduce referential inconsistencies whenever the changed data are pointed to from other segments of the database, for example a result for a test whose identifier has been deleted from the dictionary. In some cases, where it is important, the OCIS implements tools to preserve referential integrity; in other cases the OCIS provides a mechanism to accommodate those occasional referential failures that would be computationally too expensive to avoid.

A catalog of dictionaries would be beyond the scope of this section. Nevertheless, the reader should be aware that the management of such a large number of dictionaries requires considerable effort. There is a need for programs to maintain them, menus to provide access to the programs, and documentation so that the maintainers know which dictionaries are to be updated. Most difficult of all, however, is the building of a correct and complete dictionary and then keeping it up-to-date. This is commented on in Chapter 10.

Clinical Data Entry

It was briefly noted above that the clinical data entry falls into one of three categories:

Manual data entry, for example, entry by a clinical data coordinator of material taken from the medical record, or by a computer operator of data already formatted for entry.

Automated data transfer using the JHOC facilities, for example, between the Pharmacy and the OCIS, or from the Hematology Laboratories to the OCIS.

Automated data entry between the JHOC and another Hospital organization, for example, from the clinical laboratory system to the OCIS, or between the Oncology satellite pharmacy and the central pharmacy system.

In the first two categories the process is closed within the JHOC, and it is easier to define and control the software. In the third category, on the other hand, the OCIS is a secondary user of the data. The entry software must be able to recognize inconsistencies that can result from the use of two independent systems, for example, data with an inappropriate history number. Also, because all systems are subject to change, the OCIS must be able to identify changes in the data formats transmitted, for example, results reported in a new format or different units.

The problems that the OCIS faces in this third category is common to all decentralized systems that share data over a network. In some cases there are formal, low-level, institutional exchange standards. In this event, mechanisms exist to maintain the standard at a cost in responsiveness. However, when a independent system such as the OCIS is tied into a network, it is interfaced with the understanding that it will not hinder the data supplier's main mission. Therefore, the independent system must be programmed to insulate itself from changes that it cannot control. In our situation we have always had the full cooperation of the data suppliers, but, because we are dealing with the data used in clinical decision making, we have had to write programs that do not take that cooperation for granted.

Report Definition and Scheduling

Because the OCIS was designed to produce paper reports, it includes a variety of tools that automate the production and distribution of the reports. The standard processing flow is oriented around the distribution of the clinical data reports in time for morning rounds (inpatients) or an encounter (outpatients). After the database is updated from the clinical laboratory system and the pharmacy system, the requested plots and flow sheets are printed. The outputs are organized by nursing unit and outpatient clinic and delivered to the units in time for their use. Separate schedules are followed for the generation of the daily care plans, pharmacy operations, and the management of blood products.

```
                JOHNS HOPKINS OCIS       DICTIONARIES

   ABIOT        ANTIBIOTIC PROFILE    HORIZONTAL FLOW  NARROW (8.5X11)

                RKS  10/26/82         DLN  04/01/88

   FLOWSHEET OF A PATIENT'S JHOC ANTIBIOTIC HISTORY

   NUMBER  ITEM    TEXT
   ---------------------------------------------------------------
     1    *ANT     ANTIBIOTIC     CLASS OF ITEMS WITH DATA AND HEADING
     5    *DLV     DRUG LVL       CLASS OF ITEMS WITH DATA AND HEADING
```

Figure 31. Definition of a horizontal flow-sheet format.

There are OCIS system-level tools that manage the production of the reports on a predefined schedule (see Chapter 8). Additional tools are required to establish which reports the system is to produce. The clinical data coordinators have a menu that allows them to define new output formats and patient-specific report requests. We briefly describe these functions.

All plots and flow sheets are considered general reports created from the Patient Data files. Each report is given a short name and an optional description; its contents are defined using the terms in the Item Dictionary. For example, Figure 31 contains the definition for a horizontal flow sheet that displays all antibiotics (ANT) and drug levels (DLV). The dictionary terms *ANT and *DLV indicate that a heading line should be printed and that all data values in this category reported during the days covered in the report should be listed. A sample flow sheet from this definition is shown in Figure 32.

When a report is defined for a class of items, the contents of each page will vary with the patient's treatment. It is also possible to define explicitly what items are to be included in a flow sheet. For example, the flow sheets shown in Figure 32 could have been defined as

```
>ANT   This produces just the heading line
FLU    This produces the FLUCYTOSIN line
ACYC   ....
```

Of course, in the second definition, if a specified drug was not administered during the period, then a line with no values would be included. Also, if an antibiotic that was not explicitly listed was administered, then it would not be reported in the flow sheet. The vertical flow sheets are defined in a similar fashion, except, because of their limited width, the headings and generic item classes (e.g., >ANT and *ANT) are not accepted.

Figure 33 contains a definition of a plot output. Here the user must specify the items to be plotted, the letter to be used in the plot, the kind of plot (log or linear), and the scale. In addition, one must define what events are to be displayed at the bottom of the plot. In this example, MEDICATION TYPE 3 and CHEMOTHERAPY are generic terms, and the plot will include all events of that category.

```
JOHNS HOPKINS ONCOLOGY CENTER  2S        HISTORY NO: 111 11 11
                                         NAME: PATIENT,SAMPLE
                                         DATE: 07/20/88
ANTIBIOTIC PROFILE                               FILE COPY CURRENT
                                                 PAGE  1
:----------------:-------:-------:-------:-------:-------:-------:-------:
:   CURRENT      :13JUL88:14JUL88:15JUL88:16JUL88:17JUL88:18JUL88:19JUL88:
:   MANAN        :DAY  31:DAY  32:DAY  33:DAY  34:DAY  35:DAY  36:DAY  37:
:   J8410        :DAY  29:DAY  30:DAY  31:DAY  32:DAY  33:DAY  34:DAY  35:
:ANTIBIOTIC------:-------:-------:-------:-------:-------:-------:-------:
:FLUCYTOSIN GM   :       :     7:     7:     7:     7: 1.75:       :     :
:ACYCLOVIR  MG   : 1000: 1000: 1000: 1000: 1000: 1000:     :
:AMPHOTER-B MG   :   70:   70:   70:   70:   70:   70:     :
:NORFLOX    MG   :  800:  800:  800:  800:  800:  800:     :
:TICARCILLN GM   :   18:   18:   18:   18:   18:   18:     :
:TOBRAMYCIN MG   :  440:  480:  520:  520:  690:  600:     :
:VANCOMYCIN MG   : 1000: 1000: 1000: 1000: 1000: 1000:     :
:DRUG LVL   -----:-------:-------:-------:-------:-------:-------:-------:
:TICAR NOS  MCG/M:       :       :       :       : 65.0:       :     :
:TOBRA NOS  MCG/M:       :       :       :  4.3:       :       :     :
:----------------:-------:-------:-------:-------:-------:-------:-------:
```

Figure 32. Sample output from flow-sheet definition.

Figure 34 illustrates an on-line plot that was produced with that definition. Because the plot is limited to 24 lines, the plot and event portions are displayed as separate screens; in this figure the two screens are combined into a single unit.

In addition to defining the report formats, the clinical data coordinator schedules their routine production. This is done by (a) identifying a patient, (b) selecting a report format, and (c) selecting a schedule for production. Examples of schedules are every day, every Monday, and Wednesday and Friday. The bacteriology reports can be ordered on a fixed schedule or whenever they are updated.

```
          JOHNS HOPKINS OCIS        DICTIONARIES

SWP       SEMILOG PLOT OF WHITE CELL AND PLATELET DATA

          (COUNTS 100 - 1000000)

SHORT NAME: SEMILOG PLOT OF WHITE CELL AND PLATELET DATA

          XXX 01/04/82  FM  12/17/84
```
```
ITEMS PLOTTED        FROM  TO          EVENTS DISPLAYED
------------------------------------   --------------------
PLATELETS  P  LOG   100   1000000      CHEMOTHERAPY
WBC        W  LOG   100   1000000      MEDICATION TYPE 3
                                       TEMP
                                       PLT TR-TOT P
                                       WBC TRNS (VALUE)
LINES PRINTED:
1000 IN LOG SCALE FROM 100 TO 100000
20000 IN LOG SCALE FROM 100 TO 100000
```

Figure 33. Definition of a plot format.

```
1234567: SAMPLE,PATIENT

                   SEMILOG PLOT OF WHITE CELL AND PLATELET DATA
                            (COUNTS 100 - 1000000)
                     :-----------------------------------------------------:
      1000000  :                                                          :1000000
               :
       100000  :WP*                   PP*P    P*P                         :100000
               :W   P*                    P    *P P     P*                 :
               : W    P*P*P     P* P         P          P*                 :
        20000  :--W--------P-P-----------------------P----P-----P----------:
               :    *        P                       P  P                  :
        10000  :                                                          :
               :     W                                      W*W*W*W        :10000
               :      *                            *W       W*             :
         1000  :--------W--------------------------*W   W          W       :1000
               :         *             W            W------W**W*W*W--*------:
               :        *W          W   W      *         W       W *       :
               :        W*     *W      W    W                     W        :
          100  :              WW*       W*W*W                               :
               :-----------------------------------------------------------:
      CHEMO    :-----------------------------------------------------------:
      CYTOSINE:  CCC                CCC                                     :
      DANOMYCN:  DDD                                                        :CYTOSINE
               :-----------------------------------------------------------:DANOMYCN
      GENTMICN:     G G G G G G G G G G G G G G G G G G G G G G G:GENTMICN
      CARBNCLN:     C C C C C C C C C C C C C C C C C C C C C C C:CARBNCLN
               :-----------------------------------------------------------:
      TEMP    :2 2   2 2 2 1 1   0   0   0   1   1 2 0   1   0   0 1 1 0 0 1 :TEMP
      PLT TRNS:      5   5   5                     5   5       5           :PLT TRNS
      WBC TRNS:                          1   1   1   1                     :WBC
               :-----------------------------------------------------------:
      J8410   : 0   2   4   6   8   10   12   14   16   18   20   22   24   26   28 :J8410
               :-----------------------------------------------------------:
       1986   : FEB                              MAR                       :
      DATE    :15   17   19   21   23   25   27   01   03   05   07   09   11   13 :
               :-----------------------------------------------------------:
```

Figure 34. Sample output from plot definition.

All of the report definition and scheduling programs use a prompting interface so that all selections are made from the current dictionaries of valid terms.

The OCIS and the Medical Record

The ability of the OCIS to manage and maintain the patient's clinical data has been described in this chapter. The power of the OCIS raises obvious questions about the relationship between the computerized system and the formal medical record. In The Johns Hopkins Hospital, the Medical Records Department is responsible for the maintenance of a complete paper record. The fact that the JHOC duplicates much of the clinical data in that medical record does not eliminate the requirement that a paper medical record be kept. Thus, the OCIS need not maintain all of the information that would otherwise be required of a medical record.

The JHOC maintains a supplementary or local record. It consists of the patient abstract, the standard flow sheet for the entire period of treatment, optional plots, and copies of all consultation and discharge notes. (The notes are prepared by a dictation service and are not maintained as part of the OCIS database.

Perhaps the use of word processing and networking will facilitate the future integration of these notes into the OCIS database.) A hard copy form of this record is stored within the JHOC; virtually all of the information also is available on line.

The paper medical record is requested from Medical Records for all admissions and many outpatient visits. If the record is not delivered promptly, the local record is used. All required notes are entered into the medical record. If appropriate, a copy of the note is also entered into the local record. To reduce the bulk of the paper record, some OCIS printed reports can be used to substitute for individual laboratory reports.

At first glance, this may seem to be a cumbersome system. However, the reader should recognize that there is a considerable increment in system responsibility when one goes from displaying the clinical data of greatest interest to the management of a complete medical record. Moreover, it must be remembered that the JHOC is but one unit in a 1000-bed hospital; it must conform to institutional standards. Therefore, the OCIS was designed to meet the internal JHOC clinical needs in a manner that would be compatible with Hospital practices. Clinical decision making is freed from a reliance on the bulky paper record, and record delivery delays do not affect emergency admissions. At the same time, the OCIS developers and operational staff do not have to address some of the more difficult problems that confront the Medical Records Department.

5
Protocol-Directed Care
Bruce I. Blum

Introduction

This chapter discusses the use of the OCIS in the preparation of daily care plans that recommend clinical actions based on predefined protocols. There are relatively few clinical information systems that provide this type of support, and therefore this chapter addresses three issues: What is meant by protocol-directed care? What is the design of an "ideal" system? How does the OCIS support this function? The perspective is limited to the needs of the Oncology Center.[1]

The term *protocol* simply means a set of formal rules. It is frequently used in the context of diplomacy or etiquette. There also are electronic communication protocols that define the rules for interaction among devices. In the medical environment, the term may be used in a variety of ways. The following are the most common usages in the Oncology Center.

Research Protocol. The basic model for clinical research relies on an experiment in which a hypothesis is tested. An essentially homogeneous sample of patients is selected, and a formal therapeutic plan is designed; the plan changes only a limited number of variables in order to test the validity of the hypothesis. Although randomly introduced biases cannot be avoided, the protocol is designed to control potentially confounding factors, such as age and stage of disease.

One may view the research protocol as a formal algorithm for treatment. It includes the criteria for accepting a patient for treatment under the protocol and for evaluating the outcome of the treatment. The protocol typically is recorded in a document of up to 60 pages. A diagrammatic representation of the therapy organization, called the schema, is prepared to represent the salient features of the document for easy reference.

---

[1]For a more general discussion of this topic see B. I. Blum, *Clinical Information Systems*, Springer-Verlag, New York, 1986. This book also contains a chapter on the OCIS in which the database structures for the daily care plan system are described.

At the Oncology Center there are about 100 research protocols active at any time. These include cooperative national studies, in which the data are periodically transcribed and sent to a central processing facility, and local protocols that are managed within the Oncology Center. There is a Johns Hopkins protocol committee that must approve each study before it is put into clinical use.

Individual Therapy. In many cases, the essential features of a research protocol are to be followed for a patient who does not quality for admission into the study. In this case the research protocol is modified to meet the individual needs of the patient; this modification typically invalidates the use of any outcome data in the subsequent protocol analysis.

A second form of individual therapy involves the modification of standard treatment plans (as opposed to a research protocol) to accommodate individual needs.

General Clinical Support. The preceding two classes of protocol are generally restricted to antitumor therapy and responses to the side effects of that treatment. In some cases the responses to the side effects can be isolated as independent protocols. Examples are clinical responses to infection (which are almost always an integral part of a research protocol), pain, nausea, and low platelet counts (described in Chapter 7).

A generalization of the clinical support protocols are the standard treatment protocols that have been established as baseline plans for dealing with a medical problem. These problems normally are not related directly to the antitumor treatments. Most alert and reminder systems are concerned with this type of protocol.

Disease-Specific Follow-Up. There is the need for the management of long-term patient follow-up. This follow-up is related to the patient's diagnosis. Examples include 6-month chest x-ray studies for breast cancer patients and 3-month monitoring of serum protein electrophoresis for certain multiple myeloma patients.

In most clinical settings, these protocols are managed by the clinician, who draws upon memory with occasional references to a written guideline. The problems with this approach have been well documented. For example, McDonald has shown how reminders alter physician behavior, especially with respect to clinically significant changes in therapeutics; the HELP system alerts have identified life-threatening drug–drug interactions that were subsequently altered for 1.8% of the hospital's patients. Wirtshafter and Mesel implemented an algorithm-based breast cancer consultant extender that produced a 95% compliance rate from 75 local physicians, in contrast to a 64% compliance rate from the cancer center physicians.

As already described in Chapter 2, there is too much information to be managed in a stressful, time-sensitive clinical setting. The physician needs help in anticipating problems to avoid being in a position of reacting to a critical medical situation. In the case of therapeutic plans that involve the use of highly toxic drugs in combinations over an extended period of time, the physician requires tools to help ensure that the proper sequence is followed. (For example, pharmicokenetic studies have shown that some drugs should be administered in two doses a precise number of hours or days apart; failure to adhere to this schedule will diminish the response.) Finally, in managing the care of a large number of patients with similar diseases, therapies, and problems, the physician requires tools to help identify the needs of each individual patient.

There are several approaches to providing this automated support. The remainder of this chapter describes the approach taken by the OCIS. This section concludes by briefly identifying some alternative methods. First, one can formalize the protocol as an algorithm. This may be done by using a form or checklist (e.g., the initial consultant extender) or coding the protocol as a program in a special protocol language (e.g., the extension of that concept by Gams). One also can combine orders into a block to be managed as a single unit (e.g., the use of protocols in the context of compound orders with the Technicon MIS). Next, one can formalize the protocol as a sequence of (often repeated) actions and print out extended plans and schedules (e.g., the systems of R. B. Friedman at Wisconsin University and R. H. Friedman at Boston University). Finally, one can treat the issue as an artificial intelligence problem, as Shortliffe and his colleagues have done with ONCOCIN.

The constraints placed upon the OCIS approach were that it be considered first and foremost a tool for supporting medical decision making in a large clinical setting. Therefore, it had to be easy to use and learn, understandable, low in risk, and natural to both the senior faculty (the researchers who define the protocols) and the health care providers (the house staff, nurses, physician assistants, etc., who must respond to the recommendations). In summary, the support for protocol-directed care had to use proven technology and be pragmatic in the selection of functions to be implemented. The design of a daily care plan facility was not considered a research activity; there was no research financial support for it. The clinical users were not interested in medical computing; their acceptance of a product and their patience in critiquing the evolving tools were directly related to their perception of the function's utility in a clinical setting.

There is an interesting contrast between the OCIS approach and that of ONCO-CIN. In the case of the latter, there is a clinical evaluation of a system that exploits artificial intelligence techniques, adds to our knowledge of medical informatics and computer science, and has the potential for going beyond the protocols that can be reduced to algorithms. In the case of the OCIS, on the other hand, a tool was designed for a specific environment, and its utility and evaluation were constrained by the local needs of that environment. Even though the goals and techniques differ, each contributes to our knowledge.

The Overall Design

This section presents the general design of the daily care plan system. As suggested in Chapter 3, one develops a system first by building a conceptual model of how it should operate, then by translating that concept into a specific (and often incomplete) implementation, and finally by refining the model as the result of operational experience. Naturally, the process is iterative. The general design to be presented in this section is the conceptual model and its initial implementation; the topic of the next section is a description of the system as it is used operationally. There are differences between the two sections. Some parts of the conceptual model were never used in an operational setting. Some parts of the operational system (which are considered to be of great value) are not really part of the conceptual model. Thus, what follows here is limited to a systems analysis of the problem; the implementation experience is described in the next section.

When work on the OCIS first began, it was a given fact that the system would manage a clinical database that could support both the display of data and the recommendation of therapeutic actions. The early perceptions of the Oncology Center founders were that most of the clinical care in the new center either was managed by protocol or could be so organized. Therefore, a database that contained all the clinical data and the protocol rules could be referenced to print out, for each inpatient day and outpatient visit, a list of all the protocol recommended actions. The provider would then be able to base his or her orders on this plan. The following section will temper these assumptions with the results of operational experience, but for now the presentation will consider the problem from a higher, more abstract perspective on the basis of this assumption.

Organization of the Protocol

Figure 1 contains the schema for a 1976 Eastern Cooperative Group protocol for the treatment of advanced stages of Hodgkin's Disease. There is an induction phase in which the patient undergoes six cycles (repetitions) of treatment with a combination of five drugs. The note at the bottom identifies the drugs, doses, and special instructors. At the end of the sixth cycle, if there is a complete response (CR) or partial response (PR), then one of two other regimens is followed. Either the patient is treated with three cycles of four drugs or radiotherapy is begun. The final outcome is then evaluated.

In this particular schema the flow is straightforward and relatively easy to explain. Note that the therapy extends over a long period of time (6 × 28 days plus 3 × 35 days for about 9 months). Thus the physician must know what protocol the patient is on, what branch of the protocol, what cycle within the branch, and what day within the cycle. Different clinical decisions will require different knowledge of the patient's status with respect to the protocol.

Information implicit in this protocol includes the criteria for accepting a patient into the study, definitions of CR, PR, etc., for protocol evaluation, definition of the stratification process, and the therapy details referenced in section 5 of the protocol. Of considerable importance is the detailing of what should be done if the drugs produce toxic reactions. Such toxicity is common in the aggressive treatment of cancer with drugs that are used in combinations powerful enough to destroy the diseased cells. Too low a dosage will have no impact on the

S C H E M A

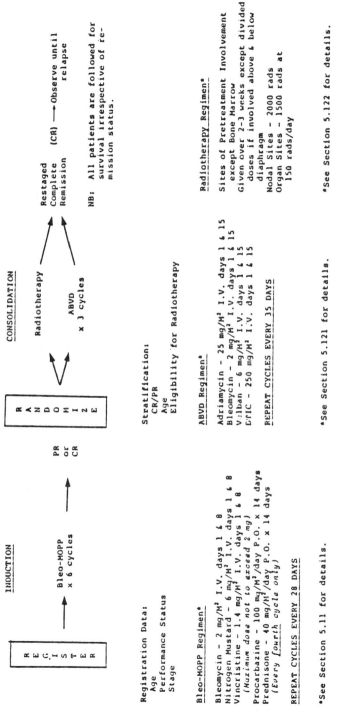

INDUCTION

REGISTER

Bleo-MOPP
x 6 cycles

PR
or
CR

CONSOLIDATION

Radiotherapy

ABVD
x 3 cycles

RANDOMIZE

Restaged
Complete
Remission (CR) ⟶ Observe until relapse

NB: All patients are followed for survival irrespective of re-mission status.

Registration Data:
Age
Performance Status
Stage

Stratification:
CR/PR
Age
Eligibility for Radiotherapy

Bleo-MOPP Regimen*

Bleomycin - 2 mg/M² I.V. days 1 & 8
Nitrogen Mustard - 6 mg/M² I.V. days 1 & 8
Vincristine - 1.4 mg/M² I.V. days 1 & 8
(Maximum dose not to exceed 2 mg)
Procarbazine - 100 mg/M²/day P.O. x 14 days
Prednisone - 40 mg/M²/day P.O. x 14 days
(Every fourth cycle only)

REPEAT CYCLES EVERY 28 DAYS

*See Section 5.11 for details.

ABVD Regimen*

Adriamycin - 25 mg/M² I.V. days 1 & 15
Bleomycin - 2 mg/M² I.V. days 1 & 15
Vilban - 6 mg/M² I.V. days 1 & 15
DTIC - 250 mg/M² I.V. days 1 & 15

REPEAT CYCLES EVERY 35 DAYS

*See Section 5.121 for details.

Radiotherapy Regimen*

Sites of Pretreatment Involvement
except Bone Marrow
Given over 2-3 weeks except divided
doses if involved above & below
diaphragm
Nodal Sites - 2000 rads
Organ Sites - 1500 rads at
150 rads/day

*See Section 5.122 for details.

Figure 1. Schema for Eastern Cooperative Oncology Group Protocol 1476.

tumor; too high a dosage may threaten the life of the patient. Consequently, toxic effects must be recognized promptly, and drug dosage adjusted accordingly.

From this brief description of the schema, it can be seen that a protocol can be decomposed into the following components:

Descriptive Information. Descriptive information is textual information about the protocol that is best maintained in a descriptive fashion. It is referenced when the protocol is first used and is consulted periodically. It is seldom used in the making of clinical decisions. (The schema is designed to provide general reminders and guidelines.)

Therapy Regimen. A therapy regimen is a summary of the treatment to be given as a block over an extended period of time. Associated with the administration of drugs is the ordering of tests to monitor the patient's status and provide early warnings of toxic reactions and responses to treatment.

Formal Rules. Formal rules is the set of rules that describe the relationships among the therapy regimens, the dose modifications in response to observed toxic reactions, the stratification criteria, etc. All formal rules, by definition, can be defined algorithmically. The therapy regimen is a special case of a formal rule; all such rules (when they reliably reflect actual practice) can be automated.

Given this representation of the protocol, it can be seen that one system design for protocol-directed care would structure its database to provide access to:

Protocol Description. Protocol description would make the protocol information available on line and in printed form. Access from the various clinical terminals would offer a valuable reference for medical decision making. In a truly closed system the protocol would be defined on the computer, and a printed listing would replace the standard document.

Treatment Sequences. Treatment sequences would contain all the therapy regimens in a formal language. They would identify what drugs to administer, what tests to order, what reminders to print, etc. The sequences would be decomposed into small cohesive blocks, and a single regimen might be expressed as more than one treatment sequence. Thus, a patient's care might be determined by multiples of such treatment sequences.

Schema. A schema is essentially a directed graph (or program) that links the treatment sequences and cycles within a protocol. At the conclusion of a treatment cycle the schema would be able to determine which treatment sequences to terminate and which options were available to the physician. Once the physician chose an option, the appropriate treatment sequences would be initiated.

Dose Modification. Criteria formalize responses to toxicity. Some criteria could be stated formally, for example, if the white blood cell count were to fall below a given value, then the dosage of certain drugs would be reduced by 50%. Other criteria would result in the printing of a warning to the physician to take some appropriate action.

Supporting Information. Identifies the contents of the clinical database that would be useful in the management of patients on this protocol. Some of this information would be presented in the form of the data displays described in Chapter 4; other information would be presented as a part of the care plan.

This is the view that the OCIS implemented in its protocol-directed care facility.

Processing Flow

The OCIS database maintains protocol descriptions containing the preceding information, together with the clinical data for each patient on a protocol. Therefore, the system should be able to access the protocol data and create a general plan for each patient. To do this, the OCIS uses the following processing flow:

Enter Patient on Protocol. The patient is entered on a protocol by means of a communication with the research office. (For individual therapy, no such coordination is required.) From the perspective of the protocol-directed care function, entering the patient results in associating one or more treatment sequences with the patient. For example, a common practice is to enter the therapy for the first cycle of treatment, a sequence for long-term follow-up, and a sequence for follow-up related to the anticipated inpatient stay. These sequences become the patient's standing orders.

Prepare Daily Care Plan. For inpatients, every morning the standing orders for each patient are processed, and a plan that identifies all therapies, tests, and reminders scheduled for that day is prepared. These are printed out in the various daily care plan formats. The processing also eliminates redundant tests. For example, if one treatment sequence requires a complete blood count (CBC) every two days (Q2D) and another requires a CBC Q3D, then the second request is never invoked. This allows physicians to define minimum criteria for each clinical situation independently and without concern for overutilization.

Review and Distribute Orders. Once the patient's treatment sequences are processed, the daily care plans are printed and distributed to the clinical areas. Several formats are provided: for the physician, for the nurses and physician assistants, for the attending physicians, and for the unit clerk. The plans represent the protocol recommendations. (The extended definition of protocol is used here; it includes inidividual therapy, clinical support, and follow-up.) The plans are amended as necessary, and the unit clerk plan serves as an order guide.

Record Actions. Because the care plan must relate to the patient's current status, it is essential that the actions of the previous plan be known before the next plan can be printed. For example, if a CBC was processed the previous day, then a sequence containing the order for CBC Q2D would not initiate a CBC order. On the order hand, of course, if the CBC was not ordered the previous day, then a request must be made for such a test order. In some cases, such as the CBC, it is possible to determine the status from the clinical data; in other cases, such as the reminder to read a skin test, a manual entry is required to close the loop.

In actual practice, as described in the following section, each morning the data coordinators enter the previous night's actions, and the plans are produced for distribution near noon. Treatment sequence changes are normally made after morning rounds and processed asynchronously. When the treatment sequences change a patient's standing orders, new plans are produced on demand.

Figure 2 represents an overview of this flow and system organization. Although the flow is quite simple, there are many problems in translating the conceptual model into operational use. The remainder of this section discusses how some of those problems were solved technically and/or operationally.

The Protocol Description

From a technical point of view, the management of the protocol description was quite simple. The development environment (TEDIUM[2]) provided a text processor and text data type; building a tool to manage the description was straightforward. The protocol was divided into the following sections:

Identification. This contains the protocol identifier, the principal investigators, and key administrative dates associated with its use. This coded information is also shared with the Research Office programs.

General Description. This is a short (one- or two-page) overview of the protocol. It serves as an abstract and simple reminder of the protocol structure.

Patient Selection. This is a text description of the selection criteria. It also includes an explicit list of exclusions.

Evaluation Criteria. This is a text description of the evaluation criteria.

Dose Modification. This is either a tabular display of the dose modification or a description of the modification. The tabular display is managed internally so that a computer program can identify the test results and drugs to be modified; by use of this information, the dose recommendations in the daily care plan can be

---

[2]TEDIUM is a trademark of Tedious Enterprises, Inc.

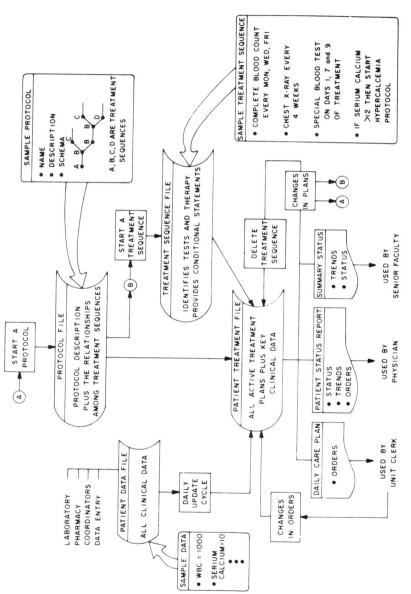

Figure 2.

Johns Hopkins Oncology Center 06/23/88

PROTOCOL DEFINITION

E5181 ADJUVANT/OPERABLE N(+)
ADJUVANT/OPERABLE N (+)

INVESTIGATORS : TORMEY,DOUGLASS M.D.
ABELOFF,MARTIN M.D.
ROSEMAN,DAVID M.D.
GILCHRIST,KENNEDY M.D.
FALKSON,GEOFFREY M.D.

ACTIVATED:
REVISED:
STATUS: ACTIVE

GENERAL DESCRIPTION for E5181 ADJUVANT/OPERABLE N(+):

An ADJUVANT CLINICAL TRIAL to COMPARE Cytoxan, Methotrexate, 5FU, Predisone, and Tamoxifen (CMFPT) to alternaing CMF(P)TH and ThioTepa, Adriamycin, Vinblastine, Halotestin and Short-versus Long-term Tamoxifen in PREMENOPAUSAL PATIENTS with OPERABLE N+ BREAST CANCER.

OBJECTIVES

To test the concept that introduction of a noncross-resistant Adriamycin containing regimen (TsAVbTH) in an alternaing sequence with CMF(P)TH will be superior to CMFPT alone.

To test across the protocol the theoretical advantage of providing exposure to an antiestrogen for prolonged periods against discontinuing its use with the termination of chemotherapy.

To compare these effects with respect to 1) decreasing the recurrence rates across time, 2) increasing survival across time, and 3) the impact of pretreatment characteristics on the above parameters.

To assess the quality of survival from performance status and toxicity analysis of the regimens.

RANDOMIZATION ARMS

1. Patients assigned to the CMFPT group will receive 12 COURSES of CMFPT followed by re-randomization to either OBSERVATION or to continue T to a total of 5 years.

CYTOXAN 100mg/m2 PO days 1-14 of each cycle as a single daily dose

MTX 40mg/m2 IV days 1 and 8 of each cycle

Figure 3a.

DOSE MODIFICATIONS for E5181 ADJUVANT/OPERABLE N(+):

RENAL 2 (RENAL DYSFUNCTION)

	MTX	CYTX	5FU	PRED	TAMO
CREATININE <1.3	100%	100%	100%	100%	100%
CREATININE 1.3 - 2.0	50%	100%	100%	100%	100%
CREATININE 2.1 - 3.5*	OMIT	100%	100%	100%	100%
CREATININE > 3.5*	OMIT	OMIT	OMIT	100%	100%

RENAL 1 (RENAL 1)

RENAL DYSFUNCTION

	ADRA	THIO	VELB	PRED	TAMO
CREATININE <1.3	100%	100%	100%	100%	100%
CREATININE 1.3 - 2.0	100%	100%	100%	100%	100%
CREATININE 2.1 - 3.5*	100%	100%	100%	100%	100%
CREATININE >3.5*	OMIT	OMIT	OMIT	100%	100%

HEM TOX 4 (HEM TOXICITY)

PLTS AND WBC DOSE MODIFICATION TABLE

	CYTX	MTX	5FU	TAMO	PRED
PLTS>100K:WBC>4000	100%	100%	100%	100%	100%
PLTS>100K:WBC2500-4000	50%	50%	50%	100%	100%
PLTS>100K:WBC<2500	OMIT	OMIT	OMIT	100%	100%
PLTS 75K-100K: WBC>4000	50%	50%	50%	100%	100%
PLTS 75K-100K: WBC 2500-4000	50%	50%	50%	100%	100%
PLTS 75K-100K: WBC <2500	OMIT	OMIT	OMIT	100%	100%
PLTS <75K:WBC >4000	OMIT	OMIT	OMIT	100%	100%
PLTS <75K:WBC 2500-4000	OMIT	OMIT	OMIT	100%	100%
PLTS <75K: WBC <2500	OMIT	OMIT	OMIT	100%	100%

CYTX TOX (CYTOXAN TOXICITY)

ALL PATIENTS SHOULD BE INSTRUCTED ON THE IMPORTANCE OF VIGOROUS HYDRATION DURING CYTOXAN THERAPY. IF HEMORRHAGIC CYSTITIS SHOULD OCCUR DESPITE VIGOROUS HYDRATION, CYTOXAN SHOULD BE STOPPED AND SUBSEQUENT THERAPY MANAGED WITH MELPHALAN 4 MG/M2 PO DAYS 1 THROUGH 5 OF EACH TREATMENT CYCLE.

HEM TOX 3 (HEM TOX 3)

	THIO	ADRA	VELB	TAMO	HALO
PLTS>100 K:WBC>4000	100%	100%	100%	100%	100%
PLTS>100K:WBC 2500-4000	50%	50%	50%	100%	100%
PLTS>100 K:WBC<2500	OMIT	OMIT	OMIT	100%	100%
PLTS 75K-100K:WBC>4000	50%	50%	50%	100%	100%
PLTS 75K-100K:WBC 2500-4000	50%	50%	50%	100%	100%
PLTS 75K-100K: WBC<2500	OMIT	OMIT	OMIT	100%	100%
PLTS<75K :WBC>4000	OMIT	OMIT	OMIT	100%	100%
PLTS<75K :WBC 2500-4000	OMIT	OMIT	OMIT	100%	100%
PLTS<75K:WBC<2500	OMIT	OMIT	OMIT	100%	100%

Figure 3b.

altered to adjust for toxicity automatically. Where a tabular display does not exist, it often is possible to recognize when a warning message should be printed.

Protocol Schema. This is a formal language that describes the treatment sequence graph. It is managed as a text program and contains operators such as STOP seq and START seq. The format was never felt to be useful by the physicians, and, given the impact of a wrong decision, it was decided not to use the schema. Thus, although in the abstract the schema could produce reliable reminders and perhaps even automated support, such a tool was considered inappropriate in the clinical environment. Consequently, the development of a schema facility was terminated.

Figure 3 contains two pages from a protocol description. With the exception of the administrative data that were required for other purposes, the concept of on-line protocol definitions never matured. There were several reasons. First, the protocol had already been prepared in a typescript form, and the on-line description was redundant. It required reentry of the text plus an additional review by the principal investigators. Second, the tools used in development were primitive when compared with those now available in personal computers. Typewriters (rather than word processors) were the standard as the system was being developed. Without a strong demand for on-line access, the tool was seen as extra work for busy people. Finally, because there were so many protocols, many had few patients on study. One might argue that this would justify the need for on-line access to seldom-used protocols; however, the users perceived the definition of the automated form of the protocol to be a lot of work with a limited payoff.

The Treatment Sequences

In some Darwinian sense the protocol descriptions (along with their automatic dose modifications and schema reminders) became extinct; the code remained, but the database atrophied. The treatment sequences, on the other hand, grew and flourished. In the very first prototypes, the treatment sequences were limited to the ordering of drugs and tests. The sequence could create orders cyclically (e.g., Q2D or Q1W), by day of week (e.g., M, W, F) or by day relative to the start of the treatment sequence (e.g., 1, 8).

The next iteration added features to deal with special situations. Because of operational considerations, for example, some labor-intensive tests might be ordered cyclically but should not be ordered on weekends or holidays. The standing orders had to accommodate this constraint. Warning messages were also added to the plans, and these were stratified by the audience (physician, nurse, physician assistant) and priority. Because many messages might be listed, there was a concern that important messages might become overlooked. These high-priority messages, therefore, were to be set aside and printed in a box.

In time, the treatment sequence functions matured. Ken Bakalar defined a language for specifying how the items were to be designated. Table 1 lists the key

Table 1. Summary of Key Repeat Mode Rules

Category	Illustration
Day of week	M T W H F S U
Odd or even day (calendar day of the month)	E (any even day), ET (Tuesday if an even day)
Cyclic	Q2D (every 2 days), Q3W (every 3 weeks)
Treatment sequence day	1, 3, 22, 56
Treatment sequence week (use with outpatients)	1W (day 1 to 7 of therapy if not done previously)
Special operators (use with cyclic or sequence day)	
* Not on weekends, use nearest weekday, e.g., *1 or *Q2D	
+ Not on weekends, order on Monday	
− Not on weekends, order on Friday	
# Order until verified, e.g., #12	
> Order until canceled, e.g., > 4	
/ Used to join conditions, i.e., and	
B or C indicates that the action begins or concludes on the given day	

definition rules, and Table 2 contains some example clauses. Liz McColligan defined a complex set of dictionaries that provided linkage between the plans and the clinical data. At the highest level, the terms used in the orders were the same, but there was a complication in going from the ordering of tests to the processing of test results. For example, a CBC includes a white blood cell count (WBC). Thus a treatment sequence for WBC Q2D should not initiate an order request if a CBC was ordered the previous (or current) day. Conversely, knowing that there is a WBC value may not provide information about the ordering of a CBC. Other

Table 2. Sample Illustrations of Repeat Clauses

Clause	Interpretation
1, 2, 3	Order on days 1, 2, 3
Q14D	Order every 14 days; this could be written Q2W
M, W, F	Monday, Wednesday, and Friday
B5/C14	Beginning on day 5, order test daily; cancel on day 14
B29/Q4W	Order test beginning on day 29 and every 4 weeks thereafter
B15/Q7D/C36;B36/Q14D	Beginning on day 15, order test every 7 days, until day 36; then order test every 14 days
*1, 3, 5	Order test on days 1, 3, and 5, except when they fall on a weekend or holiday; in that case order on the nearest working day

```
                    Oncology Information System          06/23/88
                    TREATMENT SEQUENCES

(BMT FOLT)   BMT F/U FROM DAY 0; ALL BMT'S EXCEPT AUTOLOGOUS AND AA'S

    TREATMENT TYPE                         SCHEDULE
---------------------------------------------------------------------------

    BLOOD PROCEDURES
       DIR COOMBS  (DCMB)                  *36,71,101
       SR OSMOLAL  (SOSM)                  M,H
       SR AMYLASE  (SAMY)                  M,F
       AMA&SMMSAB  (AMSM)                  *36,71,101
       ENA  (ENA)                         *36,71,101
       RBC ANTIGN  (IMGT)                  *B29/Q30D
       CYTOGENETC  (CYTG)                  *B21/T;V1
       ANTINUC AB  (ANAB)                  *36,71,101
       S IMMUN EP  (SIEP)                  *36,71,101
       RHEUM FACT  (SRF)                   *36,71,101
       DNA ANTIBD  (DNAA)                  *36,71,101

    P.A. PROCEDURES
       BM MORPH   (BMRH)                   B15/Q7D/C36;B36/Q14D
       BM CYTOGEN  (BMRY)                  *29
       BM BIOPSY  (BMBX)                   B29/Q4W

    NURSING PROCEDURES
       ECG   (ECG)                         1

    COMMENTS
       LEVEL  2    (M.D. COMMENTS)
         (1)   CHEST XRAY                  *Q7D
           CHEST X-RAY SHOULD BE SCHEDULED Q7 DAYS, OR AS CLINICALLY INDICATED.
         (2)   ABG                         Q2W
           ABG SHOULD BE DONE Q2 WEEKS, OR AS CLINICALLY INDICATED.
         (3)   ABG BMT                     1
           IT ISN'T NECESSARY TO DRAW AN ART. BLOOD GAS ON DAY OF BMT IF ONE HAS
           PREVIOUSLY BEEN DRAWN.
         (5)   BM BX PRN                   B15/Q7D/C36;B36/Q14D
           BONE MARROW BIOPSY MAY BE DONE PRN WHEN BONE MARROW ASPIRATE IS DONE

       LEVEL  3    (COORDINATOR)
         (15)  BM BX AMF                   1,4,7,10,13
           SCHEDULE AMF PATIENTS FOR BONE MARROW BIOPSY EVERY OTHER WEEK BEGINNING
           BMT DAY 14.
```

Figure 4.

dictionaries were created for text messages, and the clinical data coordinator was given the facility to define messages to be used for a specific treatment sequence.

Figures 4 through 6 contain some typical treatment sequences as they are now used. The first is the follow-up treatment for the bone marrow transplant (BMT) protocol starting on day zero. It orders blood tests and physician assist and nursing procedures. It indicates that the Direct Coombs Test (DIR COOMBS) is to be done on days 36, 71, and 101, except if they fall on a weekend, in which case the test is ordered for the nearest weekday. The Serum Osmolality (SR OSMOLAL) is to be ordered every Monday and Thursday. The treatment sequence also specifies that comments are also to be listed. Every seven days the message

    CHEST X-RAY SHOULD BE SCHEDULED Q7 DAYS, OR AS
    CLINICALLY INDICATED.

will be listed, and on day 1

```
(J8209)    START BMT DAY -1; FOR ALLOGENEIC BMT'S ON CSA STUDY

  TREATMENT TYPE                              SCHEDULE
--------------------------------------------------------------------------------

  BLOOD PROCEDURES
    BLOOD CULT   (CULB)                       Q1D

  THERAPY
    8209/CSA-P        10 MG/KG                B17/C44
      P.O. @8 A.M.
    8209/CSA-P       7.5 MG/KG                B45/C182
      P.O. @8 A.M.
    8209/CSA-I       2.5 MG/KG                2,3,4,5
      Q12 HRS CONTINUOUS I.V. START @8 AM
    8209/CSA-I      1.875 MG/KG               B6/C16
      Q12 HRS CONTINUOUS I.V., START @8 AM
    J8209/CYTX       7.5 MG/KG                3,5,7,9,11;B23/Q7D
      I.V. @8 P.M.
    METHL PRED      0.25 MG/KG                10,11,12,13,14,15,16
      I.V. Q12 HR
    METHL PRED       0.5 MG/KG                B17/C30
      I.V Q12 HRS
    METHL PRED       0.4 MG/KG                B31/C44
      I.V. Q12 H (OR MAY GIVE P.O.)
    METHL PRED      0.25 MG/KG                B45/C58
      I.V. Q12 H (OR MAY GIVE P.O.)
    METHL PRED       0.1 MG/KG                B59/C65;B66/Q2D/C74
      I.V. Q12 HRS (OR MAY GIVE P.O.)
```

Figure 5.

IT ISN'T NECESSARY TO DRAW AN ART. BLOOD GAS ON
DAY OF BMT IF ONE HAS BEEN PREVIOUSLY DRAWN.

will be printed.

The portion of the treatment sequence in Figure 5 illustrates a set of drug orders for a BMT protocol. The therapy lines include the drug name (in the internal OCIS dictionary form) and the dose. In preparing the plan, the OCIS determines the patient's weight in kilograms (or area if body surface area is specified) and computes the actual recommended dose. The plan also allows two different dose levels to be ordered. For example, CSA-P is administered at the rate of 10 mg/kg from day 17 through 44 and at the rate of 7.5 mg/kg from days 45 to 182. The therapy entry also includes a descriptive line providing administration information.

Finally, Figure 6 illustrates how the comments are used to present the dose modification information. The first message is printed starting day 1 and then daily. (The BMT sequences start on day 0.) The next block is related to the administration of the J8209/CYTX and is printed every 7 days starting on day 23. The final block is printed every day beginning on day 2 and concluding on day 5; this could also have been coded as 2, 3, 4, 5. In each case, the comment is identified by a mnemonic (e.g., AMPHOTERICIN), and the full comment is printed from the comment dictionary to make the treatment sequence easier to read.

```
                      ONCOLOGY INFORMATION SYSTEM            06/23/88
                          TREATMENT SEQUENCES

 (J8209)    START BMT DAY -1; FOR ALLOGENEIC BMT'S ON CSA STUDY

   TREATMENT TYPE                          SCHEDULE
 ------------------------------------------------------------------------
   DOSE MODIFICATIONS
     J8209     AMPHOTERICIN                    B1/Q1D
        IF AMPHOTERICIN B HAS TO BE INSTITUTED, STUDY DRUG A IS AUTOMATICALLY
        REDUCED TO 5 MG/KG P.O. QOD OR 0.625 MG/KG I.V. Q12 HR FOR 2 DOSES QOD
        (TOTAL DAILY DOSE 1.25 EVERY OTHER DAY I.V.).
        AMPHOTERICIN B IS STARTED AT A DOSE OF 0.3 MG/KG.  ON THIS DAY STUDY
        DRUG A IS GIVEN AT THE FULL DOSE.  THE FOLLOWING DAY, STUDY DRUG A IS
        OMITTED, BUT AMPHOTERICIN IS GIVEN AT A DOSE OF 0.5 MG/KG.
        THE FOLLOWING DAYS STUDY DRUG A AND AMPHOTERICIN ARE GIVEN ALTERNATING
        EVERY OTHER DAY.


     J8209     HEME STATUS                     B23/Q7D
        DOSE MODIFICATIONS FOR CYCLOPHOSPHAMIDE:
        STARTING DAY 21, THE CYCLOPHOSPHAMIDE (J8209 STUDY DRUG B) DOSE WILL
        BE ADJUSTED ACCORDING TO THE PERIPHERAL WBC: (SEE TABLE·"HEME STATUS")
        IF THE ADMINISTRATION OF CYCLOPHOSPHAMIDE POST-TRANSPLANTATION APPEARS
        TO BE CONTRAINDICATED BECAUSE OF HEMORRHAGIC CYSTITIS OR CARDIAC
        PROBLEMS, METHOTREXATE MAY BE SUBSTITUTED IN A DOSE OF 10 MG/M2/DAY.

                                         209B
 WBC > 2000                              100%
 1000 < WBC < 2000                        50%
 WBC < 1000                              OMIT


     J8209     LIVER TOX 1                     B2/C5
        IF HEPATIC IMPAIRMENT IS PRESENT, AND SYSTEMIC GVHD IS REASONABLY RULED
        OUT, THE DOSE OF CYCLOSPORINE STUDY DRUG A WILL BE REDUCED TO 1.25 MG/KG
        I.V. Q12 H. THE DOSES WILL REMAIN AT THE REDUCED LEVEL EVEN AFTER THE
        HEPATIC IMPAIRMENT HAS RESOLVED.

                                         209AI
 SGOT >= 1000 (A)                         50%
 SGPT >= 1000 (B)                         50%
 TBLI >= 4.0 (C) (1)                      50%


     (1)
        CONDITIONS (A AND C) OR (B AND C) MUST BE MET TO QUALIFY AS HEPATIC
        IMPAIRMENT FOR MODIFICATION OF STUDY DRUG A DOSE.
```

Figure 6.

The Standing Orders

Treatment sequences are independent of the patient. To be processed, the sequences must be associated with a patient. This can be done in two ways. First, a pointer to a treatment sequence can be tied to a patient. The advantage here is that the same sequence can be used for many patients, thereby saving space. The obvious disadvantage is that the sequence is associated with many patients, and therefore any changes to a treatment sequence may impact on the care of patients currently being managed with that sequence. Consequently, the system design chosen by the OCIS copies the treatment sequence to a patient treatment structure called the standing orders. These standing orders may be edited to provide individual therapy for a particular patient.

Because the patient standing orders typically are constructed from more than one treatment sequence, all order entries must identify the treatment sequence with which they are associated, along with the date on which the treatment sequence was initiated. Adding a treatment sequence to the standing orders involves the copying of all terms from the treatment sequence file to the patient standing order file while setting the start date to the current date. Stopping a treatment sequence involves going through the standing orders and deleting all entries for that sequence.

During the preparation of a patient's daily care plan, each request (i.e., statement copied from the treatment sequence) is compared with the status of that request for that patient. For example, if the standing order item is to be ordered on day 3 and this is the third day on which the treatment sequence has been active for this patient, then the item will be included in the care plan. A somewhat more complex algorithm is used for some of the other cyclic requests, and the order processing concludes with a task that removes duplicate or overlapping requests, as for example, requests for a CBC and WBC. The fact that an item has been recommended is recorded in the patient's standing orders; after validation, the fact that the item was actually ordered is also recorded. The updated standing orders are used to produce the printed daily care plans; the same information is available on line.

In addition to the treatment sequence recommendations, the patient protocol structure has the facility for maintaining a set of clinical findings, such as the cumulative doses of a drug, the last value of a test, the average of a test result over a given period, or the maximum result for a test value in some time window. When these clinical findings are requested, the daily care processing initiates the updating of the findings. (The only complicated aspect of this processing is the management of edits to the clinical database that may alter averages, maxima, etc.) The clinical findings may be listed in the daily care plan; they may also be used to recommend dose modifications, warn of excessive cumulative drug doses, or identify early trends in test results. The clinical findings functions were all implemented by Chris Brunn, but they did not seem to elicit much physician interest. Thus, although all the programs work and the outputs are included in most of the descriptive OCIS papers, this feature of the system is used only occasionally.

Outpatient Care Plans

Before describing how the system operates, the issue of outpatient care plans must be addressed. There are several technical problems that make the processing of outpatient care plans more difficult. First, the periods between events is more variable. In the treatment sequences exhibited, the granularity is one day, whereas in an outpatient setting it may be weeks or months. For outpatients, the evaluation of a Q2W criterion implies a range of 11 to 17 days, and the protocols must be able to accommodate missed appointments and delays of a week or more. This implies that the outpatient plan must be integrated with the appointment system. Also, rules for allowable visit rescheduling when therapy is in progress must be defined. Finally, the feedback and processing flow for outpatients would have to be organized differently. There are not enough outpatient clinical data co-ordinators to manage the flow as it operates in the inpatient units; the process-ing of therapy actions must be integrated with the charge capture process. For-tunately two developers, Liz McColligan and Farideh Momeni, were able to work out many of these problems, and they implemented a prototype out-patient system.

Given the OCIS orientation to patients regardless of the location of their treat-ment and the fact that many protocols integrate inpatient and outpatient care, one might think that the clinical staff would be anxious to extend the daily care plans to the outpatient clinics. In fact, most of the automated support for cancer pro-tocols developed at other institutions is restricted to outpatients. However, by dealing with the complexities of inpatient care, OCIS built a powerful system that many providers perceived to be too complex for casual use. That is, a consider-able investment in protocol definition, learning, and system maintenance is required to make the care plans effective. Just as in the case of entering the protocol descriptions, no investigator was willing to commit the time required to make the system work in an outpatient setting. As a result, the prototype was never operationally tested, and the daily care plans are restricted to the inpatient units.

If the OCIS were a research project, this lack of interest in an outpatient facility would be met with disappointment; the concept could not be validated. However, from the development perspective, the OCIS outpatient daily care plans can be viewed as one of a series of experiments in building functions that the designers hope will meet real needs. Sometimes these experiments produce operational tools for which there is no immediate demand. If the demonstrations do not cre-ate the demand, then the tools are retired. Should the demand later materialize, then the first iteration of the tools will be available. Thus, one may view the OCIS as a dynamic organism that responds and adapts to its users' needs. The discussion now turns to what the Oncology Center finds useful.

Daily Care Plan Processing

As described in the previous section, the daily care plans are processed with the following flow: a patient is entered onto a protocol, and treatment sequences are activated and deactivated as the medical decisions are made. This infor-mation is organized by patient, and the data are referred to as the patient's standing orders. Each morning, a data coordinator enters into the database any deviations from the previous day's plan, for example, orders not carried out or additional or modified orders. This is a process called "verification." Once it is complete for all patients, the daily care plans for the current day can be produced.

Figure 7 displays a two-page daily care plan for a BMT patient whose standing orders contain the following ten treatment sequences:

Treatment Sequence ID	Day started	Day number
7915 TX	05/16/88	39
BMTFOLC	05/19/88	36
BMTFOLT	05/27/88	28
BMT INT	05/16/88	39
CY4 INF	05/18/88	37
J8209	05/25/88	30
MARHARV	05/15/88	40
MAR INF	05/27/88	28
PFTS	05/15/88	40
TB14 TX	05/23/88	32

The top of the plan contains the identification, some demographic data, information used in computing the drug dose, and the names of the providers. If the census entry includes text messages (as described in Chapter 4), then these messages will be printed at the top of the page as well. The use of census text is left to the provider. On the day that the daily care plans were printed out for this chapter, 13 plans were listed for consideration. Of these, 5 had text, and four of the text fields totaled 30 lines or more in length. (The 30 lines of text contained approximately 20 separate data-flagged messages.) The providers for the patients whose plans are presented in this chapter did not take advantage of the census messages.

Below the standard heading block are printed the protocols by which the patient's treatment is being directed. These OCIS protocols represent modules of a larger integrated plan. There is no one-to-one correspondence between protocols and treatment sequences, and some protocols may not have a treatment sequence associated with them.

The next section of the plan lists the test and procedure recommendations for that day. Twelve blood and serum tests are to be ordered; there are several messages for the physician, and there are three physician assistant procedures along with a message. Because the messages are not of the first priority, they are printed in this location. When they are required, high-priority messages are printed in a box above this section.

The next section contains the recommended therapies. In this case two drugs are to be administered. The actual dose is computed by the system as a function of ideal body weight (65.8 kg, as listed at the top of the plan). Below the treatment block are the dose modification instructions. As noted earlier, even though some of the dose modifications are in the form of a table that implies the ability to adjust the dosages automatically, all modification instructions are simply text messages.

Figure 8 contains a portion of the patient's standing orders that were used to generate this plan. The standing order entries are organized by type. Each entry

```
        JOHNS HOPKINS                      HISTORY NO:
        ONCOLOGY CENTER                        NAME: Patient 1
                                           PLAN DATE: 06/24/88
        DAILY CARE PLAN                               FRIDAY     PAGE 1


   39 Y.O. W M  LYMPHOMA, NOS, BMT                 HT  172.7 CM  BSA 2.1 M2
        WEIGHTS:  ADMIN  92.7 KG   IDEAL  65.8 KG  CURRENT (06/21/88)  90.8 KG
PROVIDERS :         MARY (PRIMARY NURSE)
                    LII SHIN (ASSOCIATE NURSE)


   PROTOCOLS                                    STARTED     DAY
        J7820     CYTOMEGALOVIRUS               05/18/88    38
        J8638     IMMUNOLOGIC MONITORING BMT    05/18/88    38
        J8642     LATE TOX. FOLLOWING BMT       05/18/88    38
        J8704     EVAL. OF GVHD IN ALLO. BMT REC 05/18/88   38
        J8724     SKIN EXPLANT MODEL OF GVHD    05/18/88    38
        J8729     EFFECT OF B. MAR. ELUTR./GVHD 05/18/88    38
        J8525     BMT FOR TX OF LYMPHOMA        05/19/88    37
        J8430     PREV. GVHD CYCLOSPORIN        05/25/88    31
        BMT       SCHED BMT DAY                 05/27/88    28
                  DAY 0-J8525(CY/TBI)


TEST AND PROCEDURES:
   BLOOD AND SERUM TESTS
             HEMATOCRIT                    WBC
             PLT CNT                       WBC DIFF
             RETIC CNT                     BLOOD CULT
             TYPE&HOLDA                    SMA-12
             STAT M6                       STAT PRO TIME
             RBC ANTIGN                    PER SMEAR
   PHYSICIAN PROCEDURES CHEST X-RAY SHOULD BE SCHEDULED Q7 DAYS, OR AS
             CLINICALLY INDICATED. ABG SHOULD BE DONE Q2 WEEKS, OR AS
             CLINICALLY INDICATED. BONE MARROW BIOPSY MAY BE DONE PRN WHEN
             BONE MARROW ASPIRATE IS DONE
   P.A. PROCEDURES
             BM MORPH                      BM CYTOGEN
             BM BIOPSY
             DO NOT ORDER RBC ANTIGENS (IMGT) ON AUTOLOGOUS BMT PATIENTS
TREATMENT:
        658     MG      8209/CSA-P, BASED ON 65.8 X 10 MG/KG
        26.32   MG      METHL PRED, BASED ON 65.8 X 0.4 MG/KG
DOSE MODIFICATIONS:
   AMPHOTERICIN (AMPHOTERICIN AND STUDY DRUG A) IF AMPHOTERICIN B HAS TO BE
             INSTITUTED, STUDY DRUG A IS AUTOMATICALLY REDUCED TO 5
             MG/KG P.O. QOD OR 0.625 MG/KG I.V. Q12 HR FOR 2 DOSES QOD
             (TOTAL DAILY DOSE 1.25 EVERY OTHER DAY I.V.).
        AMPHOTERICIN B IS STARTED AT A DOSE OF 0.3 MG/KG.  ON THIS DAY STUDY
             DRUG A IS GIVEN AT THE FULL DOSE.  THE FOLLOWING DAY,
             STUDY DRUG A IS OMITTED, BUT AMPHOTERICIN IS GIVEN AT A
             DOSE OF 0.5 MG/KG.
   THE FOLLOWING DAYS STUDY DRUG A AND AMPHOTERICIN ARE GIVEN
             ALTERNATING EVERY OTHER DAY.
```

Figure 7a.

contains the order identifier, its schedule, the number of times that the order was carried out (its count or CNT), the date that it was last done (LST DONE), the day number of the treatment sequence that initiated this item, and the treatment sequence identifier.

This page of the standing orders begins with the P.A. procedures. The first procedure listed is BMRH (bone marrow aspirate for morphology or, as listed in the daily care plan, BM MORPH). This is requested by two different treatment sequences: BMT FOLT, for BMT follow up (T), and BMT INT, for BMT

```
JOHNS HOPKINS                          HISTORY NO:
ONCOLOGY CENTER                          NAME: Patient 1
                                    PLAN DATE: 06/24/88
DAILY CARE PLAN                               FRIDAY    PAGE 2
```

```
LIVER TOX 3 (LFT'S AND CYCLOSPORINE STUDY DRUG A DOSE) IF HEPATIC IMPAIRMENT
            IS PRESENT, AND SYSTEMIC GVHD IS REASONABLY RULED OUT, THE
            CYCLOSPORINE STUDY DRUG A DOSE WILL BE REDUCED TO 7.5
            MG/KG P.O.  THE DOSES WILL REMAIN AT THE REDUCED LEVEL
            EVEN AFTER THE HEPATIC IMPAIRMENT HAS RESOLVED.
                                        209AP
SGOT >= 1000 (A)                         75%
SGPT >= 1000 (B)                         75%
TBLI >  4.0 (C) (1)                      75%
```

```
(1) CONDITIONS (A&C) OR (B&C) MUST BE MET TO QUALIFY AS HEPATIC
        IMPAIRMENT FOR DOSE MODIFICATION OF CYCLOSPORINE STUDY
        DRUG A.
```

```
RENAL TOX 3 (SERUM CREATININE AND CYCLOSPORINE STUDY DRUG A DOSE) IF THE
            CREATININE RISES TO 2.2, THE DOSE OF CYCLOSPORINE STUDY
            DRUG A WILL BE REDUCED TO 7.5 MG/KG P.O.
    IF THE CREATININE RISES TO >= 3.0, THE DOSE WILL BE REDUCED TO 5.0
            MG/KG.
    IF THE CREATININE RISES TO >= 4.0, THE CYCLOSPORINE STUDY DRUG IS
            HELD UNTIL THE CREATININE LEVEL HAS RETURNED TO < 4.0.
                                        209AP
SCR >= 2.2                               75%
SCR >= 3.0                               50%
SCR >= 4.0  (1)                          OMIT
```

```
(1) HOLD CYCLOSPORINE STUDY DRUG A  UNTIL SERUM CREATININE LEVEL HAS
        RETURNED TO < 4.0.
```

Figure 7b.

Initiation. The schedule for BMRH under BMT FOLT is to begin on day 15 and then the procedure is to be ordered every 7 days until day 36, when the schedule is changed to every 14 days. (This is written B15/Q7D/C36;B36/Q14D.) The schedule under BMT INT is for the procedure to be ordered on day 2 unless that day is a holiday or weekend, in which case it is to be ordered on the working day closest to day 2. (This is written *2.)

The plan being ordered from this set of standing orders is for the following day, a Friday. As can be seen from the first line, this is day 28 of the BMT FOLT treatment sequence, and therefore the Q7D option is in effect. The BMRH was last ordered 06/17/88 and the next day (i.e., the day of the plan) is 06/24/88. This is 7 days since the last order, and a BMRH recommendation is required. The BMRY (BM CYTOGEN) is ordered because 06/23/88 is day 28 on BMT FOLT, and its schedule calls for an order on day 29 if it is not a weekend or holiday. Finally, BMBX (BM BIOPSY) is ordered every 4 weeks beginning on day 29 according to the same treatment sequence.

Notice that the P.A. procedure orders associated with BMT INT and the bone marrow harvest sequence, MAR HARV, are no longer active. These treatment sequences could be deleted without altering any future daily care plans. They are retained, however, because the providers find them helpful for documentation purposes.

```
                        ONCOLOGY INFORMATION SYSTEM
                          TREATMENT PLAN LISTING                   06/23/88
Patient 1
ORDER                     SCHEDULE          CNT LST DONE DAY#          T.SQ. ID
--------------------------------------------------------------------------------
  P.A. PROCEDURES
    BMRH                  B15/Q7D/C36;B36/   2 06/17/88  28        BMT FOLT
                          Q14D
                          *2                 3 06/17/88  39        BMT INT
    BMRY                  *29                0 05/17/88  28        BMT FOLT
                          *2                 1 05/17/88  39        BMT INT
                          1                  1 05/17/88  40        MAR HARV
    BMBX                  B29/Q4W            0 05/17/88  28        BMT FOLT
                          *2                 1 05/17/88  39        BMT INT
  NURSING PROCEDURES
    ECG                   1                  1 05/27/88  28        BMT FOLT
                          *1                 2 05/27/88  39        BMT INT
    SVUM                  *M,H              10 06/23/88  36        BMT FOLC
                          *M,H              12 06/23/88  39        BMT INT
    SVCB                  *M,H              10 06/23/88  36        BMT FOLC
                          *M,H              12 06/23/88  39        BMT INT
    SVCD                  *M                 5 06/20/88  36        BMT FOLC
                          *M                 6 06/20/88  39        BMT INT
    SVCV                  *H                 5 06/23/88  36        BMT FOLC
                          *H                 6 06/23/88  39        BMT INT
  DOSE MODIFICATIONS
    J8209   AMPHOTERICIN  B1/Q1D            30 06/23/88  30        J8209
    J8209   HEME STATUS   B23/Q7D            2 06/23/88  30        J8209
    J8209   LIVER TOX 1   B2/C5              4 05/29/88  30        J8209
    J8209   LIVER TOX 2   B6/C16            11 06/09/88  30        J8209
    J8209   LIVER TOX 3   B17/C44           14 06/23/88  30        J8209
    J8209   LIVER TOX 4   B45/Q1D            0            30        J8209
    J8209   RENAL TOX 1   B2/C5              4 05/29/88  30        J8209
    J8209   RENAL TOX 2   B6/C16            11 06/09/88  30        J8209
    J8209   RENAL TOX 3   B17/C44           14 06/23/88  30        J8209
    J8209   RENAL TOX 4   B45/Q1D            0            30        J8209
  THERAPY
    CYTX    50 MG/KG      4,5,6,7            2 05/22/88  39        7915 TX
            I.V. USUALLY GIVEN AT 4 P.M.
    TBI     300 RADS      8,9,10,11          4 05/26/88  39        7915 TX
    209AP   10 MG/KG      B17/C44           14 06/23/88  30        J8209
            P.O. @8 A.M.
            7.5 MG/KG     B45/C182          14 06/23/88  30        J8209
            P.O. @8 A.M.
    209AI   2.5 MG/KG     2,3,4,5           15 06/09/88  30        J8209
            Q12 HRS CONTINUOUS I.V. START @8 AM
            1.875 MG/KG   B6/C16            15 06/09/88  30        J8209
            Q12 HRS CONTINUOUS I.V., START @8 AM
    209B    7.5 MG/KG     3,5,7,9,           7 06/23/88  30        J8209
                          11;B23/Q7D
            I.V. @8 P.M.
    MPRD    0.25 MG/KG    10,11,12,13,14,   22 06/23/88  30        J8209
                          15,16
            I.V. Q12 HR
            0.5 MG/KG     B17/C30           22 06/23/88  30        J8209
            I.V Q12 HRS
            0.4 MG/KG     B31/C44           22 06/23/88  30        J8209
            I.V. Q12 H (OR MAY GIVE P.O.)
```

Figure 8.

The standing orders identify 10 different dose modification messages. The plan in Figure 7 lists three modification messages: AMPHOTERICIN, LIVER TOX 3, and RENAL TOX 3. The first is listed every day starting with the first day, and the other two are listed from days 7 through 44. After day 44 the modification messages LIVER TOX 4 and RENAL TOX 4 are listed. As shown in the plan, the count of these other listings is 0, and the date for last done still is blank.

The final section in this standing order page lists the therapy recommendations. The order 209AP (8209/CSA-P) is to be listed with a dose of 10 mg/kg

```
      JOHNS HOPKINS                        HISTORY NO:
      ONCOLOGY CENTER                            NAME: Patient 2
                                           PLAN DATE: 06/24/88
      DAILY CARE PLAN                                FRIDAY   PAGE 1


    16 Y.O. W M  LEUKEMIA, ACUTE MYEL - BMT        HT  182.0 CM  BSA 1.87 M2
         WEIGHTS:   ADMIN  71.6 KG   IDEAL  69.0 KG  CURRENT (06/21/88)  69.1 KG
  PROVIDERS :           MELISSA (PRIMARY NURSE)
                        BETH S. (ASSOCIATE NURSE)


  PROTOCOLS
     J8307                                     STARTED     DAY
     J7409   AUTOLOGOUS BMT/[4HC]/BM REMISS  05/06/88      50
     J7923   PHARMACOLOGY                    05/11/88      45
     J8638   AUTO/BMT-CY-BU                  05/11/88      45
             IMMUNOLOGIC MONITORING BMT      05/11/88      45
             A
     J8642   LATE TOX. FOLLOWING BMT         05/11/88      45
             CHILD
     J8809   CENTRAL IV LINES/BMT            05/12/88      44
             B
     BMT     SCHED BMT DAY                   05/20/88      35
             DAY 0-J7923(BU/CY)
```

```
TEST AND PROCEDURES:
  BLOOD AND SERUM TESTS
             HEMATOCRIT                WBC
             PLT CNT                   WBC DIFF
             RETIC CNT                 BLOOD CULT
             DIR COOMBS                TYP&HLDX48
             TYPE&HOLDA                SMA-12
             STAT M6                   AMA&SMMSAB
             ENA                       STAT PRO TIME
             STAT PTT                  ANTINUC AB
             S IMMUN EP                RHEUM FACT
             DNA ANTIBD
  PHYSICIAN PROCEDURES BONE MARROW BIOPSY MAY BE DONE PRN WHEN BONE MARROW
             ASPIRATE IS DONE CHEST X-RAY SHOULD BE SCHEDULED Q7 DAYS, OR AS
             CLINICALLY INDICATED.
  P.A. PROCEDURES
             BM MORPH                  BM CYTOGEN
          OBTAIN URINE SPECIMEN FOR URINALYSIS AND MICROSCOPIC EXAM
```

Figure 9.

from days 17 through 44 under treatment sequence J8209 (the ninth Johns Hopkins protocol to be defined in 1982). The order for MPRD (METHL PRED) is to be changed on day 31 from a dose of 0.5 mg/kg to one of 0.4 mg/kg. No other drugs are to be ordered. The standing orders provide for a message field to be printed on the daily care plan, but the message was felt to clutter the output and therefore is not printed in the final plan.

A second daily care plan is shown in Figure 9. This BMT patient is being treated with a different protocol, and there are five active treatment sequences.

Treatment sequence ID	Date started	Day number
3SGEN	05/09/88	46
BMTFOL3	05/20/88	35
BMTFOLC	05/11/88	44
CYR INF	05/14/88	41
MAR INF	05/20/88	35

```
                            ONCOLOGY INFORMATION SYSTEM
                             TREATMENT PLAN LISTING                06/23/88
Patient 2
ORDER                             SCHEDULE        CNT LST DONE DAY#           T.SQ. ID
-------------------------------------------------------------------------------------
URINE PROCEDURES
  UURC                            W                 7 06/22/88  46            3SGEN
                                  W                 6 06/22/88  44            BMT FOLC
  UPEP                            W                 7 06/22/88  46            3SGEN
                                  W                 6 06/22/88  44            BMT FOLC
  24RT                            W                 7 06/22/88  46            3SGEN
                                  W                 6 06/22/88  44            BMT FOLC
  URINE                           M                 7 06/20/88  46            3SGEN
                                  M                 6 06/20/88  44            BMT FOLC
P.A. PROCEDURES
  BMRH                            B15/Q7D/C36;B36/   3 06/17/88  35           BMT FOL3
                                  Q14D
  BMRY                            B15/Q7D/C36;B36/   3 06/17/88  35           BMT FOL3
                                  Q14D
  BMBX                            15,22,29           3 06/17/88  35           BMT FOL3
NURSING PROCEDURES
  ECG                             *1                 2 05/20/88  46           3SGEN
                                  1                  1 05/20/88  35           BMT FOL3
  SVUM                            *M,H              14 06/23/88  46           3SGEN
                                  *M,H              12 06/23/88  44           BMT FOLC
  SVCB                            *M,H              14 06/23/88  46           3SGEN
                                  *M,H              12 06/23/88  44           BMT FOLC
  SVCD                            *M                 7 06/20/88  46           3SGEN
                                  *M                 6 06/20/88  44           BMT FOLC
  SVCV                            *H                 7 06/23/88  46           3SGEN
                                  *H                 6 06/23/88  44           BMT FOLC
THERAPY
  MPRD     250 MG       1                            1 05/20/88  35           MAR INF
           I.V. ROUTE-AT BEDSIDE FOR PRN USE
  BENA     50 MG        1                            1 05/20/88  35           MAR INF
           I.V. ROUTE- AT BEDSIDE FOR PRN USE.
  PHNB     60 MG.           2,3,4,5                  4 05/18/88  41           CY4 INF
           M2 P.O. 1 HOUR PRIOR TO CYTOXAN
  THOR     10 MG.           2,3,4,5                  4 05/18/88  41           CY4 INF
           M2 I.V. 2 HOURS POST CYTOXAN AND PRN Q 6 HOURS


COMMENT
  LEVEL  0     (CRITICAL INFO)
     (5)   MAR INF3    1                             1 05/20/88  35           MAR INF
        DO NOT IRRADIATE NOR REFRIGERATE BONE MARROW
     (10)  MAR DRUGS   1                             1 05/20/88  35           MAR INF
        BENADRYL, EPINEPHERINE & SOLUMEDROL (OR SOLUCORTEF) MUST BE AT PT'S
        BEDSIDE DURING MARROW INFUSION
     (15)  EPINEPH     1                             1 05/20/88  35           MAR INF
        EPINEPHRINE 1:1000 1 ML

  LEVEL  1     (GENERAL COMMENTS)
     (1)   FURO 10-20      2,3,4,5                   4 05/18/88  41           CY4 INF
        FUROSEMIDE 10-20 MG/M2 I.V. 1&6 HR POST CYTX
     (40)  BMT FLUID1    B1/C6                       6 05/19/88  41           CY4 INF
        1000 ML D5 0.2 N.S. + 20 MEQ KCL  Q 4 HOURS
     (50)  PRN FURO      B2/C6                       5 05/19/88  41           CY4 INF
        FUROSEMIDE 10-20 MG/M2 I.V. PRN TO KEEP URINE OUTPUT AT 200 ML/HR
     (5)   MAR INF1    1                             1 05/20/88  35           MAR INF
```

Figure 10a.

As shown in the plan, there are seven active protocols. The BMT protocol is used for documentation only; it identifies the BMT day. Two protocols, J8638 and J8809, have multiple branches, and the letter identifies the protocol branch to which the patient has been assigned.

In this plan there are 19 blood and serum tests, two physician messages, and two P.A. procedures with one message. The segment of the standing orders shown in Figure 10 illustrates how the messages are organized. In this set of

```
                              ONCOLOGY INFORMATION SYSTEM
                                 TREATMENT PLAN LISTING
Patient 2                                                          06/23/88
ORDER
                          SCHEDULE         CNT LST DONE DAY#
                                                                   T.SQ. ID
-----------------------------------------------------------------------------
COMMENT
LEVEL  1     (GENERAL COMMENTS)
     MARROW SHOULD BE INFUSED I.V. WITHIN 4 HOURS OF ASPIRATION
  (10)  MAR INF2         1                  1 05/20/88  35
     SALINE INFUSION SET WITHOUT ANY IN-LINE FILTERS MUST BE EMPLOYED    MAR INF

LEVEL  2     (M.D. COMMENTS)
  (1)  BM BX PRN         B15/Q7D/C36;B36/   3 06/17/88  35
                         Q14D                                        BMT FOL3
     BONE MARROW BIOPSY MAY BE DONE PRN WHEN BONE MARROW ASPIRATE IS DONE
  (2)   CHEST XRAY       *Q7D               5 06/17/88  35           BMT FOL3
     CHEST X-RAY SHOULD BE SCHEDULED Q7 DAYS, OR AS CLINICALLY INDICATED.
  (3)  ABG               Q2W                3 06/17/88  35           BMT FOL3
     ABG SHOULD BE DONE Q2 WEEKS, OR AS CLINICALLY INDICATED.
  (4)  ABG BMT           1                  1 05/20/88  35           BMT FOL3
     IT ISN'T NECESSARY TO DRAW AN ART. BLOOD GAS ON DAY OF BMT IF ONE HAS
     PREVIOUSLY BEEN DRAWN.
  (5)  BMT ABG           5,7,9              3 05/19/88  44
     OBTAIN A BASELINE ARTERIAL BLOOD GAS PRIOR TO BMT               BMT FOLC
  (5)  MAR ABG           1                  1 05/20/88  35
     ABG PRIOR AND POST MARROW INFUSION                             MAR INF

LEVEL  3     (COORDINATOR)
  (5)  ABO INCOMP        B5/C14            10 05/24/88  44
     IF BMT RECIPIENT AND DONOR HAVE A MAJOR ABO INCOMPATIBILITY, START TX    BMT FOLC
     SEQUENCE "SEN3" ON DAY OF TRANSPLANT.
  (15)  BMT FOLC31       B1/C21            18 05/31/88  44
                                                                    BMT FOLC

LEVEL  5     (P.A. COMMENTS)
  (1)  MICRO U-A         Q7D                5 06/17/88  35
     OBTAIN URINE SPECIMEN FOR URINALYSIS AND MICROSCOPIC EXAM      BMT FOL3
  (20)  CY INF           2,3,4,5            4 05/18/88  41
     CYTOXAN IS DISSOLVED IN 250 ML D5W ADMINISTERED OVER 30-60 MINUTES    CY4 INF
  (30)  CY CARDIO        B2/C12            11 05/25/88  41          CY4 INF
     NON-SPECIFIC ST CHANGES ARE NOT UNUSUAL, BUT A DECREASE IN VOLTAGE IS
     SIGNIFICANT AND OMINOUS
  (5)  MAR ECG           1                  1 05/20/88  35
     ECG PRIOR AND POST MARROW INFUSION                             MAR INF
  (10)  MAR VS1          1                  1 05/20/88  35
     V.S. FLOWSHEET AT BEDSIDE                                      MAR INF
  (15)  MAR EQUIP        1                  1 05/20/88  35
     OXYGEN & SUCTION EQUIPMENT MUST BE SET UP IN PT'S ROOM         MAR INF
```

Figure 10b.

standing orders there are six levels of messages. Level 0 and the first of the Level 1 messages are on the first page of this standing order segment. Level 0 consists of critical information that is printed in a box at the top of the daily care plan. In this example all critical information is printed out only on day 1.

The plan in Figure 9 includes two physician messages (Level 2, M.D. comments). Each message in the standing orders is identified with a short mnemonic (BM BX PRN), and in this case the full message is printed below the status line.

```
BONE MARROW BIOPSY MAY BE DONE PRN WHEN BONE
MARROW ASPIRATE IS DONE
```

The number in parentheses to the left of the message indicates the order of the message relative to other messages of the same level when listed in a plan. The remainder of the comment order line is identical to that of the other standing order items.

```
       JOHN HOPKINS                       HISTORY NO:
       ONCOLOGY CENTER                        NAME: Patient 2
                                         PLAN DATE: 06/24/88
           PHYSICIAN ORDER GUIDE                  FRIDAY    PAGE 1


     16 Y.O. W M  LEUKEMIA, ACUTE MYEL - BMT      HT  182.0 CM  BSA 1.87 M2
          WEIGHTS:  ADMIN  71.6 KG   IDEAL  69.0 KG  CURRENT (06/21/88)  69.1 KG
   PROVIDERS :        MELISSA (PRIMARY NURSE)
                    BETH S. (ASSOCIATE NURSE)


                                              STARTED     DAY
     PROTOCOLS                                05/06/88    50
         J8307    AUTOLOGOUS BMT/[4HC]/BM REMISS 05/06/88   50
         J7409    PHARMACOLOGY                 05/11/88    45
         J7923    AUTO/BMT-CY-BU               05/11/88    45
         J8638    IMMUNOLOGIC MONITORING BMT   05/11/88    45
                  A
         J8642    LATE TOX. FOLLOWING BMT      05/11/88    45
                  CHILD
         J8809    CENTRAL IV LINES/BMT         05/12/88    44
                  B
         BMT      SCHED BMT DAY                05/20/88    35
                  DAY 0-J7923(BU/CY)


     BLOOD PROCEDURES
   :----------------------------------------------------------------------:
   :  TEST NAME        AMOUNT     TUBE         LAB        SLIP            :
   : HEMATOCRIT        3 CC       SM LAVEND(   ONC        ONCOLOGY        :
   : WBC                          SM LAVEND    ONC        ONCOLOGY        :
   : PLT CNT                      SM LAVEND    ONC        ONCOLOGY        :
   : WBC DIFF                     SM LAVEND    ONC        ONCOLOGY        :
   : RETIC CNT         3.00 CC    SM LAVEND    ONC        ONCOLOGY        :
   : BLOOD CULT                   BLOOD CULT   BACT       BACT           :
   : DIR COOMBS        3.00 CC    LAV          BLOOD BANK PT REQN,BLD BNK :
   : TYP&HLDX48        7 CC       YELLOW       BLOOD BANK BLOOD BANK      :
   :                  TYPE & HOLD X 48 HOURS                             :
   : TYPE&HOLDA        10 CC      1YELL+1LAV   BLOOD BANK BLOOD BANK      :
   :                  FOR PTS WITH ANTIBODIES;JUST CHECK T&H             :
   : SMA-12            7.00 CC    RED TOP      MAIN CHEM  BLD CHEM I      :
   : STAT M6           4.00 CC    SM RED       MAIN CHEM  EMERG CHEM      :
   :                  SEND STAT                                          :
   : AMA&SMMSAB        7.00 CC    RED TOP      GI         MISC           :
   : ENA               7.00 CC    RED TOP      BLAL 917   MISC           :
   : STAT PRO TIME     5.00 CC    BLUE         MAIN/PARK  EMERG COAG     :
   :                  NO ADD BLD NECESS IF FIBR IS DRAWN                 :
   : STAT PTT          5.00 CC    BLUE         AD SP HEM  EMERG COAG     :
   :                  NO ADD BLD NECESS IF FIBR IS DRAWN                 :
   : ANTINUC AB        7 CC       SM RED       DX IMMUNO  DX IMMUNO      :
   : S IMMUN EP        10 CC      LG RED       DX IMMUNO  DX IMMUNO      :
   :                  CHECK "IMMUNOGLOBULIN SURVEY" ON SLIP             :
   : RHEUM FACT        7 CC       SM RED       DX IMMUNO  DX IMMUNO      :
   :                  RHEUM FACTOR (RF SCREEN)                          :
   : DNA ANTIBD        1 CC       YELLOW       916 BLALOC MISC          :
   :                  1 CC IN YELLOW TOP TO DR. EVAN FARMER            :
   :----------------------------------------------------------------------:
```

Figure 11a.

In this set of standing orders, the P.A. procedure for the bone marrow biopsy (BMBX) is recommended on days 15, 22, and 29. The other two bone marrow procedures (BMRH and BMRY) are ordered every 7 days from days 15 to 36 and every 14 days thereafter. This is the same schedule for the preceding physician reminder. The result is that the suggestion that a bone marrow biopsy be ordered PRN will be printed on the same day that the marrow aspirate is to be done.

The M.D. comment, CHEST XRAY, suggests that a chest x-ray be ordered every 7 days or as clinically indicated. If there was no order in at least 7 days, then

```
      JOHN HOPKINS                          HISTORY NO:
      ONCOLOGY CENTER                         NAME: Patient 2
                                       PLAN DATE: 06/24/88
      PHYSICIAN ORDER GUIDE                          FRIDAY      PAGE 2


  BLOOD PROCEDURES
: -----------------------------------------------------------------------:
:  TEST NAME              AMOUNT    TUBE      LAB        SLIP             :
: -----------------------------------------------------------------------:
:                                                                        :
: -----------------------------------------------------------------------:
:                                                                        :
: -----------------------------------------------------------------------:
TOTAL BLOOD TO BE DRAWN:   86CC

  URINE PROCEDURES
: -----------------------------------------------------------------------:
:   TEST NAME                     CONTAINER   LAB        SLIP            :
: -----------------------------------------------------------------------:
:                                                                        :
: -----------------------------------------------------------------------:
:                                                                        :
: -----------------------------------------------------------------------:

  RADIOLOGY PROCEDURES
: -----------------------------------------------------------------------:
:   TEST NAME                                LAB        SLIP            :
: -----------------------------------------------------------------------:
:                                                                        :
: -----------------------------------------------------------------------:
:                                                                        :
: -----------------------------------------------------------------------:

  OTHER TESTS AND PROCEDURES
: -----------------------------------------------------------------------:
:   TEST NAME                     TUBE/CONT   LAB        SLIP            :
:  BM MORPH                                   ONC        MISC           :
:                       BONE MARROW ASPIRATE FOR MORPHOLOGY             :
:  BM CYTOGEN                                 ONC 3-130  SPEC "3S"      :
:                       BONE MARROW FOR CYTOGENETICS                    :
: -----------------------------------------------------------------------:
:                                                                        :
: -----------------------------------------------------------------------:
:                                                                        :
: -----------------------------------------------------------------------:


--------------------       --------------------     ------------------------------
PHLEBOTOMIST               UNIT CLERK               PHYSICIAN
```

Figure 11b.

the message is printed. If the chest x-ray is not ordered when recommended, then the message will be repeated until one is ordered. On the other hand, if the chest x-ray was clinically indicated before the end of the 7-day cycle, then the fact that it was ordered will be entered into the standing orders during the verification process. The next reminder will always be printed 7 days after the last order.

Figure 11 contains the information in Figure 9 in the form of an order guide. This is delivered to the unit clerk for the preparation of the necessary laboratory

Table 3. Number of Inpatients on Protocol*

Unit	Beds	Patients	1985	1986	1987
2 North	14	Solid tumor	103	132	126
2 South	14	Leukemia	108	76	75
3 North	22	Solid tumor	107	168	149
3 South	20	BMT	119	149	143
Peds	14	Pediatric	85	119	118
Total	84		522	644	611

*Note that the table represents the number of patients admitted to an inpatient unit who were actively on a protocol. Readmissions of the same patient are not counted. Some of the numbers have been adjusted to account for administrative changes in the unit's size and use. The relative stability since 1987 reflects the fact that, owing to the nursing shortage, fewer patients are being admitted.

slips. As shown on the first page, the test name, the amount of blood to be drawn, the tube to be used, the laboratory to which the specimen is to be sent, and the requisition slip to be used are all specified. This is followed by spaces in which additional orders may be written. At the bottom of the blood procedures section, the order guide totals the amount of blood to be drawn, in this case 86 cc.

The second page contains space for urine and radiology procedures. The P.A. procedures are listed in the final section. At the bottom are places for the physician to indicate that these tests and procedures are to be ordered, for the unit clerk to indicate that the forms have been filled out, and for the phlebotomist to indicate that the blood has been drawn.

The signed order guide is used by the clinical data coordinator to update the patients' standing orders. The OCIS maintains a verification list of all the tests and procedures that were included in the current daily care plan. Recommended tests and procedures not ordered or carried out are deleted from the list; added tests and procedures are appended to it. Once the list is correct, the plan is marked as verified, and the count and last-date-done fields of the standing orders are updated.

Evaluation

From the examples in the previous section, it is clear that the protocol-directed-care plan function of the OCIS provides useful support in the clinical management of patients treated with very complex therapies. Obviously, these therapies are used in other cancer institutions, and one cannot make the claim that an automated system is a necessary tool for these therapeutic modalities. Nevertheless, we believe that protocol-directed care enables the Oncology Center to provide aggressive therapy in a safe and controlled environment in a relatively cost-effective manner. This is only an assertion. To demonstrate this as a fact, one would have to perform a multicenter study that compared therapeutic

Table 4. Distribution of Tests Ordered during One Week in 1987

Unit	Patients	Number of Tests Ordered	
		Automated (Plans)	Written in
2 North	14	16	230
2 South	10	337	13
3 North	15	854	130
3 South	5	2652	13

regimens, operating costs, and outcomes. Because this has not been done, our evaluation is subjective.

First we observe that the system has been in daily use since 1982 and is paid for out of patient care revenues. Thus, the clinical staff and hospital administration perceive it to be useful. In the previous sections we have described how some of the original system features were abandoned and how less sophisticated tools were added. This also implies that the system has adapted to meet the needs of its users. However, it must be observed that the demand for the daily care plans is limited. Several sophisticated features of the software were left to ossify; the outpatient plans were never tested. Consequently, one may conclude that, although the tools are used routinely, there is no predisposition to rely on automated reminders.

There are some characterizing metrics that suggest the extent of the system's use. Table 3 shows the number of patients on protocol for five units. Table 4 summarizes the protocol-directed activity during one week in 1987. In the BMT and leukemia units, the care plans are used to manage most of the therapy. Few changes are made. However, in units where there is little reliance upon the protocol system, more orders must be entered manually. Of course, the units treat patients with very different types of diseases, and no comparisons among units would be valid. The table does make the point, however, that where the daily care plans are appropriate, they can be made to be complete.

What lessons does the OCIS experience offer to others who would like to formalize their therapy plans and automate part of the management of patient care? First, it must be recognized that there is a broad spectrum of protocol complexity. At the least complex level are actions such as the drug–drug interaction warnings, the Regenstrief therapy reminders, and the HELP alerts. These are highly modular and independent, each requires some physician feedback, and they are used only in exceptional situations. Studies have shown that these tools alter the physicians' actions, but they do so in the context of feedback within the standard medical decision-making process.

The OCIS inpatient protocol system, as implemented for the BMT and leukemia units, is an example of a closed approach to an automated patient management system. The full set of therapy plans must be defined for all therapeutic situations, and the system must be able to prepare complete plans every day for every clinical situation. For complex treatment modalities, as practiced in units in which the plans are relied upon, there is a major benefit in using the plans. Compliance with the protocol is ensured, training and orientation of the rotating house staff is facilitated, documentation is created automatically, and the management of many different patients using essentially the same treatment regimens is controlled. The major cost for this type of system is the heavy investment in preparing the treatment plans. Where plans are used often and over an extended period of time, the preparation cost is justified.

It is the middle level of treatment planning that has the least automation and, perhaps, the greatest need. In the case of the OCIS, the treatment plans are not used in units that treat patients with many different protocols. The cost of preparing the plans does not seem to be justified. Perhaps, if the treatment plans could be produced as a by-product of the protocol definition process, then more plans would be documented and there would be more of an incentive to use the system. Alternatively, if new reporting requirements, say for FDA or NCI, were identified and the protocol system could satisfy them easily, then the system might be perceived to be a labor-saving tool, as well as a patient management aid. Finally, if some centerwide therapeutic objectives could be formulated, then these could be independently supported by the care plan system. (In fact, this has been done with the ordering of all inpatient blood tests.)

In conclusion, this chapter demonstrates that, if an organization knows what it wants to do in specific clinical situations, it is possible to use automation to guide the process. For a set of independent actions, there are ways of producing alerts or reminders to warn of potential problems. In complex therapeutic situations it is possible to offer a daily plan based on predefined rules. These automated systems can be defined as algorithms, or they may use inference mechanisms with various degrees of complexity. Limitations to success are the tool's acceptance by the providers as a useful adjunct, the availability of broadly accepted decisions regarding what actions are appropriate in given situations, and the ease with which this knowledge can be maintained and the tool can be used. The OCIS experience illustrates that automation and the writing of computer programs are not limiting factors, except as they are affected by these constraints.

6
Pharmacy System

Patricia M. Harwood, Jean P. Causey,
and Suanne Goldberger[1]

Introduction

The Oncology Center Pharmacy operates as a satellite of the Johns Hopkins Hospital Department of Pharmacy, serving only Oncology Center patients. As part of its basic charter, the Oncology Center Pharmacy supports the clinical and research functions of the Center, as well as providing traditional pharmacy distributive functions.

Operationally, the Oncology Center Pharmacy distinguishes among three groups of patients; inpatients, outpatients receiving medications within the clinic setting (typically, chemotherapy and investigational drugs); and outpatients presenting prescriptions for take-home medications. The inpatient service includes preparation and dispensing of all inpatient medications for a 70-bed facility, and involves approximately 300 new orders and 1450 dispensed doses per day. The in-clinic outpatient service generates approximately 45 new orders and 55 dispensed doses per day. The outpatient prescription service processes approximately 60 prescriptions per day. The inpatient and the in-clinic outpatient operations are supported by the OCIS pharmacy system, which is the subject of this chapter. The outpatient prescription operation is supported by a stand-alone system not yet interfaced with the OCIS. Pediatric oncology patients are housed on the Pediatrics Units, and are served by a pediatrics satellite pharmacy, which does not participate in the OCIS pharmacy system.

[1]Patricia M. Harwood, Pharm. D., was formerly a Research Associate at The Johns Hopkins University School of Medicine, Assistant Director of The Pharmacy at The Johns Hopkins Hospital, and Director of Pharmacy at The Johns Hopkins Oncology Center.

Jean P. Causey was formerly an analyst for the Oncology Clinical Information Systems and is presently Manager of Systems and Development at the Laboratory Medicine Information Systems at The Johns Hopkins Hospital.

Suanne Goldberger was formerly a senior pharmacist at The Johns Hopkins Oncology Center Pharmacy.

All automated inpatient pharmacy systems provide functions for dose delivery and patient billing. They differ in the flexibility and sophistication of their ordering, display, and delivery functions, and in the facilities offered for administrative reporting. Clinical interfaces between pharmacy and other systems, where they exist, tend to be limited and cumbersome additions.

In relation to the "typical" pharmacy system, the OCIS pharmacy system is "unit dose" based and controls the dispensing of individually packaged and labeled doses on a 4-hour delivery cycle. It provides a full range of ordering and display functions. It supports all dosage forms, including intravenous (IV) admixtures, chemotherapy, and total parenteral nutrition, with broad flexibility in dose definition and scheduling. Finally, it offers a reasonable set of administrative tools. But the true distinction of the OCIS pharmacy system lies in its integration within the OCIS. This integration allows all subsystems to share data effectively for pharmacy, clinical, and research purposes.

From the perspective of the pharmacist, the OCIS pharmacy system is an effective tool for order-entry and unit-dose dispensing. It also provides special access to clinical information, such as patient body surface area and treatment protocol, which assists in quality control. From the perspective of the clinician, the OCIS pharmacy system is an effective source of clinically significant data and also assists in ensuring compliance with specific protocols in clinical research. This successful range of uses is the result of a system-development approach that acknowledged both the business and clinical aspects of the pharmacy's role.

Historical Background

During the initial development of the OCIS, the Oncology Pharmacy was one of three satellite pharmacies using a unit-dose computer system developed in-house for the Central Pharmacy in the early 1970s and run on an IBM mainframe.[2] During the early OCIS operations, pharmacy data were captured manually. Later, IBM programs were developed for automated extraction and posting of inpatient data from the pharmacy system to the OCIS system. This effort was successful, but fraught with frustrations, some of which are discussed below.

When it was announced that the IBM pharmacy system was to be withdrawn pending design of a new centralized pharmacy system, the OCIS and the oncology pharmacy satellite saw an opportunity to develop their own system. This new system would provide improved functionality to the pharmacy, while at the same time participating directly in the integrated OCIS project. In addition to the pharmacy dose-delivery tools, report, and displays, the new system would provide for dose acknowledgment and the accurate transfer of dosage data to the OCIS data-

---

[2]For a contemporary examination of this system see D. W. Simborg and H. J. Derewicz, A Highly Automated Hospital Medication System: Five Years Experience and Evaluations, *Annals of Internal Medicine*, 83: 342–345,1975.

base for inclusion in flow-sheet displays and in case management logic. It would further support the pharmacy by providing access to OCIS patient data, such as body surface area, protocols, and cumulative dosages. The nature of an oncology unit presents unique responsibilities to the pharmacy service and demands a special level of communication between the Pharmacy and the clinical staff. The expectation that the new system would actively support such team effort in clinical care provided the level of user motivation necessary to support the more demanding development effort involved in this integrated approach.

What follows is a more detailed history of the OCIS pharmacy system development, a description of basic system functionality and its special clinical features, a detailed discussion of the interfaces to other OCIS subsystems and Hospital systems, and notes on system effectiveness, limitations, and future plans.

The Original IBM System Interface

The original computer system used by the oncology pharmacy had been developed several years earlier by the Hospital's central information systems groups. That system used IBM 3278 screen terminals to provide basic drug-ordering functionality. It produced unit-dose dispensing envelopes, daily printed patient order profiles, and printed discharge summaries and created daily files of billing transactions for the Hospital's inpatient billing system. The system served only inpatients and shared a patient database with the inpatient admissions–discharge–transfer (ADT) system. The system ran on IBM mainframe machines (360 and 370 OS/MVS architecture). It had been the first of Johns Hopkins interactive applications. At the time of its development, the language tools available had been "macro" CICS and ALC. Database efficiency depended on creative, logically designed direct-access file structures. As a result of this design history, access to pharmacy clinical data was difficult. Access was frequently complicated by the dose-delivery bias of the system and by the Pharmacy's creative procedural solutions to limitations in the overall system's flexibility. Technically, access was limited by the requirement of relatively specialized programming skills. Politically, and justifiably, access was guarded by an organization responsible for security, stability, and production support and suspicious of "outside" efforts.

When the OCIS went into production mode in 1979, the sources of medication data were the printed inpatient medication profiles and the outpatient clinic notes. Data from these sources were manually extracted and entered by clinical data coordinators in the Oncology Center. Because of the labor involved in this form of data collection, only a limited set of drugs was targeted for collection. Because the manual effort required name recognition of targeted drugs and unit conversions of ordered dosages, data accuracy was difficult to achieve.

The first attempt at automation of data acquisition involved daily extraction of data from the IBM-based pharmacy system. This procedure included OCIS-written data extraction programs for IBM execution, an IBM job to write extracted data to tape, and OCIS in-house programs, dictionaries, and procedures to receive and process the tape. It also involved some elaborate rules and procedures for data coordinator review of the data posting and for resolution of problems. There were numerous technical and procedural problems associated with this approach to providing synchronous data between these two unique systems.

The Oncology data extraction project was granted "guest" status on the IBM mainframe, and it functioned in a reactive mode with respect to the mainframe pharmacy system. Technical information was difficult to acquire, as was advance notice of software changes. IBM program library entries were in constant danger of "cleanup" by IBM maintenance staff who were unaware of the project's legitimacy.

The development of this automated data capture involved retrofitting a data collection function onto a traditional pharmacy system in which the design of the database and of the formulary maintenance function had favored dose delivery and billing, and did not offer a clinical view of the dose data. A second development problem was the result of the use of incompatible dictionaries. Whereas the OCIS collects clinical data under mnemonic shorthand codes (e.g., PENV for penicillin-V), the pharmacy drug formulary used generic names, with modifiers for special forms, augmented by free-text drug name entry for nonformulary items and for IV admixtures. It was therefore necessary for the OCIS routines to recognize and transform that assortment of pharmacy names into the appropriate OCIS codes. Additionally, the OCIS standardizes all data values for the same item to a common unit; but the pharmacy formulary (especially the IV-admixture free-text field) presented the whole range of dosage units, including some creative ones such as "POP" (popsicle) and "HG" (a keying error intended as "MG"). It was therefore necessary for the OCIS routines to decipher and convert all units to the OCIS standards.

Intravenous admixtures posed special problems to this development effort. Because the IBM-based pharmacy system lacked any special provision for such orders, the Pharmacy was using the defined-order fields to record the IV vehicle (e.g., D5W 1000ml) and an available free-text field for entry of all remaining admixture details. This situation presented the OCIS routines with both misspellings and alternative spellings of drug names. It also presented the problem of recognizing sets of drug/dose/units text from within the free-text paragraph. This sort of problem was a "natural" for the OCIS programming language (MUMPS) using key words and character patterns for data recognition, but it still represented a significant chance for missed or misinterpreted data.

There also were questions about the internal handling of some issues ("Is the dose-not-given marker for a midnight dose recorded in the twenty-fourth marker of day 0, or in the zeroth marker of day 1?") which were never answered satisfactorily. Also, although the pharmacy system provided for negative dose acknowledgment, such entries were made by the Pharmacy on the basis of materials returned from the floors and were generally recognized to be incomplete.

Staffing and procedural issues also posed problems. Maintenance of the data extraction program and jobs on the IBM mainframe required technical skills not otherwise in use in the OCIS programming group. And, given the complex set of transformations required to map the IBM pharmacy data to the OCIS system, the daily posting run at the OCIS included a problem case report, which required data coordinator resolution.

The positive result of this interface effort was a data collection system that removed a significant burden from the data coordinators, allowed a dramatic expansion of the list of collected drugs, increased the reliability of the data, and was operationally successful, but which still required significant human tending and had potentially serious limitations due to the OCIS status as "tolerated guest" with respect to the central pharmacy system. This experience is probably typical of efforts to support dual databases between dissimilar systems on heterogeneous equipment.

The OCIS System Decision and Development

In mid-1981, the Hospital's Information Systems Department, which was responsible for the existing IBM pharmacy system, declared its intention of withdrawing that system pending design and creation of a new and improved hospital-wide pharmacy system. For the Oncology Pharmacy, this action would have meant reversion from automated unit-dose functioning to a manual cart-delivery system, with total loss of capacity for automated clinical data extraction. The Oncology Pharmacy and clinical unit staff were insistent that they could not function under such a system. Therefore, seeing an opportunity for tightly integrating the oncology clinical and pharmacy needs, the OCIS offered to develop a replacement system for the Oncology Pharmacy. The resulting OCIS-integrated pharmacy system was installed in late 1982, providing both enhanced pharmacy functionality (IV, hyperalimentation, improved profile review, active allergy checking, etc.) and direct data coupling with the OCIS clinical database. The rapid development and installation process (a total of 1.5 man-years of analyst time) was made possible by the MUMPS development environment, the experience level (in both pharmacy and OCIS systems) of the primary analyst, and the fact that an existing system was serving as a design baseline.

There were significant development and start-up problems. Procedural and style differences between the old and new systems made it nearly impossible to verify the results of parallel testing. Moreover, because the oncology pharmacy was participating in development of a local system, there was limited support from the Central Pharmacy administration, especially in the staff-intensive effort of parallel testing. These conditions contributed to a high intensity level in the preparation for production installation, but did not finally compromise the system.

There was no full-load capacity testing of the new system prior to installation. Initial installation was done on a Saturday; Sunday operations were smooth; Monday revealed nearly disastrous problems with on-line response time. This situation was eventually corrected by adjustments in the software to shift to background processing much of the intensive database activity that accompanies verification of a new order.

It was several weeks after installation before the new production job load was settled into a steady operations schedule. The pharmacy system was the first of the OCIS subsystems to require critical production work on the night shift, and night staff adjustment to the new level of responsibility required some unanticipated coaching. Again, production volume performance issues required careful scheduling adjustments.

Finally, it is worth noting that because the pharmacy system had been developed by a single analyst (a situation made possible by the MUMPS development environment), the on-call support "team" for the critical first weeks of this 24-hour system consisted of that one analyst—a point of vulnerability not adequately appreciated beforehand. Nevertheless, the initial transition to the new system was accomplished as planned, over one weekend. The system was basically stable from the start. It was performing acceptably within several weeks, and production supports and utilities, such as archiving, were in place within several months. This experience serves as a testament to the MUMPS development environment and the modular manner in which applications can be implemented.

Major Extensions

Significant system enhancements installed over the intervening five years have included antibiotic monitoring, interface to a pain management dose equivalency function, entry and review of patient protocols, automation of the cumulative chemotherapy record, and extension of the system (originally only inpatient) to include the in-clinic outpatient orders.

The extension of the system to handle in-clinic Outpatient Department (OPD) orders (primarily chemotherapy and study drugs) was a natural development. These orders normally are handled by the "inpatient side" of the pharmacy operation and share the same inventory. The extension required a special OPD perspective on dose scheduling, a separate daily "fill list," and a special interface to the OCIS Outpatient Clinic billing function.

An independent stand-alone outpatient prescription system was purchased in 1984. The decision to purchase outpatient software, rather than to attempt extension of the inpatient system, was based on several factors. The labeling, record-keeping, and cash box functions required in an outpatient prescription system suggested the need for a new, tailored system for which programming resources were not available. Meanwhile, there were affordable, off-the-shelf, fully functional prescription systems available from several vendors. Furthermore, since the outpatient prescription service is optional, the system supporting that service cannot function as the primary source for capture of outpatient medication data. Finally, the stand-alone system's lack of an automated interface to OCIS for patient identification and registration was seen as only a minor nuisance in the relatively closed population of patients being served by the system (although such an interface continues to be a long-term goal).

As OCIS began work on the pharmacy system, there was some expectation that a successful product would catch the attention of the central administration and be considered for full hospital extension. Unfortunately, since the OCIS pharmacy system was developed using a little-recognized language in a minicomputer environment, it was never considered seriously in the IBM mainframe environment outside of the Oncology Center. As a result, the Hospital had made other pharmacy commitments by the time the oncology system was successfully installed. The Hospital's new pharmacy system (cart replacement on mainframe-based software) was installed on a limited basis one year after the oncology pharmacy system. Within another 18 months, that system has been extended to all nononcology units and had incorporated full IV and parenteral nutrition functionality. But it still lacked tools for data extraction.

The Central Pharmacy–Oncology Pharmacy

As would be expected, there have been some points of uneasiness between the oncology satellite pharmacy and the Central Pharmacy administration over the use of an independent system. Once the Central Pharmacy had installed its own new system, there was a concern over the lack of consolidated departmental statistics. This concern was answered by the provision for tape transfer of such administrative data from the oncology system to the central system.

On another occasion, it was requested by central pharmacy administration that the oncology system remove the menu transaction that allowed the Oncology Pharmacy Director to update the billing algorithm without programmer intervention, on the grounds that the central system did require programmer intervention for such an adjustment. This request was successfully resisted by the Oncology Pharmacy Director.

Central Pharmacy administration regularly voices concern over staff training for the unusual oncology environment, but these concerns are related less to the differences in the user/computer interface than to the more basic differences in procedures and services.

It is frequently suggested that the central pharmacy system, having developed full pharmacy functionality, could now be substituted for the OCIS pharmacy system within the oncology satellite. Such a change would require the Oncology Center to accept a 24-hour cart replacement dose delivery system – an adjustment that has so far been resisted by the clinical units. However, the larger obstacle to system consolidation is the fact that stand-alone "full pharmacy functionality" is no longer sufficient within the Oncology Center environment. The benefits of system integration have become an essential part of the oncology pharmacy's functionality. Similarly, the benefits of access to pharmacy data have become essential to other components of the OCIS.

System Flow Walk-Through

The OCIS pharmacy computer system was developed to support the unique distribution system in the Oncology Center, as well as to provide critical drug data elements for clinical decisions. It is based on a 4-hour medication exchange cycle utilizing unit-dose envelopes, rather than the more typical 24-hour medication exchange cycle utilizing cassette drawers.

As with most pharmacy computerized systems, initial entry is triggered by a new medication order. The pharmacist evaluates the medication order and interactively enters the order into the computer system, responding to prompts for all necessary order information, such as medication and formulation selection and dose scheduling. The order-entry header includes relevant patient data, such as body surface area, allergies, diagnosis, and protocols, used in evaluation of the order. And the computer performs appropriate checks for such things as patient allergies and single doses exceeding a predetermined limit.

At the time of order entry, patient-specific single-dose envelopes or labels are printed for each STAT (immediately needed) dose or for any scheduled dose to be administered within a 20-hour future time frame. (A description of the system outputs is presented in the next section.) Orders for controlled substances (which are stored on the nursing units) do not generate an envelope or label print. Orders for a PRN (as needed) medication generate one envelope or label print, with subsequent doses generated only upon on-line request by Nursing or Pharmacy. As a quality control check, a removal notice is printed for each discontinued PRN order and for each scheduled dose to be removed from already printed fill lists.

Future scheduled doses beyond the 20-hour time frame are printed in 4-hour fill list batches (envelopes and labels) for predetermined time intervals. The batch generation process is initiated automatically, but envelope and label printing are controlled by the Pharmacy. Each envelope and label includes full order details, allowing easy pharmacy fill. Fill lists are ordered by unit, time, and patient.

Pharmacy fill list doses are filled and checked by pharmacy technicians or pharmacists before temporary pharmacy storage. Approximately two hours prior to delivery time, fill lists are checked against a batch control report to verify that all required doses are present and that all discontinued doses have been removed. Doses are then delivered to the nursing units by a pharmacy technician.

As with all medication systems, nursing verification of dose accuracy is an important step. This step is simplified because each dose is individually labeled with all pertinent patient- and drug-related information. Dose administration documentation is recorded by nurses on the medication administration record (MAR) provided by the system. Scheduled doses not administered and discontinued medications are returned to the Pharmacy.

If a PRN dose or a "starter dose" (a pharmacy item stocked on the nursing unit in limited supply for likely immediate need) is used on the floor, the nurse may use the computer to request a refill. In this case, the required envelope or label will automatically print in the Pharmacy for next-delivery fill.

On the day after each MAR use, OCIS data coordinators review the MARs for drug administration edits. Data coordinator entry of scheduled doses not given and of PRN doses given automatically adjusts the recorded drug dose in the clinical database and the patient billing record, as appropriate.

PHARMACY ENVELOPE

DEPARTMENT OF PHARMACY SERVICE
THE JOHNS HOPKINS HOSPITAL-BALTIMORE, MARYLAND

CHECK'D.
BY_____

SAMPLE, PATIENT (1111111)   2S   DOSE: 04/21/88 1000A

0032A PREDNISONE

    62.5MG   DISPENSED AS 1.25 X (50MG TAB) PO

    BID   (125 MG/DAY TOTAL DOSE)   AT: 10A 10P

    NOTE: J8802

002

☐ MEDICATION ON NURSING UNIT

RETURN ENVELOPE TO PHARMACY FOR THE FOLLOWING REASONS:

☐ (1) THIS IS A STARTER DOSE   PT'S. NAME _____
    ATTACH COPY OF ORDER SHEET   ORDER #_____TIME DOSE GIVEN:_____
☐ (2) THIS IS A "PRN" DOSE
☐ (3) THIS IS AN "ON CALL" DOSE   TIME DOSE GIVEN: _____
☐ (4) A REPLACEMENT SUPPLY IS NECESSARY
☐ (5) IF THE DOSE WAS NOT GIVEN, CHECK THE REASON BELOW:

    ☐ ORDER D/C'D BY M.D.   ☐ PATIENT ABSENT FROM FLOOR
    ☐ PATIENT REFUSED DOSE   ☐ PATIENT VOMITED DOSE
    ☐ PATIENT NPO   ☐ PATIENT DISCHARGED
    ☐ PATIENT TO O.R. - ALL ORDERS D/C'D.

    ☐ OTHER - PLEASE SPECIFY_____

    ☐ IV FLUID D/C'D: APPROX._____ ML INFUSED

ES600000093   JHH-27-020X REV. 1/77

Figure 1. Pharmacy envelope.

The order-processing flow described above is supported by an array of background tasks and maintenance functions involving the OCIS operations staff, the Pharmacy, and others. OCIS operations initiate the daily batch processing, which produces reports such as the nursing MAR and the hard-copy profiles, the inpatient billing tape, and the discharge summaries and archive tapes, as well as the daily update of the OCIS patient database with medication data. The Pharmacy has the responsibility and the necessary tools for maintenance of the dictionaries, from frequency code definition, to charging algorithm, to drug-stocking formulary. The data coordinators have the responsibility for maintaining the inpatient census and the Pharmacy/OCIS dictionary linkages, and for entering dose administration information from the MAR. Both the Pharmacy and the Nursing Units have the necessary tools for printing and displaying alternative views of the patient medication profiles, and for generating refill envelopes and labels.

PHARMACY LABEL

```
DEPARTMENT OF PHARMACY SERVICE
THE JOHNS HOPKINS HOSPITAL

     SAMPLE, PATIENT    (1111111)        2S  04/21/88 0100P
     0094A  GENTAMICIN
     140MG/3.5ML  =  3.5ML X  ( 40MG/1ML INJ )  IV MNB
     IN D5W    50ML                               EXP: 24HR
     Q6H
     TIME CHANGED
     LS600000054                                        005
```

Figure 2. Pharmacy label.

Outputs Related to Dose Delivery

The pharmacy system prints a large number of outputs and reports. Those related to the dose delivery functions include:

Envelopes. Special-stock unit-dose envelopes are printed for all required doses other than small or large volume parenterals (Figure 1). Full order detail, dose time, and patient identifier information is printed. Printing is done in the Pharmacy. Single envelopes are printed immediately in response to order-entry transactions or special requests. Fill list batches are printed at approximately 4-hour intervals approximately 20 hours prior to administration time (with the long lead time allowed to prevent shortage situations should a prolonged down time occur).

Labels. Small and large volume parenteral labels are printed for each dose required (Figure 2). Scheduling of print and handling of labels are essentially identical to the same procedures for envelopes.

Batch Control Lists. Batch control lists are printed lists, organized by floor, of all future scheduled doses within the specified 4-hour batch time (Figure 3). They are requested by the Pharmacy and printed in the Pharmacy approximately 2 hours before delivery of doses to the floor. Envelopes and labels are listed separately in 1-hour segments, with discontinued doses so marked. This listing is the final quality control point used by the Pharmacy to verify the contents of the 4-hour batched doses.

Discontinued Order Notices. Discontinued medication orders are printed automatically in the Pharmacy, prompting removal of prepared doses from the dose fill lists and eliminating preparation of future doses. One notice is printed per dose and includes sufficient detail to locate the discontinued medications.

BATCH CONTROL LIST

BATCH-CONTROL		ENVELOPES		3S		08/10/88 05A		
	TIME	PATIENT		ORD	MED	DOSE	RP	DISP
1	0500A	PATIENT, ONE (1111111)		0234A	TICARCILL	VOL	1GRAM	
2	0500A	PATIENT, NINE(9999999)		0140B	TICARCILL	VOL	1.4GRA	
3	0500A	PATIENT, SIX (6666666)		0330A	TICARCILL	VOL	3GRAM	
4	0500A	PATIENT, FOUR(4444444)		0455A	AMIKACIN	VOL	650MG	

BATCH-CONTROL		LABELS	3S			08/10/88 05A		
	TIME	PATIENT		ORD	MED	DOSE	RP	DISP
1	0500A	PATIENT, TWO (2222222)		0143B	MICONAZOL	MNB	130MG	
2	0500A	PATIENT, FIVE(5555555)		0332A	VANCOMYCI	MNB	500MG	
3	0500A	PATIENT, ONE (1111111)		0085A	VANCOMYCI	MNB	500MG	
4	0500A	PATIENT, THREE(333333)		0485A	CO-TRIMOX	MNB	360MG	

Figure 3. Batch control list.

Floor Discharge Notices. The Pharmacy automatically receives computer-printed notification of patient discharges as they are entered by data coordinators on the units. This notification alerts the Pharmacy to the need to discontinue all medication orders (referred to as a pharmacy discharge) after verification that the patient has indeed left the nursing unit. Discontinued medication notices are printed as a result of this pharmacy discharge. This action synchronizes pharmacy orders with the inpatient census and also provides a secondary check on patient discharges.

Patient Profile Outputs

In addition to managing the preparation and distribution of the drug doses, the pharmacy system must maintain drug profiles for every patient treated at the Oncology Center. A variety of profile formats are available:

Full Current Profile. A full current profile is a printed or screen listing of recently expired, current, and future orders, including, for each order, full detail and projected dose administration schedule (Figure 4). A daily printout of all patient profiles serves as the backup reference document for the Pharmacy and the Nursing Units.

Abbreviated Profile. An abbreviated profile is a screen or printed listing of

```
OCIS PHARMACY MEDICATION PROFILE    3S  PATIENT,FOUR (7778884)
FOR 05/11/88
HT: 185.0 CM    WT: 71.6 KG        BSA: 1.92 CM2      AGE:15  RACE:W  SEX:M
DIAG: LEUKEMIA, ACUTE MYEL - BMT   PROT: J8307 (05/06/88)  AUTOLOGOUS BMT/[4HC
                                         J7409 (05/11/88)  PHARMACOLOGY
                                         J7923 (05/11/88)  AUTO/BMT-CY-BU
                                         J8638 (05/11/88)  IMMUNOLOGIC MONITOR
                                         J8642 (05/11/88)  LATE TOX. FOLLOWING
------------------------------------------------------------------------------
0015A CO-TRIMOXAZOLE DOUBLE STRENGTH                  START: 05/09/88 1000A
      ORDERED AS: SEPTRA-DS

      160MG   DISPENSED AS   ( 160MG TAB )   PO

      QDW ( MON TUE WED )   AT:  10A

      DOSES FOR 05/11:  10A
------------------------------------------------------------------------------
0024A MORPHINE                                        START: 05/10/88 0314A
                                                      END:   05/10/88 0829A
 D/C
      6MG/.6ML   DISPENSED AS  .6ML X  ( 10MG/1ML INJ )   IM   / MONU

      ON-CALL                                         FOR 1 DOSES
                                                      EXP:   24HR

      DOSES GIVEN  (MOST RECENT DAY) -
      05/09/88 0630A
------------------------------------------------------------------------------
0024B MIDAZOLAM                                       START: 05/10/88 0314A
      ORDERED AS: VERSED                              END:   05/10/88 0830A
 D/C
      2MG/.4ML   DISPENSED AS  .4ML X  ( 5MG/ML INJ )   IM   / MONU

      ON-CALL                                         FOR 1 DOSES
                                                      EXP:   24HR

      DOSES GIVEN  (MOST RECENT DAY) -
      05/09/88 0630A
------------------------------------------------------------------------------
0046A TYLOX                                           START: 05/09/88 0303P
                                                      END:   05/12/88 0302P

      1    DISPENSED AS   ( 1  CAP )   PO   / MONU

      PRN PAIN   Q4H

      DOSES GIVEN  (MOST RECENT DAY) -
      05/09/88 0900P
------------------------------------------------------------------------------
      ... CONTINUED~
```

Figure 4. Full current profile.

orders, one line per order, with the on-line option of expanding any selected order to full profile format (Figure 5).

History. As with the medication profiles, both full and abbreviated formats are available as a screen listing, and both may be printed on request. Full order detail and history and a full history of doses given and omitted are shown on the full-format history. The abbreviated history is similar to the abbreviated profile, one line per order, but includes all expired orders.

PHARMACY LISTING (SHORT FORMAT)

```
PHARMACY ORDERS DISPLAY   (SHORT-FORMAT)   3S SAMPLE,PATIENT   3333333

ORDN   MEDNAME          DOSE        FRM   #/RT  SCHED      START   T-TM

0012A LORAZEPAM         2MG         TAB   PO          S    02/23/88  600A X

0017A MORPHINE          5MG/.62ML   INJ   IM               02/23/88 0119P X

0018B ALLOPURINOL       300MG       TAB   PO    QD    S    02/23/88 0800A X

0022B MORPHINE          5MG/.62ML   INJ   IV    Q4H  P  P  02/23/88 0221P X

0023A STREPTOKINASE 30000U/3ML      INJ   IV          S    02/23/88 0300P X

0026A PHENYTOIN         500MG/10ML  MNB   IV          S    02/23/88 0400P X
```

Figure 5. Abbreviated profile.

MAR (Nursing Medication Administration Record). The MAR is a printed 24-hour time-line display of all ordered medications, with asterisks marking scheduled doses (Figure 6). All dose markings are signed by Nursing as given or not given, and all nonscheduled doses given are marked and signed. This document serves as the authoritative record of medication administration and the reminder of scheduled doses to be given. Printed by the OCIS as part of the daily batch work, the report covers the 24-hour time period from 4:00 A.M. through 3:59 A.M. The MAR includes current and future orders and lists separately scheduled large volume parenterals, all other scheduled orders, and nonscheduled orders. Blank lines and blank forms are provided for write-in of new orders and new admissions.

Special Clinical Functions and Tools

The following special reports and displays contribute to the clinical functions of the pharmacy system:

Pain Management. Cancer patients frequently present pain management problems requiring diligent follow-up for adequate control of the pain. Utilizing core system resources, clinicians can consistently and accurately convert from one pain management medication to another or change the route of administration. They may also use this tool in speculative consideration of unusual dosage and scheduling alternatives. The pharmacy staff uses this system to cross-check medication orders. Additionally, the Pharmacy utilizes a pain management report to identify patients with pain management difficulties as evidenced by frequent

THE JOHNS HOPKINS ONCOLOGY CENTER MEDICATION ADMINISTRATION RECORD   PRINTED: 3:31 PM 04/11/88   FOR 24HR STARTING 4AM 05/11/88

FLOOR: 3S   PATIENT: PATIENT,FOUR (7778884)   SEX: M   AGE: 15   WT: 71.6   ADMIT-DATE: 05/04/88   PAGE: 1

PROTOCOL: J8642 (05/11/88) J8638 (05/11/88) ...   DIAGNOSIS: LEUKEMIA, ACUTE MYEL - BMT

```
------- SCHEDULED DOSES -------
ORD#   MED                    DOSE/VOL      FORM #/RT TIMG  04 05 06 07 08 09 10 11 12 01 02 03 04 05 06 07 08 09 10 11 12 01 02 03

0015A CO-TRIMOXAZOLE DOUBLE   160MG         TAB  PO  QDW                 *<<                                                   .DC
   ORDERED AS: SEPTRA-DS

0051B PHENYTOIN              350MG          CAP  PO  Q6H       *         *<<                                                   .DC
   ORDERED AS: DILANTIN

0052B PHENYTOIN              350MG          CAP  PO  QD
   ORDERED AS: DILANTIN                                                 >>*                                                   >>

0061A BUSULFAN              70MG            TAB  PO  Q6H    V                          *                    *

--------- PRN/ON-CALL ---------

0046A TYLOX      / MONU 1                   CAP  PO  Q4H  P

0049A NEOSPORIN TOPIC / BULK 1APPLN         OINT TOP                               *

0063A DIPHENHYDRAMINE       25MG            CAP  PO  Q4H  N                 .>.

------ NEW ORDERS ------
ORD#   MED                    DOSE/VOL      FORM #/RT TIMG  04 05 06 07 08 09 10 11 12 01 02 03 04 05 06 07 08 09 10 11 12 01 02 03
```

ORD#   MED   DOSE/VOL   FORM #/RT TIMG   04 05 06 07 08 09 10 11 12 01 02 03 04 05 06 07 08 09 10 11 12 01 02 03

[* MARKS DOSE IN HOURLY TIMESLOT FROM 04 =(4:00-4:59AM) THRU 03 =(3:00-3:59AM) OF THE FOLLOWING DAY.   >> & << MARK START & END]

THE JOHNS HOPKINS ONCOLOGY CENTER MEDICATION ADMINISTRATION RECORD   DATE: 05/11/88   PAGE: 1   MARK IF THERE IS A NEXT PAGE: (*)

FLOOR: 3S   NAME: PATIENT,FOUR

* * * COPY FOR MEDICAL RECORDS * * *   J.H.H. 777-88-84

Figure 6. Nursing Medication Administration Record (MAR).

```
JOHNS HOPKINS OCIS              ANTIBIOTIC USAGE LISTING

------------------------------------------------------------------
3S
------------------------------------------------------------------

PATIENT,FOUR

        DRUG                  DOSE      SCHEDULE   START DATE/TIME
1 CO-TRIMOXAZOLE DOUBLE  STRE160MG     QDW        05/09/88  1000A
2 NEOSPORIN TOPICAL          1APPLN               05/09/88  0800P

JOB COMPLETED   2:29 PM
```

Figure 7. Antibiotic usage listing.

drug, dosing, and schedule changes and/or inadequate dosing adjustments (from IV to PO). This daily report identifies all patients receiving pain medication. Pharmacists, in conjunction with the pain management team, follow up on patients requiring special attention. (Targeted pain medications are defined by a subdictionary under Pharmacy control.)

Antibiotic Screening. Similar to the pain management report, antibiotic screening identifies patients receiving specific antibiotics that are identified in a subdictionary under Pharmacy control (Figure 7). Patients receiving inappropriate drug combinations and/or doses are targeted for follow-up by a pharmacist or microbiologist. Drugs and doses are checked to ensure appropriateness on the basis of culture and sensitivity data. This report prints daily as part of the OCIS batch work. Patient-specific details include drug, dose schedule, route, start date, and patient location. Again, this is only possible through the tight integration of the clinical and pharmacy systems.

Chemotherapy Card. The chemotherapy card is designed to automate by patient and drug all chemotherapy and investigational drug doses administered. This record reflects date of administration, dose, volume, and form and calculates cumulative doses for medications defined in a subdictionary. The system capably tracks medication usage regardless of patient location (whether inpatient or outpatient). This function can be used to facilitate audit inquiries, which are frequent when dealing with investigational drugs. Figure 8 displays the chemotherapy history for the drug cytarabine for a SAMPLE, PATIENT.

Administrative Outputs

Specialized administrative reports and functions were developed to support administrative functions within the Pharmacy. Prior to implementation of these functions, no comparable system existed, and many man-hours of manual labor were required. The administrative functions are described below:

CHEMOTHERAPY CARD

```
 PATIENT NAME : SAMPLE,PATIENT              HISTORY NUMBER : 2331399

   ** CYTARABINE **                                         2S
=====================================================================
| DATE |    DOSAGE    |INFUSION MEDIUM|   NOTES/ADMIXTURES   |ACKNL DISP|
=====================================================================
07/13/88|1066MG/21.32ML| 500ML OF D5W | [1000A]- PROTOCOL 8410A |  * |    |
---------------------------------------------------------------------
07/14/88|1066MG/21.32ML| 500ML OF D5W | [1000A]- PROTOCOL 8410A |  * |    |
---------------------------------------------------------------------
07/15/88|1066MG/21.32ML| 500ML OF D5W | [1000A]- PROTOCOL 8410A |  * |    |
---------------------------------------------------------------------
```

Figure 8. Chemotherapy card.

Statistical Report. Daily and monthly counts of orders entered, doses, and types of doses dispensed are included in this report (Figure 9). Daily, monthly, and yearly volume and mix changes can be easily identified and evaluated. The report is compiled automatically and prints on demand by the pharmacy.

Selected Drug Use Statistics. Drug usage by unit is based on a pharmacy-defined drug subdictionary. It prints monthly on Pharmacy demand. The report assists in allocating and tracking drug usage by nursing unit. Through links with the core database, drug usage reporting by diagnosis, protocol, and/or many other patient-related variables is also possible, and identification of the drug in the sub-dictionary is not required. These special reports require interaction with the OCIS operators, and turnaround time varies, depending on system demands.

Discharge Summary/Outpatient Clinic Reports. These reports facilitate answers to billing inquiries, whether they are from a third-party insurance carrier or from a patient. Immediately upon discharge, a complete medication history with billing information is printed. The full-profile history is archived to tape, and retrieval tools are available. After discharge, the on-line inpatient gross billing information by discharge date is available. Full billing disclosure after discharge can also be obtained from archive.

Outpatient clinic billing information is available on-line, detailing drug, dose, route of administration, number of doses administered, and billed amount. This function is of immediate value, since many claim requests are received from the clinic area.

Billing Report. The billing report is a printed listing of the daily billing tape that has been sent to the Inpatient Billing Office. The tape and report are produced as part of the OCIS daily batch work.

Dictionary Listings. Multiple utility tables, including form, route, order-entry stocking codes, solution vehicle codes, shorthand drug codes, formulary listings,

PHARMACY SERVICES

GENERAL STATISTICS FOR OUTPATIENTS

PERIOD	TOTAL	ENV	LAB	HYL	INJ	MJB	MNB	OE
07/01/88	29	16	13	0	14	1	12	0
07/02/88	4	2	2	0	2	0	2	0
07/03/88	0	0	0	0	0	0	0	0
07/04/88	0	0	0	0	0	0	0	0
07/05/88	63	33	30	0	31	5	25	0
07/06/88	68	39	29	0	36	3	26	0
07/07/88	9	6	3	0	6	0	3	0
07/08/88	17	7	10	0	7	0	10	0
07/09/88	4	3	1	0	1	0	1	0
07/10/88	17	6	11	0	5	6	5	0

Figure 9. Statistical report.

etc., are maintained by the Pharmacy. Access to utility tables is authority code protected. Screen or printed listings are available on request.

Formulary Inquiry and List. Screen display of formulary names and details may be requested by full or partial formulary name or number. (Formulary number is based on the ASHP formulary classification code with modification within the Pharmacy.) A full printed listing is available on request by formulary number or by name with cross-reference to formulary number. Both show full drug detail. Access to full formulary listing and the capability of modification are authority protected. Figure 10 shows a formulary display dictionary for vancomycin with available stockings, cost algorithm, and the OCIS dose equivalent.

External Interfaces

As stated above, the OCIS pharmacy system and the OCIS core system benefit mutually by the integration of the two. This integration can be described in terms of specific interfaces, some providing supporting functionality from the OCIS core to the pharmacy subsystem (e.g., patient identification, census, and data) and others providing patient medication data from the pharmacy subsystem to the OCIS core. Each of these interfaces is discussed in some detail below. Additionally, there are interfaces to provide OCIS pharmacy billing and administrative data to remote systems. These are also detailed below.

Patient Census. All pharmacy functions make use of the OCIS-maintained current inpatient census. A patient must be admitted to a nursing unit before order entry can occur. Because the data coordinators who maintain the census are not available on a 24-hour basis, and because the first point of a clinical system

FORMULARY DISPLAY FOR PHARMACY

```
┌─────────────────────────────────────────────────────────────────────┐
│                                                                       │
│   OCIS PHARMACY      FORMULARY DISPLAY                 03/24/88        │
│                                                                       │
│   081821                  0. VANCOMYCIN              1. VANCOCIN       │
│                                                                       │
│   USABLE IN ADMX                                                      │
│                                                                       │
│   OCIS DATA EQUIVALENT:              VAN    MG                        │
│                                                                       │
│   STOCKINGS                                                           │
│     FRM    QTY               RTE   COST  F BK MAXD MINWT EXP  OCIS-VAL │
│                                                                       │
│   1. CAP  125 MG             PO    00401 Y N                    125   │
│   2. INJ  500 MG/10ML        IV    01483 Y N                    500   │
│                                                                       │
│                                                                       │
│   (Q)UIT  (E)DIT  (L)IST                                             │
│                                                                       │
└─────────────────────────────────────────────────────────────────────┘
```

Figure 10. Formulary display dictionary for *vancomycin*.

encounter for an emergency admission is likely to be a pharmacy order, the pharmacists have access to a rudimentary admit function within the census system. Subsequent to admission, discharge and transfer functions in the census subsystem generate messages within the Pharmacy, but do not directly affect pharmacy processing. The Pharmacy executes independent transfer and discharge functions appropriate to its own management of dose delivery. Outpatients are registered by the Pharmacy for order entry from the existing OCIS patient database.

Patient Demographics and Clinical Data. The pharmacy system acquires patient data such as name, body surface area, age, sex, diagnosis, and protocol history from the OCIS core database for display within the pharmacy system.

Patient Protocols. Some drugs are dispensed only against a protocol. Because it is common practice for a protocol to be initiated by the concurrent presentation of the protocol document and the associated drug order at the Pharmacy desk, the Pharmacy has access to the protocol subsystem for protocol-start entry and review.

Body Surface Area. Consistency and accuracy in calculating body surface area (BSA) are key elements in correct patient dose determination, particularly for chemotherapy dosing. The OCIS pharmacy system is linked with a core system resource allowing efficient and accurate BSA calculations, which are utilized when cross-checking chemotherapy dosing. Both height and weight, required for BSA calculation, are displayed from the core database, but both can be overridden as needed. Once calculated, the BSA is then used for dose calculation based on a specified dose per square meter.

Cumulative Dose Reporting. Cumulative dose reporting is a function currently under development. When installed, it will provide patient cumulative dose information in the order-entry transaction for medications that have recommended lifetime cumulative limits.

Patient Allergies. This function provides for the entry of patient allergies to specific drugs or to groups of drugs, along with explanatory notes. These allergy declarations are automatically reviewed during order entry, and an alert is displayed, with override required, if the order appears to be in conflict with an allergy.

Other Patient Data. All other patient data included in the OCIS core database are available for pharmacist on-line review, as needed, from the standard OCIS inquiry menus.

Medication Data. The medication data interface involves extraction and posting of dosage data; the internal linkage between the pharmacy drug formulary and the OCIS data element dictionary; the electronic mail utility, which helps to ensure dictionary synchrony; and the data entry function, which acknowledges actual dose administration.

Medication data are extracted from the orders file and passed to the OCIS patient database by a batch job. The first portion of the data extraction process reviews the orders for each patient and the applicable dose acknowledgments (scheduled doses not given, or PRN doses given). This determines the total daily dosage of each drug. The dosage value is given in standard OCIS dictionary units and the drug mnemonic key. The second portion of the data interface actually applies these values to the patient database. Normally, this data update run is made daily, shortly after midnight, for the preceding day. Dose acknowledgments received after data posting will increment or decrement the patient data value at the next update run.

The conversion of the dispensed pharmacy drug stocking to the OCIS data element equivalent is accomplished by the maintenance of linkage information in the pharmacy drug-stocking dictionary. For each possible pharmacy dispensing unit, the equivalent OCIS code and unit-adjusted value is kept. These formulary fields are maintained by the supervisor of data coordinators. There is an automatic electronic message generated to the mailbox of that supervisor if these required fields are missing at order entry (typically, after a new item has been added to the formulary) or at daily data extraction.

As previously described, acknowledgment of PRN doses given and of scheduled doses not given, based on the medication administration record (MAR) nursing notation, is entered by the data coordinators.

Billing and Administrative Data. Inpatient billing charges are generated from patient pharmacy orders daily (reflecting doses actually administered) and passed to the Hospital inpatient-billing system on magnetic tape. Included in this run are charges for the second prior day, as well as late acknowledgment adjustments to earlier days. Similar data are passed, on a separate tape, to the Central Pharmacy's administrative system for use in statistical analysis.

Technical and Operational Issues

System development always involves choices among the sometimes contradictory goals of efficiency, maintainability, simplicity, timeliness, robustness, and integrity. In the case of the OCIS pharmacy system, integrity and operational robustness were generally favored. The result has been a relatively steady, dependable system. But there are also negative aspects to these choices.

On-line response time was a near-crisis problem in the initial days of production. This problem was relieved by the transfer of much of the new-order update process into "background mode" so that the user does not wait for completion. However, response time is still uncomfortably long at some points of flow when the general computer load is near capacity. At several points in time, this problem has been relieved by computer system upgrades. Unfortunately, such increases in capacity have been absorbed by the addition of new (non-pharmacy) functionality to the system, with eventual reversion to preupgrade performance. More computing power is presently being added to manage response time effectively. (See Chapter 9.)

Pharmacy system processing is a heavy consumer of machine cycles. This fact forces some processing into off-shift batch mode (data extraction, billing, MAR setup, etc.), when other schedules or real-time handling might better serve the OCIS applications.

The OCIS patient medication data acquired from the pharmacy system lags reality by up to 24 hours, since data are not posted to OCIS until after scheduled administration time, in a batch run that executes shortly after midnight. Additionally, modifications to reported doses (scheduled doses not given, PRN doses given) are entered by the data coordinator from the MAR during day shift, for the previous day and are therefore not posted to OCIS until 24 to 48 hours after the fact. This means that medication data appears on the flow sheets before it has been adjusted for PRN and omitted doses. Of course, the data will normally have incorporated all such adjustments by the time of the next flow-sheet printing, and in the interim, the providers do have access to the paper MAR. Prospective data posting was considered while the system was in development, but was rejected at that time as introducing significant complexity (both technical and procedural) and prime-shift operating load. Certainly, the system would provide more timely data with more timely posting.

The extraction of dosage data for billing is also a batch operation. To avoid significant percentages of transaction adjustments, it also waits until the day after data coordinator dose acknowledgments are entered. This flow adds one extra day of lag to the billing process. Because the decision was made to allow dose acknowledgment corrections at any time (not "closing" dose history at some arbitrary time), the resulting program complexity has so far discouraged the good inclination to tighten the billing cycle.

Future Possibilities

Some attractive functionality, such as drug/drug interaction and inventory control, was deliberately deferred by the development team on the basis of past experiences with these topics and on the expectation that later Central Pharmacy developments would provide direction and tools. Specifically, it was hoped that the Central Pharmacy would approach its formulary by subscription to a commercially available drug products dictionary with built-in drug/drug interaction data. In fact, the Central Pharmacy maintains its own formulary and has developed its own limited drug/drug system; so it appears that the OCIS pharmacy system will likely also build its own in-house version of drug/drug at some time in the future.

The development team concurred in omitting inventory control from the initial system, owing largely to the relatively high percentage of fractional doses dispensed in the oncology setting and the absence of clear rules for inventory effect of such doses. Automation of general inventory management still appears to be a low-priority item for the pharmacy. On the other hand, it has been deemed appropriate to develop special programs for the management of investigational stocks, which are generally closely audited by the suppliers and dispensed only against specific studies. At the time of initial development, only simple reminder messages and study number prompts were included in the system.

There is pharmacy interest in changes in fill list handling to produce dose preparation efficiencies. One specific suggestion would group IV dose labels so that like formulations could be batched at the mix station.

The actual pharmacy distribution system, with its 4-hour delivery cycle and unit-of-use envelopes and labels, is relatively expensive in terms of materials and labor. Although the system could be modified to a more typical 24-hour cart replacement model, this option has so far been rejected in the Center because of space constraints and primary-care nursing responsibilities.

Evaluation and Summary

Although no formal evaluation of the pharmacy system has been conducted, the computer system is viewed as an integral part of both the pharmacy operation and the OCIS clinical database. Purely from the viewpoint of accessible current and historical data retrieval, the system provides timely review of clinical and administrative data important to the overall efficient functioning of the Pharmacy

and the Oncology Center. Computerization of medication records, label generation, formulary updates, billing, and statistical data saves the pharmacy approximately three to five full-time equivalents. The value of the inpatient clinical data
interface with the Pharmacy, which supports relatively high-level personnel, is
difficult to quantify.

Overall, the pharmacy system has received high marks in terms of thorough-
ness of functionality (see Chapter 9). The order-entry flow is considered to be
logical, friendly, and easy to learn. System speed has often been an issue, and it
has been addressed by increasing the main processor capacity. Prolonged and
unscheduled downtime has been an exceedingly rare event during the past 5
years. This is partially due to a semi-fault tolerant system, which is being
improved (see Chapter 9).

The interface with the clinical database cannot be underestimated. From the
pharmacy perspective, review of drug therapy appropriateness based on protocol
eligibility, metabolic functions (renal, liver, etc.), and concurrent therapy is
exceedingly efficient. The pharmacist can independently access this information
from any computer terminal within the Center. From the clinical and administrative perspective, drug administration can be plotted as a function of various physiological responses, better enabling the physician to assess an individual's
response to specific drug therapy, prospectively or retrospectively. Pharmacist
access to pharmacy functions from terminals in the clinical areas promotes an
unusual degree of interaction with the clinical staff. The result is a rapid response
to needs, with dose-delivery materials automatically generated in the Pharmacy
in response to transactions from the floor. Internal and external (FDA and NCI)
audits are simplified and reflect an accurate accounting of each patient's medication drug usage. Finally, as a result of this system, third-party billing audits are
simplified, information can be supplied with minimal personnel effort, and challenges or payment denials have been minimized. This last element, which is due
to the integration of clinical, pharmacy, laboratory testing, and research data,
could easily pay for the total system's yearly operation and development costs.

7
Hemapheresis System
Hayden G. Braine, M.D.[1]

Introduction

Historically, the major transfusion requirements for cancer treatment have been for blood and plasma products used in surgery. The relatively long storage time of these products, 35 days for red cells and 1 year for fresh frozen plasma, have made management of inventories of these products amenable to relatively simple data systems. Many hospital blood bank inventory systems have been developed to handle these products. Likewise, systems for the management of the large-scale donor center manufacture and testing of blood components are also available. However systems to assist in the management of platelet concentrates with 1- to 5-day storage times have not been so well developed.

Platelets are small cellular fragments that circulate in the bloodstream. They are primarily responsible for controlling bleeding by initiating thrombosis. Deficiencies in platelet numbers usually result in an increased risk of spontaneous or posttraumatic bleeding. Prior to the development of platelet transfusion therapy, 50% of the patients treated for acute lymphocytic leukemia died of hemorrhage; with effective platelet transfusion technology this was reduced to less than 5%.

Effective platelet transfusion therapy has also allowed the development of intensive curative treatment regimens in many other hematopoietic malignancies. The development of these treatment regimens has increased the use of platelets dramatically in the last decade. In general, most platelet transfusion support has been concentrated in tertiary care hospitals; in 1980 1000 such tertiary centers accounted for two-thirds of the platelet transfusions in the United States.

[1]Hayden G. Braine, M.D., joined the Oncology Center in 1976 and established the Hemapheresis and Transfusion Service. During its inception, Dr. Braine initiated work on the automation of this service and its integration with the OCIS. Dr. Braine is an Associate Professor in Oncology with a special interest in the transfusion of cancer patients. He holds joint appointments in both Medicine and Laboratory Medicine at Johns Hopkins, and is presently the Director of the Hemapheresis and Transfusion Services at the Center.

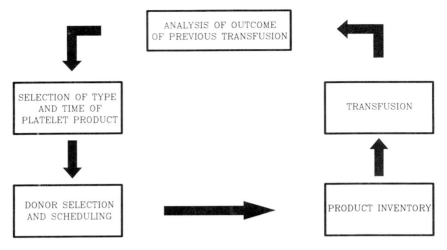

Figure 1. Platelet transfusion planning flow.

The JHOC administers 7900 platelet transfusions annually. This chapter describes the systems used to manage the JHOC platelet transfusion service.

System Overview

Management of patient platelet transfusion requirements is a repetitive cycle of six sequential steps (Figure 1). The challenge in this flow is to match the clinical transfusion requirement with product availability. When only 5 or 6 patients are being supported at one time, conventional manual methods of information flow can support timely decision making. However, the JHOC services daily over 50 patients potentially requiring a platelet transfusion. These patients are geographically distributed in five inpatient services and three outpatient departments. In this setting, computer systems are essential for the accurate formatting of data for timely and appropriate decisions.

Step 1. Analysis of Transfusion Outcome

There are two major considerations in evaluating the outcome of a platelet transfusion: the extent to which the patient's platelet count is increased (increment) and the length of time the transfused platelets persist in the patient's circulation (survival). The observed increment (posttransfusion platelet count − pretransfusion platelet count) can be normalized for the number of platelets transfused (# of units) and the volume of the patient's vascular system [estimated by the patient's body surface area in square meters (m²)]:

JOHNS HOPKINS OCIS
PATIENT TRANSFUSION DATA   04/08/88
  HEIGHT: 155CM   WEIGHT: 64.7KG   BSA: 1.69M2   HNO: NAME: 0+   D.O.B.:07/04/24   LOCATION:3NN
63 WF WALDENSTROM"S   LOCI: A3,24 B51,7 BW4,6
VINC/BLEO (111987)
ADRIA/VP16 (122387)
TAKES 8,11,18,21,22,35,44:   AVOID 1,32,57,62 (032988)
PROMACE/CYTOBAM (011388)

LEUKO.POOR PLTS. (032188)

DATE	PD	TIME	PL (K)	WBC X100	HC	INCREM/HR	#U	LE9	HLA	MATCH/V	A	TEMP	B/I	ABO/RES	PRODUCT	COMMENT
02/24/88	43	910A	12	402	32											
		1200P					P12	0.6	A29,30 B7, BW6,6	11000/-	1	36.9	2/0	0	SS17648PAB	
02/25/88	44	100P	9	284	28	-403	/1									
		705A	5	247	25	-940	/19									
							P8		A3,24 B7,22 BW6,6	30100/-	1	36.5	2/0	A	R2444PX0 PL 732	AMICAR
		1100A														
		1250P	73			14110	/2									
		730P	64	302	26	12243	/9									
02/26/88		655A	51	283	24	9545	/20					36.7	2/0			

Figure 2. Sample comprehensive platelet transfusion history.

$$\frac{\text{(platelet increment) (m}^2\text{)}}{(\text{\# of units})} = 10,000.$$

Thus, immediately after the transfusion, 1 unit of platelets should raise the platelet count of a 1 m^2 patient by 10,000 platelets/mm^3. By normalizing the post transfusion platelet count in this manner, the outcome of platelet transfusion can be compared among various patients of varying sizes receiving varying doses of platelets. Using a definition of 1 platelet unit as 5.5×10^{10} platelets, our "normal" posttransfusion increment is $10,000 \pm 5000$ (± 1 SD).

By monitoring patients' platelet counts in relation to transfusion, we can determine whether we have achieved the desired platelet count and, after considering the number of units transfused, whether the observed increment in platelet count was that which was expected. Failure to achieve the expected immediate posttransfusion increment can result from several factors, including formation of antibodies to tissue (HLA) antigens on the platelets, organomegaly, or intravascular coagulation.

Similarly, survival of transfused platelets can be calculated: 18 to 24 hours after the transfusion the corrected increment should be greater than 2500. Failure to observe a normal posttransfusion platelet survival can be caused by a variety of clinical variables, including fever, infections, and bleeding.

The complex clinical and laboratory database required to interpret logically the posttransfusion platelet increment and survival is organized and maintained on line in OCIS as "the platelet transfusion history" (Figure 2). Pertinent data for evaluating platelet transfusion outcome include each patient's peak daily temperature (TEMP) and bleeding and infection status (B/I). Comments on other clinical variables, such as splenomegaly or disseminated intravascular coagulation, are noted in the "header" or margin, that is, in the upper left-hand corner or right-hand margin of the report. Product variables that affect transfusion outcome, such as ABO type (ABO), storage age (A), HLA type, and white cell (LE9) and platelet content (#U), are displayed. Posttransfusion corrected platelet increments are calculated for each transfusion and formatted with the clinical and laboratory information.

The example shown in Figure 2 is that of a 63-year-old white woman with Waldendrom's Macroglobulinemia. She was treated with combination chemotherapy on 13 January 1988 and was on protocol day (PD) 43 posttherapy on 24 February 1988. At 9:10 A.M. her platelet count (PL) was 12,000/mm^3, white count (WBC) 40,200/mm^3, and hematocrit (HC) 32%. At 12:00 P.M. that day she received 12 units (P12) of platelets with HLA type A29, A30, B7, BW6, 6. One hour later her platelet count was 9000/mm^3, an obvious failure. At 7:05 A.M. the next day her platelet count was 5000/mm^3, and at 11:00 A.M. she received a second transfusion of 8 units of platelets with HLA type A3, A24, B7, B22, BW 6, 6. Two hours (12:50 P.M.) after transfusion her platelet count was 73,000/mm^3. This gave a normalized platelet increment of 14,110 two hours after the transfusion (14,110/2). Clearly a successful transfusion. Data not shown in this example implicated antibodies to A29 and A30 as the cause of the first transfusion failure.

```
JOHNS HOPKINS OCIS                                              03/16/88
  MATCH FOR 1234567                    PATIENT, A
        A ANTIGENS: 3,30
        B ANTIGENS: 18, 8
        BW VALUE REQUIRED:NONE   REJECT ANTIGENS:   NONE
```

	MATCH INDEX	DONOR ID	LAST DONATION	BLD TYPE	SITES A	A	B	B	BW	CM	NAME
					3	30	18	8			
A											
	40000		04/13/87	O+	3	19	8	18	6,6	−	
B1U											
	31000		03/15/88	B+	3	30	8		6,6	+	
B1X											
	30100		02/18/88	O−	3	31	8	51	6,4	−	
	30010		(FROZEN)	O+	1	3	8	18	6,6	+	
	30010		01/20/87	O+	1	3	8	18	6,6	+	
	30010		08/11/87	AB+	3	32	18	62	6.6	+	
	30010		11/25/87	A+	3	32	18	39	6,6	+	
	30010		01/26/88	O+	1	3	8	18	6,6	+	
	30010		03/08/88	O+	1	3	8	18	6,6	+	
B2UX											
	21100		12/26/87	A+	32		8	51	6,4	+	
	21100		02/22/88	O+	3		35	18	6,6	+	
	21100		03/02/88	A−	3		35	18	6,6	+	
	21010		02/02/88	O−	3	25	18		6,6	+	
	21010		02/11/88	A+	3	26	18		6,	+	
B2X											
	20110		01/21/87	O+	3	33	14	35	6,6	−	
	20110		09/01/87	A−	3	32	51	49	4,4	+	
	20110		10/22/87	A+	1	3	35	8	6,6	+	
	20110		01/02/88	O+	31	25	8	35	6,6	−	
	20110		01/20/88	O+	1	3	8	35	6,6	−	
	20110		02/05/88	O−	1	32	8	35	6,6	+	
	20110		02/10/88	O−	1	3	8	35	6,6	+	
	20110		02/15/88	A−	1	31	51	8	4,6	−	

Partial HLA matching program for patient with HLA Type A3, A30, B18, B

Figure 3. Partial listing from HLA matching program. This list contains donor matches for a patient with HLA Type A3, A30, B18, B8.

MON 04/04	TUE 04/05	WED 04/06	THU 04/07	FRI 04/08	SAT 04/09
800 A2,31 B62,57 BW64 0+ C-	800 A3,28 B44,7 BW46 AB+ C	830 A2,3 B14,44 BW64 0+ C- H	800 A1,2 B8, BW66 0- C- H	800 A3,32 B18,39 BW66 A+ C+ H	730 A, B, C BW
800 A3,24 B35 BW66 AB- C- H		800 A1,26 B8,45 BW66 0+ C+			730 A, B, C BW
800 A2,24 B7,47 BW64 0+ C-	800 A3, B7,35 BW66 A- C+ H	800 A11,26 B38,44 BW44 B- C+		800 A1,2 B5,8 BW46 0+ C-	730 A2,24 B7,62 BW66 0+ C-
800 A1,9 B44,17 BW44 0- C+	800 A1,29 B8,44 BW64 0+ C		830 A2,9 B44,22 BW46 0- C+	800 A1,2 B8,62 BW66 B+ C-	730 A, B, C BW
800 A1,28 B8,71 BW66 0+ C+ H	800 A29,30 B7, BW66 0+ C- H		830 A1, B8 BW66 A+ C- H		730 A2,9 B44, BW44 A+ C-
830 A28,31 B51,18 BW46 C	800 A3,26 B18, BW6 A+ C+ H	830 A1,3 B7,14 BW66 0+ C-	830 A3,24 B35,44 BW64 0+ C- H	830 A2,9 B14,62 BW66 B+ C+	730 A, B, C BW A- C
830 A3,9 B7,8 BW66 A+ C+ H	830 A2,3 B35, BW66 AB+ C-	830 A2,29 B8,14 BW66 A+ C-	830 A3,24 B7,49 BW64 0+ C+ H	800 A3,25 B44,18 BW46 B- C-	
	830 A2,24 B62,37 BW64 0+ C+	830 A3, B7,44 BW64 A- C+			
	800 A1,2 B8,44 BW64				

Figure 4. Sample morning donor room schedule. This is the schedule for the week of 4 April 1988. Ten cell separators are available. Donors (indicated by their HLA type) are scheduled to arrive between 7:30 A.M. and 8:30 A.M.

JOHNS HOPKINS OCIS   DONOR SCHEDULE   04/07/88

MATCHES	MON 04/04	TUE 04/05	WED 04/06	THU 04/07	FRI 04/08	SAT 04/09
3N BW46 A3,24B51,7	800 A3,24 B35, BW66 AB- C-			830 A3,24 B35,44 BW64 O+ C-		1100 A3,11 B7,8 BW66 O- C-
3N BW46 A3,24B51,7	830 A3,9 B7,8 BW66 A+ C+			830 A3,24 B7,49 BW64 O+ C+		
2S BW64 A1,B8,57		200 A1,31 B51,8 BW46 A- C-			800 A3,32 B18,39 BW66 A+ C+	
DECEAS BW46 A2,19B5,??	200 A2,30 B62,18 BW66 A+ C-					
DECEAS BW66 A1,2B8,62		800 A1,2 B8,44 BW64 C				
DECEAS BW66 A1,2B8,62		110 A3,11 B51,7 BW46 B+ C+				
HOME BW66 A1,11B8,35				830 A1, B8, BW66 A+ C-		
HOME BW46 A20,36B53,35		800 A3, B7,35 BW66 A- C-		1230 A3,25 B51,49 BW44 B+ C-		
3S BW64 A11,11B35,44		100 A3,11 B41,52 BW64 B- C-				
HOME BW66 A3,30B18,8		800 A3,26 B18, RW66 A+ C+			100 A26,32 B38,62 BW46 A- C-	

Figure 5. Sample schedule for HLA matches. Patient's (names deleted) location and HLA type indicated on left hand column.

Step 2. Selection of Platelet Products Required

Each week a transfusion plan is established for all patients on platelet transfusion support. Frequency of transfusion requirement, product type (concentrates made from a single donor by apheresis or 6 to 10 units pooled from individual units of whole blood), HLA type, and CMV serology are considered. From these individual projections a master transfusion plan is prepared. Special requirements for products without risk for cytomegalovirus are also considered.

Step 3. Donor Selection

The JHOC maintains a volunteer blood donor program of over 1200 members. Individual donor files are maintained and include information on HLA, ABO, and Rh type; cytomegalovirus serology; donation history, and availability for donations.

Patients requiring specific HLA types are matched with available donors (Figure 3). In this example a patient with HLA type A3, A30, B18, B8 is found to have two excellent matches (A and B1U) and many close matches (B1X, B2UX, and B2X). (Donor names and IDs have been deleted.) Subprograms then display the schedule for the hemapheresis donor room (Figure 4) and the transfusion coordinators (Figure 5).

Step 4. Platelet Production

In order to support the platelet transfusion needs of the JHOC, the Hemapheresis Center operates a large platelet collection program. Platelets are harvested from donors using blood cell separators; each donation produces 8 to 10 units of platelets during a 2- to 3-hour donation.

Each product prepared is entered into the hemapheresis database and includes data on the product's unique identifying number, volume, platelet content, white cell content, HLA type, red cell type, machine operator, and cell separator number. This database is then used for generating productivity statistics of the Hemapheresis Unit, as well as assisting in preventative maintenance of the cell collection equipment. Data collected on each cell separator are used to calculate average platelet yields and operating efficiency. (Figure 6). In the report shown, one can see that the CS3000 cell separators consistently produce fewer numbers of platelets (ranging from 3.8 to 4.1×10^{11}) with a lower collection efficiency (ranging from 41% to 44%) than the Model-30 system, in terms of both absolute yield (ranging from 4.5 to 4.9×10^{11}) and collection efficiency (ranging from 56% to 58%).

Step 5. Inventory

All platelet concentrates produced are entered into a master on-line inventory (Figure 7). This is then used by the clinical transfusion coordinators to assign

JOHNS HOPKINS OCIS
09/02/87

PLATELET YIELD – ALL 08/01/87 TO 08/31/87
(PI,PII,WC DONATIONS NOT INCLUDED)

MACH. NAME	#	#DONS.	AVE. PLT. COUNT (X 10") PER DON.	STD. DEV.	PLT. EFF.	STD. # DEV.	
CS 3000	1070	8	3.9	0.7	0.41	0.06	8
CS 3000	1159	19	4.2	0.9	0.44	0.05	19
CS 3000	1247	24	4.4	0.9	0.43	0.04	20
CS 3000	1605	31	3.8	1.0	0.40	0.04	30
CS 3000	1609	30	4.2	1.1	0.42	0.07	22
CS 3000	1613	41	3.8	0.8	0.43	0.05	38
CS 3000	1615	40	4.1	0.9	0.42	0.05	36
MODEL 30	1520	NOT USED					
MODEL 30	130	NOT USED					
MODEL 30	238	NOT USED					
MODEL 30	498	12	4.7	1.2	0.57	0.06	12
MODEL 30	590	25	4.8	1.2	0.58	0.08	25
MODEL 30	739	24	4.9	1.5	0.57	0.09	24
MODEL 30	975	9	4.5	1.0	0.56	0.06	8
-50	1090	NOT USED					
-50	1555	16	3.5	1.0	0.42	0.13	16

Figure 6. Platelet yield and operating efficiency by machine.

products to recipients for final transfusion assignment. The inventory also operates as a central quality control step. All products, each assigned a unique sequential number, remain in inventory unless assigned to one of five outcomes:

1. Transfused into a patient, in which case the data are entered into the patient's database and used to generate transfusion history data, as well as a billing file for administrative purposes.
2. Used for quality control and destroyed.
3. Destroyed because of a positive serology for hepatitis, AIDS, etc.
4. Outdated and destroyed. Data in this and the previous category are reported monthly.
5. Frozen for future use, in which case the product is entered into a master inventory of frozen platelet concentrates; this frozen inventory is also searched for each HLA matching program ordered.

EXPIRES 04/07/88

PRODUCT	TIME	UNITS	LE9	VOL	RECIPIENT	BT/CM	HLA
R24714P	950A	8		287	_____	O+/	A28,19 B7,40 BW6,6
R24717PX0	145P	6		135	_____	B+/-	A25,31 B18,60 BW6,6
R24718P	200P	9		279	_____	O+/	A2,11 B8,14 BW6,6
SS18189PX	1053A	6.73	0.3	221	_____	O+/+	A1,26 B8,45 BW6,6
SS18191PAB	1115A	5.09	0.6	142	_____	A-/+	A3, B7,44 BW6,4
SS18192PAD	1135A	6.18	0.04	430	_____	A+/-	A2,29 B8,14 BW6,6
SS18193PX	145P	8.73	0.5	223	_____	A+/+	A1,2 B17,62 BW4,6
SS18194PX	144P	8.36	0.3	222	_____	A+/-	A2,11 B44, BW4,4

EXPIRES 04/08/88

PRODUCT	TIME	UNITS	LE9	VOL	RECIPIENT	BT/CM	HLA

EXPIRES 04/09/88

PRODUCT	TIME	UNITS	LE9	VOL	RECIPIENT	BT/CM	HLA
R24699PY0	1105A	11		222	_____	A+/-	A29,31 B22,44 BW6,4
R24701PY0	225P	5		160	_____	O+/-	A2,3 B35,60 BW6,6

EXPIRES 04/10/88

PRODUCT	TIME	UNITS	LE9	VOL	RECIPIENT	BT/CM	HLA
R24710PY0	255P	6		180	_____	B+/-	A2,3 B7,8 BW6,6

EXPIRES 04/11/88

PRODUCT	TIME	UNITS	LE9	VOL	RECIPIENT	BT/CM	HLA
R24713PY0	945A	6		215	_____	A+/-	A1,24 B18,37 BW6,4
R24715PY0	1026A	9		219	_____	B+/-	A2,24 B13,27 BW4,4

EXPIRED   Master Inventory

Figure 7.

With this control step any delay in data entry or other nonstandard outcome is rapidly known: Products not assigned a destination are easily detected as they remain in inventory. Similarly, products not entered into the system are detected, as a sequential number is missing.

```
                          TRANSFUSION PLAN

     SAMPLE,PATIENT -  1212121      HOME        M-2/ACUTE MYEL LEUK

                     ** PREFERRED RED CELLS **

     1. IRRADIATED (TO PREVENT GVHD)
     2. LEUKOCYTE POOR (TO REDUCE RISK OF FEBRILE TRANSFUSION REACTION)

     warning:  THIS TRANSFUSION PLAN MAY BE 72 HOURS OLD. IF THERE HAS
     BEEN A CHANGE IN CLINICAL STATUS OR A TRANSFUSION REACTION, THIS PLAN
     MAY HAVE BEEN VERBALLY ALTERED.  IF THERE ARE ANY QUESTIONS, CALL THE
     BLOOD BANK (6580) OR DR. PLATELET (5020).
     -------------------------------------------------------------------
                          ** COMMENT **

     SUGGEST PREMED WITH ACETAMINOPHEN (031387)
     ===================================================================


                     ** PREFERRED PLATELETS **

     1. ABO COMPATIBLE (EXCEPT EMERG, PLT TR MUST BE ABO COMPAT OR
        RESUSP IN SALINE AFT REMOVING PLASMA)
     2. IRRADIATED (TO PREVENT GVHD)
     3. LEUKO POOR/LEUKOTRAP

     warning:  THIS TRANSFUSION PLAN MAY BE 72 HOURS OLD.  IF THERE HAS
     BEEN A CHANGE IN CLINICAL STATUS OR A TRANSFUSION REACTION, THIS PLAN
     MAY HAVE BEEN VERBALLY ALTERED. IF THERE ARE ANY QUESTIONS, CALL THE
     BLOOD BANK (6580) OR DR. PLATELET (5020).
     -------------------------------------------------------------------
                          ** COMMENT **

     SUGGEST PREMED WITH ACETAMINOPHEN (031387)
     ===================================================================


               ** JHOC TRANSFUSION REACTIONS SINCE MARCH, 1985 **
               SAMPLE,PATIENT - 1212121      M-2/ACUTE MYEL LEUK

                     ** RED CELLS -- REACTIONS **
```

PRODUCT	DATE	MODIFICATION	REACTION	PREMEDI-CATION
RED CELLS	07/23/87	LEUKOCYTE POOR	FEBRILE: FEVER	ACETAMIN DIPHENHY

```
                     ** PLATELETS -- REACTIONS **
```

PRODUCT	DATE	MODIFICATION	REACTION	PREMEDI-CATION
PL APH(AGE:1)	03/04/87	NONE	FEBRILE: CHILLS	ACETAMIN DIPHENHY
PPC (AGE:5)	03/12/87	NONE	FEBRILE: FEVER	ACETAMIN DIPHENHY
-SUGGEST PREMED WITH ACETAMINOPHEN (031387)				
PPC (AGE:4)	04/11/87	NONE	FEBRILE: FEVER	ACETAMIN DIPHENHY
PL APH(AGE:1)	05/06/87	NONE	FEBRILE: CHILL	ACETAMIN
PL APH(AGE:1)	06/30/88	NONE	FEBRILE: CHILLS	ACETAMIN

Figure 8.

Step 6. Transfusion

All platelet products produced locally or ordered from other bloos centers are stored in the Hospital's Central Blood Bank. The patient's individual physician is responsible for ordering the transfusion of the product and specifying any secondary processing, such as leukocyte depletion to prevent febrile transfusion reactions. To assist the physician in ordering platelets, on-line files are maintained with specific recommendations for transfusion (Figure 8). Files also include transfusion reaction history and recommendations for any pretransfusion medications needed.

Step 7. Reanalysis of Transfusion Outcome

With completion of each transfusion, analysis of the outcome is again reviewed as in Step 1. Unexpected outcomes are then identified and alternate transfusion approaches ordered.

Quality Control of Platelet Transfusion Outcome

The American Hospital Commission (AHC) requires review of all transfusions on a regular basis. At the JHOC's current rate of nearly 8000 transfusions per year, this would be a logistical nightmare. However, with daily review of the computer-based transfusion histories, the AHC standards can be met in a timely manner. More important, modification of transfusion practice can be achieved in real time rather than retrospectively.

Transfusion practices are also traditionally monitored by review of departmental utilization statistics over time. However, departmental trend analyses have two major deficiencies: First, they do not adjust utilization for volume. A doubling of platelet utilization could be accounted for by a doubling of use per patient or a doubling of the number of patients transfused. Second, utilization statistics do not address the question of the quality of care. Platelets are transfused to prevent or stop bleeding. In order to evaluate the appropriateness of a given number of transfusions, one must consider whether hemostasis was maintained.

To address this problem, we have implemented the case-adjusted statistical evaluation (CASE). Patients are grouped by diagnosis and treatment; for example, all patients with acute myelocytic leukemia (AML) treated with a particular combination of drugs are grouped, and then daily platelet counts, along with platelet transfusion and bleeding status data, are acquired from the OCIS database. Mean daily platelet counts, the mean number of units of platelets transfused per patient per day, and the mean bleeding status of the group are reported. Trends of higher platelet counts with fewer transfusions and less bleeding would be desirable. For this evaluation all patients are scored daily on a scale of 0 to 4 (Table 1) for bleeding status.

If comparisons among patient populations are to be made, platelet transfusion requirements must also be adjusted for patient size: Larger patients require more platelets than smaller patients. This can be accomplished by dividing utilization by mean patient size (m^2). Figure 9 displays the quality control report for adult patients undergoing induction chemotherapy (Ac-D-AMSA) for acute myelocytic

Table 1. Bleeding and Infection Status Codes

Code	Grade				
	0	1	2	3	4
Bleeding status	No symptoms	Petechia	Epistaxis, venipuncture sites	More than 1 unit per day due to hemorrhage	Life-threatening symptoms
Infection status	No symptoms	Complete response—on antibiotics, afebrile, sites stable	Partial response—on antibiotics, previous plus culture now, or decreasing T max	No change	Progression

JOHNS HOPKINS OCIS   02/27/88
01/01/84 TO 12/30/87 -- POPULATION OVER TIME -- RUN CODE:1
POPULATION OVER TIME FOR REM. INDUC. OF AML W/AC-D-AMSA (J8410) -- 01/01/84 TO 12/30/87

YEAR BEGINNING	TR: ALL DAYS (BSA>0) U/BSA/PT	PTS	WBC LT 500 (BSA>0) RDNGS	PTS	BLEEDING (ALL & ACUTE) MEAN	S.D.	RDNGS	PTS	INFECTION (ALL & ACUTE) MEAN	S.D.	RDNGS	PTS	AV U/A ACUTE DAYS PTS	*	S.D.
01/01/84	125.6	33	692	33	0.4	0.7	1347	33	1.6	1.1	1347	33	33	*	3.6 2.8
					0.5	0.8	651	33	1.9	1.1	651	33	33		
01/01/85	100.7	39	809	38	0.5	0.8	1460	39	1.7	1.2	1461	39	39		3.4 2.5
					0.5	0.8	720	38	2.0	1.1	720	38	38		
01/01/86	89.5	74	1581	74	0.5	0.8	2798	74	1.4	1.2	2798	74	74		2.7 1.4
					0.5	0.8	1450	74	1.7	1.1	1450	74	74		
01/01/87	99.4	51	1118	51	0.4	0.7	1930	51	1.6	1.2	1930	51	51		2.9 2.1
					0.5	0.8	1025	51	1.9	1.2	1025	51	51		

Figure 9. Case report for patients treated for AML with chemotherapy regimen 18410 1984-87. Data on first line of each year includes all data points: Data on second line includes data only for days WBC <500/mm^3.

JOHNS HOPKINS OCIS   02/27/88
01/01/84 TO 12/30/87 -- POPULATION OVER TIME -- RUN CODE:1
POPULATION OVER TIME FOR REM. INDUC. OF AML W/AC-D-AMSA (J8410) -- 01/01/84 TO 12/30/87

BLEEDING AND INFECTION
ALL DAYS & ACUTE DAYS
FREQUENCY DISTRIBUTIONS

BLEEDING: READINGS/PATIENTS

		0	1	2	3	4
01/01/84:	ALL DAYS	956/33	218/31	162/28	11/6	/
01/01/85:	ALL DAYS	1007/38	256/35	182/31	13/5	2/2
01/01/86:	ALL DAYS	1799/73	619/70	331/54	48/12	1/1
01/01/87:	ALL DAYS	1319/51	386/44	200/37	23/6	2/2
01/01/84:	ACUTE DAYS	434/31	115/27	100/23	2/2	/
01/01/85:	ACUTE DAYS	500/36	112/28	101/25	6/4	1/1
01/01/86:	ACUTE DAYS	902/68	340/58	192/43	15/7	1/1
01/01/87:	ACUTE DAYS	704/49	190/36	112/32	17/5	2/2

INFECTION: READINGS/PATIENTS

		0	1	2	3	4
01/01/84:	ALL DAYS	167/29	606/33	318/32	120/21	136/33
01/01/85:	ALL DAYS	219/34	534/38	409/38	124/30	175/39
01/01/86:	ALL DAYS	608/66	1211/71	520/69	209/48	250/72
01/01/87:	ALL DAYS	341/42	828/51	281/45	262/43	218/51
01/01/84:	ACUTE DAYS	17/6	275/31	200/28	70/18	89/29
01/01/85:	ACUTE DAYS	16/7	251/34	262/37	81/27	110/36
01/01/86:	ACUTE DAYS	126/33	705/65	321/58	142/39	156/63
01/01/87:	ACUTE DAYS	67/18	458/48	181/41	184/41	135/44

Figure 10. Individual bleeding and infection profiles: number of days at each score/number of patients. Acute days are days WBC <500/mm^3.

leukemia (AML). From 1984 to 1987 total platelet use per patient per square meter fell from 125.6 to 99.4 units pt/m²; at the same time the mean bleeding score for all hospital days remained unchanged at 0.4 ± 0.7 (1 SD). Such "average" bleeding scores, however, could mask a small number of serious bleeding episodes. In Figure 10 data are reported by individual bleeding score: Of the 51 patients hospitalized for a total of 1930 patient days in 1987, all 51 had at least 1 day of grade 0 bleeding, and life-threatening bleeding (grade 4) was limited to 2 patients, each having 1 day of potentially life-threatening bleeding. Only 6 of 51 patients experienced grade 3 or worse bleeding.

Such data still are not controlled for the actual need for platelet transfusion. In general, patients receiving intensive treatments for hematologic malignancies develop thrombocytopenia as the result of bone marrow failure. It is during these periods of marrow failure that platelet transfusion is routinely required to prevent hemorrhage. Therefore, one would like to evaluate platelet utilization on the basis of platelet transfusion need or, in the case of patients treated for hematologic malignancies, on the degree and duration of marrow failure. In theory, the degree and duration of marrow failure could be estimated by measuring the number of days a patient has a platelet count below a given number. However, this is not a true estimate of platelet transfusion need, as platelet transfusion abolishes thrombocytopenia. Therefore, we have used the daily white blood cell count, which is not affected by transfusion, to estimate days of bone marrow failure. Following chemotherapy, when patients have fewer than 500 leukocytes/mm³ (termed acute days), they usually have severe enough marrow failure to require platelet transfusion. The platelet utilization per patient can then be corrected for the days of marrow failure by dividing platelet use by patient days of fewer than 500 leukocytes.

Controlling for such "acute days" of aplasia, we note that the average number of units of platelets used per patient per square meter per day on which the white blood cell count is less than 500 has fallen from 3.6 ± 2.8 (1 SD) in 1984 to 2.9 $\pm$ 2.1 in 1987 (Figure 9). Again, the mean bleeding score remained unchanged at 0.5 ± 0.8, and the incidents of serious (grade 4) bleeding were few in number: In 1987, 2 patients out of 51 at risk experienced one day each of grade 4 hemorrhage (Figure 10). Thus it would appear that improved transfusion efficiency (fewer units) has been achieved without significantly increased toxicity (grade 3 or 4 hemorrhage).

Conclusion

Traditionally blood banking medicine has concentrated on product quality, serologic matching, and inventory control. Increasingly, however, blood banking is becoming a complex transfusion science, with increasingly effective transfusion options being applied to complex medical treatments. This requires that an accurate and timely database be maintained in order that appropriate decisions be made and that an ongoing evaluation of transfusions be performed to ensure the delivery of the right care.

In the early 1970s platelets were selected only with regard to how many units were needed. Inventory was usually low and triage of units was common. Transfusion monitoring was limited to evaluation of next-day platelet counts.

Today's platelet transfusion science delivers a safer and more effective product. Concentrates prepared by hemapheresis can be HLA matched to the donor. Secondary product washing and/or leukocyte depletion can reduce the risk of transfusion reaction. Serologic screening can reduce the risk of disease transmission. Effective use of this powerful tool is one of the challenges of transfusion medicine in the 1990s. The availability of a timely and accurate laboratory and clinical database and an ongoing evaluation of transfusion practices are essential. In the case of JHOC, an expansion of OCIS to meet these special needs has allowed us to provide effective service to a large number of patients at a reasonable cost using limited resources.

8
General Administrative Functions

Sara J. Perkel,[1] Gloria Stewart, Lisa Lattal,
Linda M. Arenth, Catherine Kelleher,
Anne Kammer, Bruce I. Blum, Gary L. Kinsey,
Farideh Momeni, and Alan W. Sacker

The administrative component of the Oncology Center has been a major advocate of the OCIS since its inception. Although the initial funding mechanism for OCIS was from a grant, central core funds procured by the oncology administration have provided the majority of developmental and maintenance activities for the past decade. In fact, the Hospital components of OCIS are a direct responsibility of the Center's central administration. As described in Chapter 1, during the planning stages of the Oncology Center building in 1975, it was recognized that computer-managed medical data would be of major benefit in providing high-quality care for cancer patients. OCIS was established with that as its fundamental mission.

As the OCIS began to take shape, it became apparent that the data that were being collected and used for patient care had secondary or "spin-off" uses. Generally, these secondary uses of the OCIS database were in the areas of general administration and research. Two of these secondary uses have been described in detail in Chapters 6 and 7, that is, the pharmacy and blood products systems. These two functions have become integral components of OCIS from both an administrative and clinical care perspective.

A wide variety of other administrative functions, which play a varied role in primary clinical care activities, have been directly integrated into OCIS. However, all of these functions are an essential ingredient in the primary purpose of the Oncology Center, that is, to provide the highest quality care possible to its patients. There is a natural relationship between administrative, clinical, and research activities in a setting such as the Oncology Center, which OCIS has helped to facilitate.

These secondary functions of OCIS include monitoring the patient load of the Center through patient census data and patient mix trends. The inpatient census

---

[1]Sara Perkel, M.B.A., joined the Center in 1983 as the assistant administrator of Oncology. In 1987 she assumed the position of Administrator of Oncology and became fiscally responsible for OCIS operations.

provides an instantaneous picture of bed occupancy, the units that are at highest occupancy, the potential supply needs, and an understanding of the personnel needs for a particular day. On the more demanding and turbulent OPD facility, the projected visits allow administration to be aware of an overload situation and alert other associated areas to potential problems.

Another function is to provide data for personnel and other resource-forecasting activities. As discussed later in this chapter, it is extremely important from an administrative perspective to have the ability to project future needs. Such projection capabilities allow facilities to gear up to meet future demands before they occur. One example of forecasting is based on the fact that the primary treatment of cancer patients is increasingly being provided as an outpatient service. The percentage of outpatient to inpatient facilities will have to be adjusted for in the near future. Another trend noted is that inpatients have become increasingly acute over the past several years. Thus, the nurse-to-patient ratio must be adjusted accordingly.

Data routinely collected by OCIS also allow central administration to respond quickly to data and statistical requests made by the Hospital's central administration and various federal agencies. Additionally, as most procedures and patient charges are captured directly by OCIS, there is an accurate means of documenting services to auditors from both third-party payors and various federal agencies, such as NCI and FDA.

In the following sections of this chapter, examples of these secondary uses in individual functional areas are provided. The authors of the following sections in this chapter are the individuals who have developed and/or are the primary users of these functions. Information on these authors is provided at the beginning of each section. It should be pointed out that there are numerous additional spin-off functions of OCIS that have not been described in detail.

Inpatient Admission, Discharge, Transfer (ADT) Scheduling[2]

The Johns Hopkins Oncology Center (JHOC) contains 70 beds in four inpatient nursing units. There also is a 14-bed Pediatric Oncology Unit residing in the Children's Center of the hospital. OCIS is used to schedule the admissions and discharges for these units. The formal admission process, however, is managed by the central hospital ADT system. In this section we describe how OCIS is used to schedule JHOC inpatient resources and how inpatients are entered into the OCIS database.

The Inpatient Scheduling System

OCIS maintains an on-line scheduling system for oncology inpatient admissions. A physician schedules an admission for a patient with the Oncology Admitting

---

[2]Gloria Stuart is the author of this section.

Office, and the admissions officer enters the data into OCIS. This schedule is available on-line to all users. This allows physicians, nurses and administrative personnel to view expected admissions for each unit. Figure 1 shows a schedule of expected admissions. It is sorted by date of admission and displays patient history number, name, inpatient unit, and reason for admission.

The use of the OCIS inpatient scheduling function is restricted to the Department of Oncology Admissions and OCIS clinical data coordinators. New patients can be scheduled for admission without a medical record number by the automatic generation of a unique temporary "dummy number" through OCIS. When the patient is actually admitted to an inpatient unit, OCIS will insist that a valid medical record number be entered before the admission can be completed.

OCIS Admission/Discharge Function

Each inpatient admission in the Oncology Center and Pediatric Oncology is entered into the OCIS census. These entries are maintained by the clinical data coordinators assigned to the inpatient units. When a patient is physically admitted to a bed on an inpatient unit, the data coordinator enters the admission into OCIS. If the patient is listed on the OCIS scheduled admit list, the coordinator transfers the name from the schedule to the inpatient census, making any corrections to the date, reason for admission, or the location displayed on the scheduled admission list. The coordinator will also enter the expected length of stay (LOS), which is based on documentation from the physician. Long stays are entered as 15 days and are modified when the estimated LOS reaches 14 days or less; OCIS automatically subtracts days for an estimated LOS of 14 or less. This listing of LOS assists the physicians in planning bed utilization. Naturally, the coordinator can modify the estimated LOS at any time should the discharge planning data change.

As noted in Chapter 6, the OCIS pharmacy applications are tied to the OCIS census. Because no orders can be entered into the system if the patient is not on the OCIS census, oncology pharmacists have been provided with admissions capabilities as well. However, the data coordinator is responsible for seeing that the census entry is correct.

Upon patient discharge, the coordinator enters the date of discharge, as well as the patient status (discharge, transfer, expired). It should be noted that, although the census/pharmacy admission is tied, the census discharge does not result in a pharmacy discharge, since this would stop active pharmacy orders currently running. Instead, the pharmacy receives an electronic message that a census discharge has occurred. Pharmacy verifies that this information is correct and then initiates a pharmacy discharge that stops the active pharmacy orders. This is an important quality control measure to ensure that critical medications are not interrupted in the event of a discharge error by the clinical data coordinator. In addition, no census discharge is processed until the patient has physically left the inpatient unit.

As stated earlier, the main Admissions Department of the hospital maintains a separate system that also records all admissions and discharges for the entire

SAMPLE: SCHEDULED ADMITS

```
JOHNS HOPKINS OCIS        OUTPATIENT TERMINAL        01/22/87

           SCHEDULED ADMISSIONS IN CHRONOLOGICAL ORDER

DATE        UNIT    HIST NO    NAME
01/11/87    3S      2222222    PATIENT,A      COMMENTS
01/12/87    PED     4566666    PATIENT,B      AUTO-BMT;CR2
01/13/87    3S      9900987    PATIENT,C      I-131
            3S      5656565    PATIENT,D      DONOR:PATIENT,SISTER
            PED     4444444    PATIENT,E      CHEMO/PA
01/17/87    2S      1555565    PATIENT,F      CHEMO/PA
            3S      9999999    PATIENT,G      AC-D-AC  AUG.(J8410-B
            3S      4321212    PATIENT,H      BMT-CML
            3S      3332222    PATIENT,I      BMT
01/21/87    2N      2222455    PATIENT,J      BMT-LYMPH
            2N      9876542    PATIENT,K      CHEMOTHERAPY
                                             CHEMOTHERAPY
```

Figure 1. Schedule of expected admissions.

hospital. There are several reasons for this duplication. All inpatient billing is the responsibility of the central hospital systems; naturally, they need the admission and discharge data to support this function. From the JHOC perspective, the inpatient census establishes a central link for many of the internal operations of the Center. We have seen that a patient must be entered into the OCIS census before any pharmacy orders can be entered into the system. A unit-specific on-line census is available to all users throughout the Oncology Center. This serves as a patient locator; a physician can access any terminal in the Center and view the number of patients on a given unit at that time (or their clinical data). Finally, the OCIS census provides a mechanism for recording the dates of all admissions and discharges for a historical review by patient, unit, diagnosis, protocol, etc.

The standard format for the unit census is the inpatient OCIS home screen shown in Chapter 4. This menu sorts the patients' names alphabetically and displays medical record number, date of admission, and estimated LOS. In addition to the on-line census, there are a number of census reports generated on a daily basis.

The admitting census is generated at 11:30 P.M. each day. It is a snapshot of the census for the Center at that time. More than 60 copies of this report are produced for use by health care professionals throughout the Center. The admitting census is sorted by inpatient location and displays history number, name, diagnosis, admission date, and estimated length of stay for the current inpatients. In addition, the report lists scheduled admissions for each unit sorted by date. A sample is shown in Figure 2.

As discussed in Chapter 4, the OCIS inpatient census serves a number of other important functions. The admission data are kept on line for a historical perspective. Because the data are patient specific and on line, the census allows a physician to review immediately the data of the last admission for his patient, as well as the number of days of hospitalization. The census also contains other helpful information, such as outpatient visits and protocol history.

To illustrate how the clinical and administrative functions are linked, consider this example. It is common JHOC practice to administer chemotherapy in an outpatient setting and delay admission until such time as a toxic reaction develops. This approach improves the patient's comfort and also reduces the cost of treatment. Naturally, the technique requires planning. The on-line census is one tool that aids the physician in this planning process. If a patient is hospitalized for low blood counts following an earlier course of chemotherapy, the physician can review the census to determine the number of days following chemotherapy that the admission occurred and the length of stay. This information can be used when planning another course of the same chemotherapy. The patient's response can be anticipated, and an admission can be scheduled to reserve a bed.

Support to the Outpatient Department (OPD)[3]

The Outpatient Department (OPD) is a significant and growing component of patient care at the Oncology Center. During its early development it became obvious that in order for OCIS to be effective, it was essential to incorporate functions for the OPD. The close links between the inpatient units and the OPD have grown over time as a result of the increasing importance of ambulatory care in the treatment of cancer.

Structure and Flow

The basic functions of the Center's OPD are similar to those of other ambulatory areas. Patients come to the OPD to see their physicians, to get treatment, and to have blood or radiology tests. Like many ambulatory care areas, there is a great deal of diversity in its functions and in the duties of its staff. The diversity of activity, combined with a patient load that approaches capacity, creates an obvious need for automation wherever possible. Additionally, there is a need for each of the automated functions to be integrated and to run in real time, which is essential for the OPD environment. As with any OPD, communication between providers is a critical element in effective and efficient patient care.

The Johns Hopkins Oncology Center OPD is a busy clinical area with two practice sites. The consultation service is located in a geographically separate office building and serves new patient consultations and breast cancer programs. OPD

---

[3]This section was written by Lisa Lattal, M.H.A., J.D., who joined the Oncology Center in 1986 as the Ambulatory Services Manager. She has over 10 years experience in ambulatory health care facility management. She has participated in the ongoing development of the outpatient functions of OCIS over the past several years.

```
JOHNS HOPKINS OCIS                    ADMITTING CENSUS            05/11/88

2N  INPATIENT CENSUS X8910  -  SOLID TUMOR SERVICE

 1  7779994   PATIENT,FIVE        8  222   LEUKEMIA, ACUTE LYM      05/11/88
 2  7779992   PATIENT,THREE       4  213   LUNG, ADENOCARCINOMA     04/27/88
 3  7778882   PATIENT,TWO         3  222   LEUKEMIA, ACUTE MYEL - B 05/04/88

2N  SCHEDULED ADMISSIONS X8910  -  SOLID TUMOR SERVICE

 1  05/14/88  7779992  PATIENT,THREE          LUNG, ADENOCARCINOMA  CHEMOTHERAPY
                       243-4260

3N  INPATIENT CENSUS X8915  -  SOLID TUMOR SERVICE

 1  7779996   PATIENT,SIX        14  314   BREAST CARCINOMA         05/11/88

3N  SCHEDULED ADMISSIONS X8915  -  SOLID TUMOR SERVICE


2S  INPATIENT CENSUS X8880  -  LEUKEMIA SERVICE

 1  7778883   PATIENT,THREE      15  267   M-6/ACUTE MYEL LEUK      05/08/88
 2  7779991   PATIENT,TWO         7  277   BREAST CARCINOMA         05/05/88

2S  SCHEDULED ADMISSIONS X8880  -  LEUKEMIA SERVICE

 1  03/25/88  7777777  TEST,PATIENT           M-5/ACUTE MYEL LEUK  TEST OCIS
                       955-6865

3S  INPATIENT CENSUS X8995  -  BONE MARROW TRANSPLANT SERVICE

 1  7778884   PATIENT,FOUR       15  375   LEUKEMIA, ACUTE MYEL - B 05/04/88
 2  7778881   PATIENT,ONE        15  374   GASTRIC CARCINOMA        05/11/88

3S  SCHEDULED ADMISSIONS X8995  -  BONE MARROW TRANSPLANT SERVICE
```

Figure 2. Scheduled admissions for each unit sorted by date.

provides examination rooms for physician and nurse visits, and includes a large infusion area for the administration of intravenous treatments and the carrying out of nonsurgical procedures. Both locations together see approximately 26,000 patient visits annually and service 50 physicians.

The primary administrative functions of the OPD include patient registration, appointment scheduling, flow tracking and control, charge capture, resource utilization monitoring, and forecasting future requirements. The OCIS serves to automate and integrate these functions. By doing so, it provides an essential component in the efficient operation of an OPD—communication.

The Johns Hopkins Oncology Center OPD depends heavily on OCIS for the administrative and medical components of patient care. OCIS terminals have been located in strategic places to facilitate the retrieval of this information. All clerical employees have OCIS terminals at their workstations. Several are spread throughout the physician/nurse work space, which is the staff's base of operations while they see patients. Terminals are also located throughout nursing areas and in ancillary departments. The general availability of data services throughout the OPD helps improve staff members' efficiency.

All patients are preregistered in OCIS prior to their first encounter with the OPD. Demographics, insurance information, and preliminary clinical data are collected in the preregistration function. Patients are registered into OCIS at each visit. The scheduling function is the master patient and physician tracking system. Patient visits to physicians and other providers, laboratory tests, radiology tests, and outpatient procedures are all integrated in the OCIS schedule system.

The schedule and registration information is used as a guide to track and control patient flow. Patient flow-tracking forms are printed and appointment history records are maintained. The collected data are used for charge capture, and statistical and documentation purposes. Charge capture is the process whereby a day's activity is translated into billing information. Charges are collected on a patient-specific basis and are distributed to all appropriate billing offices. The collection of all these data provides a substantial database that can be used for monitoring resources and forecasting future needs.

Patient Registration

The OCIS allows for two types of registration. The first of these is a new patient preregistration. This is done by the new patient referral coordinator for every patient who is new to the OPD. The second type of registration is a return registration. This is the routine registration that occurs every time a patient comes to visit the OPD and is checked in by a registrar.

New Patient Pre-registration. All patients referred to the OPD for the first time are screened by the referral coordinator, who reviews the patient's basic referral data and schedules a preliminary appointment for physician consultation. After the referral coordinator has determined that a patient is eligible to be seen at the JHOC and will be scheduled for an appointment, the pre-registration is then begun.

Because the time between appointment scheduling and when the appointment takes place is relatively short, pre-registration information is collected by telephone and directly entered into the database. The availability of pre-registration information avoids a protracted on-site interview at the time of the first visit. It also allows the referral coordinator to assign a hospital history number prior to the visit. The basic demographic, insurance, and referral information collected is also used in clinical decisions, billing functions, and research concerning the patient population.

Insurance information and primary diagnosis and histology information are routinely collected for new patients as part of pre-registration. The referral coordinator also obtains the reason for the consultation in the patient's or the referring physician's own words. Data on referring physicians are collected including the physician's name, hospital number if any, and mailing address to which copies of medical records should be sent.

Specific diagnosis-related data may be requested of the patient. Such items are identified in a "Diagnosis Data Requested" section. Examples include a referring

```
JOHNS HOPKINS ONCOLOGY CENTER              DATE OF INITIAL REFERRAL
NEW REFERRAL REQUEST FORM

TEST,PATIENT - 7777777
                                           DOB: 10/10/40  SEX: M  RACE: CAUCASIAN
1201 S. COURT HOUSE, BALTIMORE, MD  21218PHONE:
MARITAL STATUS: SINGLE                     SPOUSE:
MOTHER:                                    FATHER:
------------------------------------------------------------------------------
INSURANCE INFORMATION
EMPLOYER:
                                           INSURANCE CO.:

EMPLOYER'S ADDRESS:                        INSURANCE ADDRESS:


EMPLOYER'S TELEPHONE:                      POLICYHOLDER:
EMPLOYEE:                                  POLICY #:
                                           PLAN #:            GROUP #:

SECONDARY INFORMATION:
--------------------
EMPLOYER:
                                           INSURANCE CO.:

EMPLOYER'S ADDRESS:                        INSURANCE ADDRESS:


EMPLOYER'S TELEPHONE:                      POLICYHOLDER:
EMPLOYEE:                                  POLICY #:
                                           PLAN #:            GROUP #:
------------------------------------------------------------------------------
PRIMARY DIAGNOSIS:          HISTOLOGY:          DATE:
                                                ROUTINE ____    URGENT ____
REASON FOR CONSULT:
------------------------------------------------------------------------------
REFERRING PHYSICIAN:
    ---- NO REFERRING PHYSICIANS ----
------------------------------------------------------------------------------
DX DATA REQUESTED:    _____  REFERRING PHYSICIAN LETTER  RECEIVED: _____
                      _____  TREATMENT RECORDS           RECEIVED: _____
                      _____  HOSPITAL MEDICAL RECORDS    RECEIVED: _____
                      _____  PATHOLOGY SLIDES            RECEIVED: _____
                      _____  X-RAY FILM                  RECEIVED: _____
                      _____  SCAN FILMS                  RECEIVED: _____
                      _____  JHH CHART                   RECEIVED: _____
                      _____  JHH X-RAY                   RECEIVED: _____
------------------------------------------------------------------------------
APPOINTMENT DATE:           TIME:              JHOC:
```

Figure 3. On-line New Patient Referral Form.

physician letter, treatment records, hospital medical records, pathology slides, x-ray film, scan films, Johns Hopkins Hospital chart if any, and Johns Hopkins Hospital x-ray if any. This section allows the referral coordinator to keep track of when this particular information was requested and when it was received. It also provides control so that the Center knows when or if it has received items belonging to a patient for review by the physicians.

Finally, the pre-registration includes the date and time of the patient's first appointment and the name of the physician the patient is scheduled to see. This is done through OCIS using the scheduling system.

Pre-registration data are retrievable on line and in hard copy. The on-line function is called the "New Patient Referral Form." The data collected can be viewed in its entirety on an OCIS screen. In the hard-copy format, the information is printed on a single page (Figure 3). The form can be used by the referral coordinator to document the receipt of requested data and is also included in the new patient's medical record. In this way the consulting physician has the benefit of all of the information gathered previously by the referral office.

Return Registration. The second type of registration is performed when the patient comes to the OPD. Each registrar receives a daily hard-copy schedule, produced by OCIS. The schedule shows those patients expected for appointments on that particular day, and which provider the patient is scheduled to see. The registrar verifies that the demographics and insurance information are correct, and updates any changes. The registrar completes the process by filling out any necessary forms, indicating in OCIS that the appointment has been kept.

Automated Scheduling System

The OCIS provides an automated scheduling system that allows multiple users to schedule appointments and multiple viewers to view these schedules simultaneously. It permits on-line scheduling and instantaneous changing.

Scheduled Items. Every time a patient has an appointment to see a physician, and every time the patient is scheduled to come to the OPD to see a nurse, have a procedure done, receive chemotherapy, or have another test, the patient's encounter is scheduled into OCIS.

Schedules are created in a variety of ways. The registrar or referral coordinator enters into OCIS the patient's name, who he or she is to see, and the date and time of the appointment. The registrar also schedules any anticipated laboratory tests and x-rays or other radiology services that the physician has ordered for this patient.

By using this system, the registration staff can anticipate the patient's arrival and paper work can be prepared prior to the patient's visit. When the patient comes to check in, the registrar can view the list of tests that have been ordered for that patient, compare it with the completed forms, give the paperwork to the patient, and direct the patient to the next stop.

A registrar who wants to make an appointment for the given patient will, upon selecting the appointment function, be given a choice of the site at which the patient is to be seen. These choices include each of the ambulatory care delivery sites. A registrar in one delivery site can schedule a return appointment for the same or a different service location within the Oncology Center. This prevents the patient from having to walk to the area where the next appointment will be, and it also reduces the amount of interdepartmental telephone activity that would be required to schedule appointments in multiple sites.

Within each department, appointments are organized by clinics. A "clinic" is a way of classifying patient appointments on the basis of the service to be received or the type of provider. For example, a clinic may include only those patients who are scheduled to see a physician during their visit, or only patients who are scheduled to see a nurse or a physician assistant. This allows an administrative segregation of visit types, which is useful as a base for statistical reporting and resource use analysis.

Scheduling Authority. Input to an automated scheduling system is carefully controlled. In contrast to viewing the automated scheduling system, the input function has a higher possibility of error. Input of patient appointments into the scheduling system is limited to specially trained and supervised members of the registration and referral staff. Although nurses and physicians can view the appointment system in any one of a number of ways, they are not permitted to enter appointment data into OCIS.

Patient convenience may be enhanced by having a registrar schedule all appointments and ancillary tests. During the encounter, the follow-up actions are recorded. This includes the time of the next visit plus any tests to be completed prior to the time the patient returns. The registrar coordinates the scheduling of these activities in a way that is most convenient for the patient. For example, if the patient prefers, all tests and appointments can be scheduled on the same day. After an appointment is scheduled, OCIS lets the registrar select a printed appointment reminder slip. This slip is usually generated so that the patient will have a written record of the date and time of the next appointment.

Schedule Framework. OCIS allows the user to create a framework in which to schedule by entering certain parameters into the system, including the physician baseline schedule, vacations, and holidays. The registrar can enter a physician's preformatted schedule preferences, which will be retained for all future scheduling until they are changed. (Quite often the physician's other commit-

```
                    ONCOLOGY INFORMATION SYSTEM              11/02/88
                       APPOINTMENT SYSTEM
                        MEDICAL ONCOLOGY

*** BASE LINE SCHEDULE FOR  DOCTOR,WILLIAM P. MD
DAY                    FROM         TO
-------------------------------------------------------------------
MONDAY             8:30 AM   12:00 PM
                   1:30 PM    4:00 PM
FRIDAY            10:00 AM   11:30 AM
                   1:00 PM    4:00 PM

--- VACATION/ABSENCE SCHEDULED FOR DOCTOR,WILLIAM P. MD
FROM       TO        DAY     START TIME   END TIME   C.ID  COMMENT
-------------------------------------------------------------------
11/22/88   11/22/88  ALL       9:00 AM     2:00 PM   WPM  PDQ MTG
12/21/88   12/30/88  ALL       8:00 AM     5:00 PM   WPM  VACATION
01/12/89   01/14/89  ALL       8:00 AM     5:00 PM   WPM  GOG MTG, DENVER
01/24/89   01/24/89  ALL       9:00 AM     2:00 PM   WPM  PDQ MTG
02/28/89   02/28/89  ALL       9:00 AM     2:00 PM   WPM  PDQ MTG
03/06/89   03/24/89  ALL       8:00 AM     5:00 PM   WPM  EORTC/VACATION
03/21/89   03/21/89  ALL       9:00 AM     2:00 PM   WPM  PDQ MTG
04/25/89   04/25/89  ALL       9:00 AM     2:00 PM   WPM  PDQ MTG
05/21/89   05/28/89  ALL       8:00 AM     5:00 PM   WPM  ASCO/AACR
05/30/89   05/30/89  ALL       9:00 AM     2:00 PM   WPM  PDQ MTG
```

Figure 4. Automated scheduling system appointment entry screen.

```
                    ONCOLOGY INFORMATION SYSTEM                  11/02/88
                         APPOINTMENT SYSTEM
                         MEDICAL ONCOLOGY

SCHEDULED FOR   (ONC)   BEGINNING: 11/02/88   (WED)

  DATE      TIME      NAME                        HIST #   PROVIDER
--------------------------------------------------------------------------
11/02/88
             8:00 AM/K PATIENT,JOHN               654589   DOCTOR,ONE.
             8:30 AM/K PATIENT,SARA               798745   DOCTOR,TWO.M.D.
             8:30 AM/K PATIENT,GLORIA             2245171  DOCTOR,THREE,M.D.
             9:00 AM/K PATIENT,NICK               449459   DOCTOR,FOUR,M.D.
             9:00 AM    PATIENT,GARY              1014584  DOCTOR,THREE,M.D.
             9:15 AM/K PATIENT,DENA               544554   DOCTOR,ONE.M.D.
             9:30 AM/K PATIENT,FARIDEH            2344501  DOCTOR,TWO.M.D.
            10:00 AM    PATIENT,ALAN              1484552  DOCTOR,ONE.M.D.
            10:30 AM    PATIENT,MIKE              845308   DOCTOR,TWO.M.D.
            10:30 AM    PATIENT,CHRIS             1045515  DOCTOR,THREE,M.D.
            10:30 AM/K PATIENT,DAVE               2314525  DOCTOR,ONE.M.D.
            11:00 AM/K PATIENT,DONNA              674557   DOCTOR,FIVE,M.D.
            11:00 AM    PATIENT,KAREN             794511   DOCTOR,TWO.M.D.
```

Figure 5. Automated scheduling system schedule view by clinic for specific day.

ments leave a very limited number of time slots in which to see patients.) OCIS allows the permanent recording of these baseline schedules and then permits the registrars to make adjustments for changes as needed. Data entered into the baseline schedule include the days and time blocks on which the provider is available, and the amount of time he or she wants to allocate for each type of visit (Figure 4).

If a provider intends to take a vacation, that fact is entered into his or her OCIS schedule. The supervisor responsible for dictionary maintenance can block out all the appointments previously open for that provider during the time of absence. A registrar cannot schedule a patient to see the physician because the days of absence are already blocked off on the computer. The use of this approach avoids a situation in which one registrar is aware that a provider will be gone on a certain day but forgets to pass that information on to other co-workers.

The ability to format a schedule also allows the registrars to close off available appointments because of a hospital holiday. The supervisor enters into OCIS that a particular day is an OPD holiday. The system will automatically close out appointments for all providers for that day. This feature prevents the need to close out individually appointments for each of 40 or 50 available providers.

Use of Schedule. All OPD users of OCIS have access to viewing the scheduling system. Users have the option of viewing the schedule by physician, patient, or clinic. Within these categories, viewers can examine the schedule for a particular day, a particular period of time, or from the beginning of the patient's history at the center. There is also an option for a print function in case a hard copy of the schedule is needed.

```
JOHNS HOPKINS OCIS                    UNIVERSAL TERMINAL        11/02/88

APPOINTMENTS SCHEDULED FOR PATIENT,MAUREEN    (2848164)
BEGINNING: 10/23/88 (SUN)
 DATE      TIME       TYPE       CLINIC  PROVIDER      COMMENTS
----------------------------------------------------------------------
10/27/88  10:30 AM/K PRIMARY      OPD      NURSE
          10:15 AM/K LAB          DIFN     HEME-8

10/29/88   9:00 AM/K PRIMARY      OPD      NURSE
           8:45 AM/K LAB          DIFN     HEME-8

10/31/88   9:00 AM/K PRIMARY      OPD      NURSE
           8:45 AM/K LAB          DIFN     HEME-8

11/01/88  10:00 AM/K PRIMARY      OPD      NURSE
           9:45 AM/K LAB          DIFN     HEME-8
          12:00 PM/K XRAY         CXR

11/03/88  10:00 AM   PRIMARY      ONC    DOCTOR,FOUR M.D.PER NANCY
           9:45 AM   LAB          BNMARA     CULURN   DIFN    HEME-8   LYTES
                                  MAGNS      MIC UR    SMA-12  URINAL
```

Figure 6. Automated scheduling system search by patient appointments.

In viewing the schedule by clinic, the user is given a choice of ambulatory area to be viewed and is then asked to input the name of the desired clinic schedule. Then, in response to prompts, the user would tell OCIS to display those patients scheduled for the selected clinic on the selected date. The screen will show a list of the patients with an appointment in that clinic for the particular day selected (Figure 5). As can be seen, the screen shows the patient's name, history number, time of appointment, clinic, and provider.

This option also allows the user to determine whether a patient kept any scheduled appointment. A "kept" appointment is designated by a "K" before the patient's name. A "no show" is designated by the absence of the "K." Schedules are maintained on OCIS permanently in an interactive mode. A viewer can search back several years to see whether a particular patient kept a particular appointment (Figure 6).

The schedule view option also allows users to examine schedules by provider. To see a list of patients scheduled for a provider on a particular date, the user would look in the scheduling system under the provider's name for the date in question. The OCIS screen will show a listing of scheduled appointments, including the time and the patient's name and history number (Figure 7).

OCIS also permits viewing of a patient's past and future schedules. This can be selected as a full list of all of the appointments the patient has ever had in the OPD, or as a short schedule beginning from whatever day the user specifies. This option provides a history of the patient's ambulatory activity at the center.

Links of Schedules with Other Areas. An important feature of the scheduling system is its ability to link with other parts of OCIS. Two primary linkages are those with charge capture and medical records.

```
                    ONCOLOGY INFORMATION SYSTEM              11/02/88
                         APPOINTMENT SYSTEM
                         MEDICAL ONCOLOGY

SCHEDULE FOR DOCTOR,MARTIN M.D.   (F34345)
BEGINNING: 11/02/88 (WED)
 DATE      TIME      NAME                        HIST #   CLNC  COMMENTS
------------------------------------------------------------------------
11/02/88  8:30 AM/K  PATIENT,JOE                 798738   ONC
          9:00 AM/K  PATIENT,SAM                 449129   ONC
          9:15 AM/K  PATIENT,CATHY               543254   ONC   PT REQUEST F/U
         11:00 AM/K  PATIENT,JOE                1611810   FON   F/U

11/04/88  8:00 AM    PATIENT,SARA               2351246   FON   NEW

11/09/88  9:00 AM    PATIENT,GLORIA             2334250   OPD
          9:15 AM    PATIENT,FARIDEH            2205177   ONC
         10:00 AM    PATIENT,MIKE               2348656   FON   NEW
         11:00 AM    PATIENT,SETH               1896203   FON   F/U WITH PATTI
```

Figure 7. Automated scheduling system search by physician appointments.

The linkage with charge capture allows the registrars to process patient charges accurately. The day after a patient's visit, OCIS will automatically transfer to charge capture the data on all patients who have kept their appointments. The charge capture registrar then edits this information and adds any additional data in order to complete the charge capture process.

Likewise, the Medical Records Department is sent information from the scheduling system. Medical Records will receive a daily list of those patients scheduled for visits. This serves as the basis for their chart-retrieval function. OCIS also prints a sign out slip which Medical Records can use to inform the medical records clerk which provider has the chart and when it was requested.

These linkages help to expedite communications within the center. The automatic flow of information eliminates the need for a staff member to remember how to communicate these data. Since both functions are of a relatively detailed nature, the automated transfer feature helps to reduce the incidence of error by eliminating the chance of transfer mistakes.

Routine Reports

The OCIS produces a number of routine statistical reports. These allow administration to have accurate information on the volume and distribution of patients within the department. They allow a knowledgeable viewer to look at the distribution of patients and appointments, and determine whether there are any irregularities, and they provide an archival database from which future budgets, volumes, and financial projections can be determined.

Clinic Statistics. The OCIS system produces a clinic statistics report on a daily, monthly, and cumulative fiscal year-to-date basis (Figure 8). This report shows

```
                    JHOC OUTPATIENT CLINIC STATISTICS              11/01/88

                                                    MONTHLY TOTALS FOR:  09/88
     ------------------------------------------------------------------------------
                       : SRG : ONC : BLP : SIM : OPD : COL : BCS : OTC : TOTAL
                       :     :     : BRC :     :     :     :     :     :
                       : 373 : 375 : 376 : 377 : 379 : 380 : 381 : 383 :
     ------------------------------------------------------------------------------
           VISITS:
                 NEW       0    51     0     0    35     1     0     6  :   93
                 RETURN    0   627     0     0   977     0     0   213  : 1817
                 ----------------------------------------------------------------
                 TOTAL     0   678     0     0  1012     1     0   219  : 1910

                 WALK INS  0    77     0     0   180     0     0    24  :  281
     ------------------------------------------------------------------------------
414    5         SIMPLE    0     0     0     0    35     0     0     0  :   35
414 9900         NO CHARGE 0     0     0     0   525     0     0   219  :  744
414 3790         W/ PROC   0     0     0     0   426     0     0     0  :  426
414 3797         RET W/O PROC 0   0     0     0    26     0     0     0  :  426
414 3799         BMT W/ PROC  0   0     0     0     0     0     0     0  :   26
                 ----------------------------------------------------------------
                 TOTAL     0     0     0     0  1012     0     0   219  : 1231
     ------------------------------------------------------------------------------
     ------------------------------------------------------------------------------
5010002          THECAL    0     0     0     0     2     0     0     5  :    7
5010101          CHEM/SIMP 0     0     0     0    50     0     0    11  :   61
5010104          CHEM/INTE 0     0     0     0    50     0     0    18  :   68
5010105          CHEM 60+  0     0     0     0   129     0     0    54  :  183
5010201          HEP PUMP  0     0     0     0     9     0     0     1  :   10
5188000          OLP       0     0     0     0     0     0     0     8  :    8
5188004          OPARACENT 0     0     0     0     0     0     0    11  :   11
5188008          OTHROCN   0     0     0     0     1     0     0     1  :    2
5188016          OASP/CY   0     0     0     0     0     0     0     1  :    1
5188020          OASP BXBM 0     0     0     0     0     0     0    55  :   55
5188040          SK BX     0     0     0     0     1     0     0     9  :   10
5188105          OAMPHO    0     0     0     0     4     0     0     0  :    4
5188110          OLYTE DR  0     0     0     0    25     0     0    27  :   52
5188112          OORAL/NON 0     0     0     0     5     0     0     2  :    7
5188114          OIM/NON   0     0     0     0     2     0     0     3  :    5
5188116          OIV/NON   0     0     0     0    36     0     0    28  :   64
5188160          OPLT/TRAN 0     0     0     0    52     0     0     5  :   57
5188164          ORBC #1   0     0     0     0    84     0     0     3  :   87
5188165          ORBC+     0     0     0     0    86     0     0     0  :   86
5188215          OHEP PUMP 0     0     0     0    13     0     0     3  :   16
5188220          OSK TEST  0     0     0     0     0     0     0     1  :    1
5188230          OCATH     0     0     0     0     2     0     0     1  :    3
5188236          ODRESS    0     0     0     0     3     0     0     0  :    3
5188238          OECG      0     0     0     0     0     0     0     1  :    1
5188300          OHICKPRO  0     0     0     0   101     0     0    28  :  129
5188302          OINFUSPRT 0     0     0     0    26     0     0    12  :   38
                 ----------------------------------------------------------------
                 TOTAL     0     0     0     0   681     0     0   288  :  969
JOB COMPLETED    2:08 PM
END OF JOB
```

Figure 8. Outpatient daily statistics report by patient by clinic.

the number of patients who have visited the OPD during the period of time covered in the report, and categorizes these visits by clinic, by new and return patients, and by scheduled or walk-in patients.

The clinic statistics report also breaks down visits by charge category and enumerates procedures. This again is separated by clinic. Procedures and visits are categorized by hospital revenue and procedure code. In this way department activity can be expressed in terms of billable procedures. This is useful in examining volume and revenue potential. It is also valuable in spotting charge capture problems or changes in practice that may not be evident in any other form.

Outpatient Daily Statistics. This report is also produced on a monthly basis. It shows a breakdown of patients by clinic, and by new and return patients for each day of the month. From this report, the manager can see on one page and in one place a comparison of the new and return patients by day. This allows the manager to look for trends on new and return patients and also allows trends in the clinic population to be determined.

Daily Scheduled Show/No Show Report. The daily scheduled show/no show report gives information by day on the percentage of patients who did not keep their appointments. The report is broken down by clinic and further by new and return patients. The report gives the percentage of kept appointments for both new and return patients, and also the number of unscheduled visits. It totals the number of patients scheduled in clinic on a particular day and those who actually arrived for their appointments, and gives the percentage of patients who kept appointments. This report is issued daily and is also aggregated at the end of each month. It is a valuable tool for tracking problem areas or aberrations on the basis of type of patient visit.

New Patient Report. The new patient report is issued daily and shows the names of new patients who are scheduled for OPD appointments. These new patients are grouped by consulting physician. Appointment times and Hopkins history numbers are also shown. This report is a communication device that informs the physician, medical records, and administrative personnel what patients are new to the department and are scheduled for an appointment on a given day. This report is derived from input to OCIS by the new patient referral coordinator.

Clinic Summary Report. The clinic summary report is used primarily by the registration supervisor and the registration staff to assess the distribution of patient appointments for a particular day (Figure 9). It is printed by clinic, and shows the number of patients who are appointed during particular time slots. The registration supervisor can use this report to determine patient load for staff scheduling and to see when there may be periods of high or low registrar utilization. This report is also useful as a double check on the registrars to be sure that there are not more patients scheduled than the number of exam rooms available. By reviewing this report several days in advance, the registration supervisor can ensure an appropriate distribution of appointments throughout the day and correct any problems before they impact that day's operations.

Patient Flow Control Tracking

The OCIS produces or works with a series of patient-specific forms that aid in patient flow control, tracking, and documentation. These forms are the routing form, the encounter form, the charge voucher, and the documentation label.

```
JOHNS HOPKINS OCIS
        JOHNS HOPKINS ONCOLOGY CENTER -- OUTPATIENT APPOINTMENTS        11/01/88
CLINIC: MEDONC

11/02/88 (WED)
MORNING


             NUMBER OF PATIENTS SCHEDULED FOR THIS DAY: 83

               MORNING TOTAL:                    54

               AFTERNOON TOTAL:                  33

                    NUMBER OF PATIENTS WITH BOTH
                    MORNING AND AFTERNOON APPOINTMENTS
                                                 4


         MORNING HOURLY SCHEDULE
            AUXILIARY APPOINTMENTS ONLY
                       8 AM      1
                       9 AM      3
                      10 AM      5
                      11 AM      2
            AUXILIARY WITH PRIMARY APPOINTMENTS
                       8 AM      9
                       9 AM     14
                      10 AM     10
                      11 AM      5
            PRIMARY APPOINTMENTS
                       8 AM      3
                       9 AM     13
                      10 AM     14
                      11 AM     13


         AFTERNOON HOURLY SCHEDULE
            AUXILIARY APPOINTMENTS ONLY
                      10  PM     1
                      12  NOON   1
                       1  PM     2
                       2  PM     1
                       4  PM     1
            AUXILIARY WITH PRIMARY APPOINTMENTS
                      12  NOON   4
                       1  PM     5
                       2  PM     1
            PRIMARY APPOINTMENTS
                      12  NOON   4
                       1  PM    12
                       2  PM     7
                       3  PM     4
```

Figure 9. Outpatient clinic summary report by day.

The routing form is used as the source document for billing. One routing form is generated by OCIS for each scheduled patient visit (Figure 10). Basic demographic information is printed at the top of the form, including the patient's JHH hospital number, date of birth, and date of visit. At the bottom of the form is the patient's diagnosis. The rest of the routing form consists of a list of procedures and visit types. These are categorized and labeled by hospital revenue and procedure code, and include a text description. If a patient is a walk-in, a blank routing form is used, and the patient identifiers are hand entered.

The Routing Form follows the patient through his or her entire visit in the OPD. Each provider who transacts a billable encounter with the patient indicates this on the routing form by placing a check next to the service provided. At the

```
                        ONCOLOGY CENTER OPD ROUTING FORM

    DATE OF SERVICE  12/26/88              NAME   PATIENT,TWO

    PRO FEES BILLING#                      JHH#    -777-9991

    PHYS  DOC,NOBODY (F0001)               BIRTHDATE  01/01/27
================================================================================
     OUTPATIENT PHYSICIAN SERVICES    :    OUTPATIENT VISIT (414)
                                      : ( ) BREAST LESION EVAL VISIT    3765
    [[CHECK ONE]]      [[CHECK ONE]]  : ( ) BREAST SELF EXAM VISIT      3796
    ( ) MED ONC        PATIENT IS:    : ( ) BREAST SURVEILLANCE SERV.   3792
    ( ) BREAST CONSULT ( ) NEW        : ( ) VISIT W/ PROCEDURE          3790
    ( ) POLYPOSIS      ( ) FOLLOW-UP  : ( ) LIMITED VISIT W/O PROCEDURE 3797
    ( ) IMMUNOTHERAPY  ( ) FOLLOW-UP,EXT: ( ) INTERMEDIATE VISIT        3795
    ( ) BMT                           :         ( ) NURSE PRACTIONER
    ( ) HEENT                         :         ( ) PHYSICIAN ASSISTANT
                                      :         ( ) OTHER:............
    ( ) PSYCHIATRIC    ( ) INDIVID 50 M :
        CONSULT        ( ) INDIVID 25 M : ( ) LAB/X-RAY ONLY            9900

================================================================================
                     ONCOLOGY CHEMOTHERAPY (501)

    ( ) IM/IV - SIMPLE (0-15M)     0101   ( ) INTRAHEPATIC PUMP          0201
    ( ) IV - INTERMEDIATE (16-59M) 0104   ( ) INTRAVENTRICULAR (OMMAYA)  0001
    ( ) IV - COMPLEX               0105   ( ) INTRATHECAL                0002
                CHEMO HOURS:.........    ( ) ORAL                       0103

================================================================================
                     ONCOLOGY PROCEDURES (518)

    ( ) PLATELET TRANSFUSION        8160   ( ) EKG                        8238
    ( ) RBC TRANSFUSION - 1ST UNIT  8164   ( ) URINARY CATHETER INSERTION 8230
    ( ) RBC TRANSFUSION - ADD UNIT  8165   ( ) ENEMA ADMINISTRATION       8234
                                           ( ) THERAPEUTIC DRESSING       8236
    ( ) FLUID/ELECTROLYTE THER - IV 8110
    ( ) ADMIN MEDICATION - ORAL     8112   ( ) SKIN BIOPSY                8040
    ( ) ADMIN MEDICATION - IM       8114   ( ) INTRAVENTRIC (OMMAYA) SPEC 8210
    ( ) ADMIN MEDICATION-IV         8116   ( ) LUMBAR PUNCTURE            8000
    ( ) AMPHOTERICIN INFUSION       8105   ( ) PARACENTESIS               8004
    ( ) INTRADERMAL SKIN TESTS      8220   ( ) THORACENTESIS              8008
    ( ) INTRAHEPATIC PUMP INFUSION  8215   ( ) SIGMOIDOSCOPY              8012
    ( ) ADMIN INFLUENZA VACCINE     8310   ( ) CYST ASPIRATION            8016
    ( ) INFUSAPORT PROCEDURE        8302   ( ) BONE MARROW ASPIRATE/BX    8020
    ( ) HICKMAN CATHETER PROCEDURE  8300   ( ) FEEDING TUBE INSERTION     8305

================================================================================



    DIAGNOSIS: BREAST CARCINOMA


    PROVIDER SIGNATURE:.............................

JOB COMPLETED   2:54 PM
END OF JOB
```

Figure 10. Outpatient routing form for scheduled patient visits.

completion of the patient's visit, the physician signs the routing form to signify that the services indicated have indeed been performed. Routing forms are gathered at the end of the day for input into OCIS charge capture.

Encounter forms are clinical documentation forms that are not generated by OCIS but instead are preprinted. They are used as a source document for the capture of clinical information to be input into OCIS. An encounter form is prepared for each patient visit. It is used by the clinical providers to record clinical data such as medication, chemotherapy orders, and vital signs. At the completion of a patient's visit, the encounter forms are gathered for input into OCIS by a data coordinator. After these data are input, the encounter form becomes a part of the patient's medical record.

The OCIS will print patient billing information onto hospital charge vouchers. Billing information is processed through OCIS by the charge capture system. One type of hard-copy output from charge capture is a printout of billable charges on a standard Hopkins hospital charge voucher. In this way the OCIS-generated output can be integrated directly into an existing hospital system for processing by the Outpatient Billing Department. The printing of charge vouchers also introduces another check into the accuracy of patient bills. After charge vouchers are printed, the registrar who entered the billing data is able to review the work by inspecting the charge vouchers before they are forwarded to the billing department. This allows the registrar to catch errors before they are printed on bills and sent to insurers or patients. Errors are corrected in OCIS, and corrected vouchers are then printed.

OCIS also produces various labels which are placed on encounter forms to ensure complete documentation. They are used to record information on the administration of platelets and red blood cells. By using these labels, the provider is reminded of which pieces of data are needed to properly document the procedure that is taking place. These labels help ensure consistency and completeness in documentation. They are affixed by hand onto the patient's encounter form. Although the label is printed blank, and does not capture any patient data from OCIS, the use of the label ensures that the appropriate information has a better chance of being captured.

Charge Capture

The OCIS charge capture function allows for the computerized collection and recording of patient charges incurred in the OPD. It also maintains an on-line record of past charges so they can be referenced in the future.

Patient charge information is retrieved in two ways, directly through OCIS and from OCIS-generated hard copy. The charge capture program is linked to the patient scheduling system. As described above, when a patient presents for a scheduled appointment, the registrar signals this to OCIS through an appointment-kept flag. OCIS then transfers its data about this appointment directly to charge capture. The charge capture registrar is presented with baseline data that list the patient's scheduled appointments and any laboratory tests, x-rays, or procedures that were ordered. If a patient appeared for an appointment and tests were ordered, OCIS presumes that these tests were carried out. Any variations from this can be recorded in the charge capture editing process.

The charge capture function is a mixture of editing and data entry. The registrar views each patient's account and then adjusts it as necessary to be sure it is correct. For example, if the patient was scheduled for a Heme-8 lab test, but the laboratory informs the registrar that the test was canceled, it is then deleted from that patient's list of charges. This is the editing function.

The data entry function consists of entering any additional charges incurred by the patient and not included on the patient's original list of charges. The primary source documents for this are the routing form and an OCIS list of pharmacy charges. As described earlier, the routing form is the patient-specific document used by the physician and nursing staffs to record billable services. The charge capture registrar examines each completed routing form and the pharmacy charge list for additional charges, and will then input this information into OCIS so that the patient's charge record is complete and accurate. When one patient's record is complete, the registrar will then move to the next patient and repeat the same procedure.

In order for this system to work successfully, all faculty and staff members must be conscious of the importance of accurate and complete charge capture. This requires education. The provider is expected to document his or her services clearly and accurately. The laboratory must remember to inform the charge capture registrar if a scheduled test is canceled. Likewise, each frontline registrar must be compulsive about accurately recording whether patients have or have not appeared for their scheduled appointments.

This system does have some checks built in. The list of drug charges generated by OCIS from input by the pharmacy provides a check for recording the administration of chemotherapy, which is the most costly procedure. By using this type of check system, the chances of missing important charges or incorrectly charging for services that were not delivered are minimized.

After all the charges for a given day are put into the system, OCIS will print the data gathered in charge capture in two formats. One format is for hospital billing and the other is for professional fee billing. The hospital billing data are printed on individual hospital charge vouchers, as described above. The professional fee billing data are printed in report format, listing all patients to be billed, all billable procedures that may have a professional fee component, the name of the provider, and patient identifiers. The Professional Fee Billing Office can then use this report as the basis for issuing bills for physician services.

The database created by charge capture is an extremely valuable tool. It is used as the source for multiple operational statistics. In addition, the lists of billed patient procedures are stored in OCIS. If there is a problem with a patient bill a staff member can view on line a copy of the patient's outpatient charges incurred on a particular day (Figure 11). This provides a rapid response to patients and assists in maintaining quality control.

Resource Forecasting

The database collected by OCIS provides a wealth of historical information for use in resource forecasting. In addition to the standard reports, data can be arrayed in any number of ways by writing a program in OCIS. Using these historical data, the manager can prepare more educated forecasts of future patient volume.

```
                    ONCOLOGY INFORMATION SYSTEM
                       MEDICAL ONCOLOGY                    11/02/88

PATIENTS' OTHER CHARGES LISTING


     DATE   ENC.TYPE    ENC.UNIT   PROC.CODE    FIN.CODE   CLN   PRICE
-------------------------------------------------------------------------

2118083 - PATIENT,LINDA
    10/26/88        CLINIC: 279    FIN CD: CIC

            (DIFF-EFFECTIVE 3/15/85)
                C          OUTPAT     4973890

            (HEME-8)
                C          OUTPAT     4973022

            (BLOOD DRAWING)
                C          OUTPAT     4970080

                C          OUTPAT     4143790

            (GUEST TRAY)
                C          OUTPAT     4030700

            (PLATELET PROCESSING CHARGE)
                C          OUTPAT       4814280

            (PLATELET PROCESSING CHARGE)
                C          OUTPAT       4814280
```

Figure 11. Outpatient charge capture report for individual patient.

For example, in planning the number of physicians scheduled to see new patients for the coming fiscal year, OCIS provides historical data about the number of new patient visits for the past several years. It refines the data by breaking down new patients into individual clinics and reports what percentage of scheduled new patients did not show up for their appointments. Using these data, the manager can predict trends and obtain an estimate of the required staffing.

The Acuity of the Illness Classification System[4]

The changing environment of health care funding has been influential in stimulating hospitals to manage their resources better. Information systems provide a tool for this. Prospective payment systems, the decreasing length of inpatient stay, and a shift toward a higher proportion of more severely ill hospitalized patients emphasize the need for better tools to project long-term use of resources and to manipulate day-to-day adjustments in patient care staffing.

---

[4]The author of this section is Linda M. Arenth, M.S., who joined the Oncology Center as Director of Nursing in 1974. In 1976 she began the development of the oncology patient classification system. In 1987 she became Vice-President for Nursing and Patient Services at The Johns Hopkins Hospital.

The number of nurses needed to staff a hospital unit is based on the number of patients on that unit and the severity of their illness. When planning for a new cancer center began, nursing recognized a need to gather data that would be useful in planning long-term staffing strategies and also in managing current staff resources.

The oncology patient classification system (OPCS) was developed to address the need for a quantifiable measure of the special-care needs of patients admitted to the Oncology Center and to address limitations in available patient classification instruments. Primarily, these instruments did not reflect the special requirements for patient care associated with current cancer therapies. Additionally, they tended to be specific for an institution, generally for medical–surgical patients, and focused on tasks.

Through a retrospective review of patient experience, it was concluded that the primary determinant of oncology patient care needs was the type of treatment and its associated clinical course. A secondary factor was the extent of disease and its associated physiological impairment. The intent of the OPCS was to capture the special-care needs of patients such as the needs associated with severe bone marrow aplasia following bone marrow transplantation or intensive chemotherapy treatment, untoward effects of chemotherapy or radiation therapy, the evaluation of new drug or radiation therapies, and severe disease.

Patient care requirements vary by the type and phase of treatment. Levels of care required during different phases of hospitalization are often predictable and directly related to specific times following treatment-induced toxicity such as lowered white blood count or platelet depression. Clinical experience provided the basis for designing this classification system which relates care requirements to resource utilization. Further, the OPCS provides a practical method of forecasting and monitoring patient requirements for nursing resources.

The OPCS categorizes patients by acuity of illness and divides the associated intensity of nursing services into five levels of care using a simple data collection instrument. It contains 41 critical indicators which are descriptive phrases of the clinical conditions or support situations that have the greatest impact on nursing resources and for which there are predictable sequences of nursing interventions. The critical indicators were defined by a panel of experts. Standard nursing hours per patient day (NHPPD) were assigned to each level of care. These were based on standard NHPPD for patient classification categories of care reported in the literature and an estimation of the nursing resources required for each. Patients are concurrently categorized every 24 hours on the basis of an assessment of their clinical situation.

The critical indicators are defined on a single, easy to use form. They are grouped into five levels of severity, categorized from grade 1 (minimal severity—patients ambulatory and able to care for themselves, but hospitalized for protective isolation) to grade 5 (maximum life support—patient in cardiovascular collapse requiring intravenous pressors and external ventilator support). To determine the level of care, beginning with the highest level of nursing care (category V), the nurse checks the first appropriate indicator on the classification instrument. The overall level of care is determined by the highest level of care in which an indicator is checked. Implicit in the categorization scheme is the assumption that indicators within and below each level of care may also be applicable, but checking multiple indicators is not necessary and does not change the designated level of care. Reliability has been demonstrated by a consistently high level of agreement between two nurse raters. The medical record provides supportive documentation for the assigned level of care. Content validity was established by a panel of nursing experts. Physicians provided supportive information relative to medical practice.

After four years experience, an evaluation of the system was undertaken to provide further evidence of the instrument's validity. A criterion-related approach was taken. This involved a concurrent audit comparing observed nursing time and effort using work measurement methods and nursing hours established for each level of care in the classification instrument. The results indicated that the mean nursing hours observed for each level of care were not significantly different from the standard nursing hours of care, with the exception of category V. The variance observed in category V reflected the groupings of multiple activities that occur when patients are classified as intensive and is related to limitations of the work measurements.[5]

Since its inception, the OPCS has provided a simple, reproducible, and reliable method for categorizing patients each day according to their use of nursing resources. A summary of monthly data available through OCIS is illustrated in Figure 12. Monthly and year-to-date statistics on census, acuity, and occupancy rate are compared with those for the same month in the prior year and the year to date. NHPPD can be computed by multiplying the average acuity score by 4.

We believe that the OPCS provides a better indication of actual requirements for patient care resources than other systems that do not account for the variations in patient acuity that we have observed with cancer treatment. Of specific concern is patient classification by diagnosis-related groups (DRGs), the basis for hospital case mix management under Medicare prospective payment. Variations in patient acuity and the greater use of hospital resources that may occur during the treatment phase of hospitalization are not fully accounted for in the DRG payment rate.

Classification data from our experience with patients on treatment protocols reflect utilization of patient care resources and permit one to predict the care (costs) required for future patients. The OPCS has contributed to the effective management of patient care resources and can be used to reflect case mix severity, nursing utilization and productivity, resource utilization, program and budget planning, and nursing and hospital costs. The applicability of the system to oncology practice in other clinical settings has been demonstrated with modifications, when indicated, to reflect differences in protocols and practice.

---

[5]L.M. Arenth, The Development and Validation of an Oncology Patient Classification System, *Oncology Nursing Forum*, 12:17–22, 1985.

	TOTALS: 06/87			TOTALS: 06/86		
	TOT CEN	AVG ACC	OCC %	TOT CEN	AVG ACC	OCC %
2N	352	2.84	83.8	335	2.80	79.8
2S	401	3.34	95.5	268	3.16	63.8
3N	582	2.90	88.2	461	2.70	85.4
3S	462	3.25	77.0	418	2.90	87.1
CENTER	1797	3.08	85.6	1482	2.86	79.7
PED	283	2.87	67.4	350	2.85	83.3

	FISCAL YEAR TO DATE			FISCAL YEAR END 06/86		
	TOT CEN	AVG ACC	OCC %	TOT CEN	AVG ACC	OCC %
2N	4037	2.72	79.0	4427	2.72	86.6
2S	4748	3.34	92.9	4449	2.98	87.1
3N	5965	2.75	77.8	5029	2.74	88.9
3S	5907	3.08	84.8	18997	2.88	88.5
CENTER	20657	2.97	83.1	18997	2.88	88.5
PED	3434	2.80	67.2	3736	2.86	77.7

Figure 12. Nursing patient classification system monthly statistics.

A Resource Management, Forecasting, and Reimbursement System[6]

Background

Since 1985, personnel at the Oncology Center have been developing a case mix database and analysis system. The system was established in response to specific internal resource management needs and to the hospital regulatory environment. In regard to management, in the early 1980s administrative personnel began using personal computers and associated financial application packages, such as Lotus 1-2-3, to forecast and manage resources at the Center. Over time, it became apparent that a more sophisticated database and analytic system would be useful in future planning efforts.

Concurrently, a substantial growth in hospital costs prompted a series of federal, state, and third-party-payor efforts to control inpatient costs through prospective per case reimbursement for hospital stays. Of the federal strategies, the most controversial has been the use of the Yale ICD-9-CM diagnosis-related

[6]This section was authored by Catherine Kelleher, Sc.D., M.P.H., M.S.N., who joined the Oncology Center in 1986 as a faculty member. Her primary research interest has been in the development of inpatient, outpatient, and episode-of-care classifications for cancer patients.

group (DRG) classification for payment of inpatient services used by Medicare beneficiaries. The DRG payment scheme was approved by Congress in 1983 with a three-year national implementation period. Passage of this legislation stimulated many state and third-party payors to begin experimentation with DRG payment for beneficiary groups of all age ranges.

Since their implementation, DRGs have not been found to account for much of the variability in use of resources by acute care inpatients. As a result, government and third-party payors continue to experiment with modifications of the original methodology. They also increasingly fund research designed to develop severity-of-illness adjustments and to identify other characteristics to be used in conjunction with DRGs to account for variability in inpatient use of resources.

The Oncology Center case mix system is specifically designed for management and health services research applications. The primary management goal is to identify patient and provider characteristics that can be used to pinpoint deficiencies in quality and efficiency of care, and to forecast resource requirements. The research goal is to develop policies and recommendations for reimbursement methods that will yield more equitable compensation for oncology patient care. The specific policy research includes the development of models for payment of inpatient care on a per stay basis and investigation of approaches for capitation payment inclusive of inpatient and outpatient services over defined periods of time.

Data Sources and Structure

The database used by this system is a composite of information from a variety of institutional sources. The major data elements available through the case mix system are displayed in Table 1. The sources include The Johns Hopkins Hospital billing and discharge abstract systems, and data from the OCIS. The OCIS supplies a significant portion of the clinical data.

The database structure mimics the OCIS in that cross-sectional and longitudinal analyses can be done at patient and population levels. The primary unit of data collection is the patient rather than a specific element of patient care. This provides flexibility in the use of the database.

Merging selected subsets of data from the OCIS and other hospital information systems was not the only option in designing the case mix system. Among the alternatives was the selection of one or more of the financial and utilization management packages currently available on the market. These packages were developed in response to the evolving hospital regulatory climate and the need to collect data to go beyond DRGs in attempts to understand what drives length of stay and costs.

Use of ready-made packages was not an attractive choice owing to the numerous shortcomings of most that were available. First, they were narrow in focus and not easily adapted to broader applications. Second, they were not easily modified to permit collection of additional data items found to be important in explaining use of resources. Third, they appeared to be marketed with built-in

Table 1. Variables, the Johns Hopkins Oncology Center Inpatient Case Mix Analysis System

Variables	Source*
Resource variables	
Length of hospital stay	
Charges adjusted to cost and for inflation	A/O
Total for the hospital stay	B
Subsets of the total for hospital stay (room and board, supplies, pharmacy, blood products, laboratory, etc.)	B
Patient clinical variables	
Age	A/O
Admission urgency	A
Repeated admissions	
First Johns Hopkins Oncology Center admission	O
Number of Johns Hopkins Oncology Center admissions in the past 6, 12, 18, 24 months	A/O
Diagnosis	
ICD-9-CM diagnos(es) for the hospital stay	A
ICD-9-CM diagnosis-related group (DRG) for the hospital stay	A
ICD-0 diagnosis for the primary cancer	O
Nursing levels of care[†]	
Admission	O
Clinical course	O
Discharge	O
Toxicity-of-treatment indexes[‡]	
Admission	O
Clinical course	O
Discharge	O
Severity-of-illness indexes	
Patient management categories (PMCs) for the hospital stay	A
Systemetrics computerized disease stag(es) for the ICD-9-CM Diagnos(es) for the hospital stay	A
Centralized cancer patient data system (CCPDS) stage for the primary cancer diagnosis	O
Discharge disposition	A
Patient personal variables	
Sex	A/O
Race	A/O
Marital status	A/O
Home–hospital distance	A/O
Payment source	A/O
Hospital variables	
Fiscal year of discharge	A/O
Admission day of the week	A/O
Discharge day of the week	A/O
Admission transfer status	A/O
Protocol status	O

obsolescence because they were regularly superseded by updated versions claiming to take advantage of state-of-the-art improvements in monitoring methodology. Fourth, they did not integrate easily with existing data systems.

In contrast, the basic design of the OCIS was well suited to our needs despite the fact that its installation predated the onset of cost containment concerns. Because it was conceptualized to support medical decision making by minimizing the need for the medical record in conventional hard-copy format, the OCIS on-line data set was substantially more comprehensive than that required by the special-purpose data collection tools critiqued above. In addition, the OCIS data set was also easily linked with other standard data sources available throughout the institution, including the hospital discharge abstract and billing files listed as sources in Table 1.

Information in Table 1 suggests that only one-third of the data items are uniquely from the OCIS. However, most of the items obtained from the hospital discharge abstract file are also available via the OCIS, a circumstance providing the opportunity for data validity checks between the systems. More important, short of a detailed medical record review, the data attributed to the OCIS in the table are only available from this source. It is these particular data that have the most exciting potential to produce new models of hospital resource use by oncology patients.

Preliminary Results

As this book is being written, data analysis is in its early stages and has been limited to data obtained from inpatient hospital stays. A number of pilot studies are underway using selected Oncology Center inpatient discharge data sets to develop models to be tested across multiple fiscal years. Among the findings to date are those using fiscal year 1985 discharges to test the explanatory power of unique data from the OCIS for length of stay.

One of the goals of the case mix system is to develop a toxicity index that can be used to predict inpatient resource utilization. In the preliminary development of this index, five values for each of the 18 clinical parameters being considered for inclusion in the toxicity index were tested through bivariate regression for their ability to explain variation in the natural logarithm of length of stay

---

◀ Footnotes to **Table 1**.

*A: Johns Hopkins Hospital discharge abstract files; B: Johns Hopkins Hospital billing files; O: oncology clinical information system (OCIS).

†Daily nursing care levels are obtained from the Johns Hopkins Oncology Center Department of Nursing oncology patient classification system. For each day of stay, except the day of discharge, the patient is assigned a level of care at midnight for the previous 24 hours.

‡Temperature and 17 laboratory parameters are to be created for inclusion in the indexes. Laboratory parameters to be tested include white blood count, neutrophil count, platelet count, hematocrit, hemoglobin, bilirubin, SGOT, SGPT, alkaline phosphatase, blood urea nitrogen, creatinine, sodium, potassium, chloride, carbon dioxide, calcium, and albumin.

Table 2. Percent Variance Explained for the Natural Logarithm of Length of Stay, Significant Bivariate Regression on Temperature, and Laboratory and Nursing Variables: The Johns Hopkins Oncology Center, Fiscal Year 1985*

Values[†]	N[‡]	First (%)[§]	Last (%)	Min (%)	Max (%)	Min (%)
WBC	1385			1	1	6
NEUT	1317		2	8		7
PLATE	1385	3	9	23	.50+	25
HCT	1385	2	.45+	24	11	53
HGB	1385	2		22	12	52
TEMP	1397	2	3	25	52	63
BUN	1390		7	6	17	30
CREAT	1390		2	3	8	23
ALB	1297		6	24	3	54
SGOT	1278	.32*	1	3	7	12
SGPT	1291	1	4	22	14	20
ALK PHOS	1291		5	3	13	36
BILI	1316		5	1+	11	16
CAL	1339		2	26	6	36
NA	1385		23	13	52	
K	1385	2	33	29	48	
CL	1385	1	30	13	56	
CO2	1385		.35*	21	19	55
Nursing[‖]	1407	3	8	4	38	32

*In fiscal year 1985 there were 1488 discharges; 81 discharges consisting of 54 bone marrow donor admissions and 27 same-day admissions and discharges were eliminated from the analytical data set because their hospital stays were considered atypical from the remaining discharges. In the analytic fiscal year 1985 data set, all cases totaled 1407, the solid tumor set totaled 1121, and the lymphoma and leukemia subset totaled 286.

[†] WBC: white blood cell count; NEUT: neutrophil count; PLATE: platelet count; HCT: hematocrit; HGB: hemoglobin; TEMP: temperature; BUN: BUN; CREAT: creatinine; ALB: albumin; SGOT: SGOT; SGPT: SGPT; PHOS: alkaline phosphatase; BILI: bilirubin; CAL: calcium; NA: sodium; K: potassium; CL: chloride; CO2: carbon dioxide.

[‡] For each toxicity and nursing parameter tested, the actual number of cases having values for it is shown.

[§] Only percentages that are significant are reported. Unless indicated, the p value for the percentage $= .000; + = .01; * = .01 < p \le .05$. All p values are 2-tailed.

[‖] A daily nursing pattern-of-care variable was also tested and explained 36% of the variance. See the section on preliminary results by Catherine Kelleher in the text for a description of the variable.

(Table 2). Five values for each of these parameters were selected as those most likely to give insight into inpatient clinical course. They were the first value, the last value, the minimum value, the maximum value, and the difference between the maximum and the minimum value.

One major finding was that, across all 18 parameters, the first value of the stay explained little or no variance for the natural logarithm of length of stay. This finding is in striking contrast to other derangement indexes, which attempt to get first-day data in order to capture severity of disease before onset of therapy intended to normalize the imbalance. All other values for the clinical parameters were found to provide better explanatory power. The value that provided the greatest explanatory power was the difference between the maximum and minimum for the stay (Table 1). These results suggested that costly physiological abnormalities were largely treatment induced.

A second finding of interest in Table 1 is that selected abnormalities considered resource intensive, such as low white blood cell count, do poorly in explaining variation in the natural logarithm of length of stay because they are just too common in our inpatient mix. In addition, although not shown in Table 1, when correlations were calculated between the 18 clinical parameters being considered for inclusion in the toxicity index, many were found to serve as proxies for each other, including parameters of different organ systems as physiological functions became increasingly deranged.

The above findings were also consistently observed when controlling for diagnosis by stratifying discharges into solid tumor and systemic (leukemia and lymphoma) cases. These results indicate that, for oncology patients, treatment may be an important determinant of length of stay. In addition, the high correlation among the 18 parameters suggests that it will be possible to simplify the toxicity index to a handful of indicators.

Findings for daily nursing acuity ratings obtained from a five-level ordinal rating nursing classification instrument used routinely at the Oncology Center are also displayed in Table 1. These daily nursing ratings are summarized into six variables. Five of the six are constructed in a fashion identical to the temperature and laboratory values (first, last, minimum, maximum, and maximum–minimum values for the stay). The sixth, the daily-nursing-pattern-of-care variable, was designed to capture instability of clinical course. For this sixth variable the daily ratings were used to construct a set of dummy variables that capture patterns of nursing care over the entire hospital stay. Data were coded to reflect a steady care pattern; a steady increasing care pattern; a steady decreasing care pattern; and a fluctuating pattern. Because of the difficulty in determining valid cut points using data of a continuous nature, no attempts were made to construct instability-of-clinical-course counterparts from the temperature and laboratory values.

Results indicated that the nursing, temperature, and laboratory data generally had similar explanatory power. Exceptions were the minimum nursing value for the stay with its relatively poor performance, and the daily-nursing-pattern-of-care variable, which shows promise owing to its high explanatory power.

Projected Activities

Without the OCIS, the preceding analyses would probably have never been undertaken or would have met with massive resistance owing to the cost of data retrieval from the medical records and the lack of a guaranteed payoff of a data set highly explanatory of differences among patients in length of stay and costs.

Results encourage continued effort toward building a toxicity index and examining how nursing acuity is related to toxicity of treatment. Relationships of the toxicity and nursing variables with others listed in Table 2 will also be explored. Anticipated final products include the identification of the minimum data set required for internal planning and management of inpatient resources, and the formation of a set of inpatient reimbursement models to validate in other oncology treatments facilities so as to make policy recommendations for inpatient payment reform.

Analysis of outpatient resource use is expected to begin in the near future. Expected activities include comparison of similarities and differences in inpatient and outpatient use of services, and investigation of patterns of substitution and cycling between inpatient and outpatient care. Among the long-term plans are linkage of the inpatient and outpatient case mix databases to begin work on development of capitation payment models and to assist administration in resource management and identification of quality-of-care issues.

Tumor Registry System[7]

As has been previously described, planning and prototyping activities for the OCIS began while the Oncology Center building was being designed and constructed. The patient management system that has evolved from these initial planning activities is enormous in both scope and complexity. However, the foundation for this patient management data system began many years before during the early stages of the Hospital Cancer Registry.

The Johns Hopkins Hospital Tumor Registry was formed in the early 1950s. Even in this early stage, records in the partially computerized registry contained the basic information deemed necessary to complete the patient management profile. In the early 1960s this system was converted to a completely manual system utilizing a card file referred to as "Info-Dex." As the number of patients increased, it became increasingly difficult to manage and utilize this database effectively. Data retrieval became a tedious task.

In 1968, the system was again partially automated by the entry of selected data onto key-punched cards for computer processing. This provided a mechanism for accessing registry data and generating reports in batch mode using a remote computer facility. This method allowed improved search and information retrieval techniques, and remained in effect until 1975.

The construction of The Johns Hopkins Oncology Center was preceded by the development of a Cancer Center Provisional System (CCPS). The CCPS fulfilled

---

[7]This section was written by Anne Kammer, A.R.T., C.T.R., who has been in the health care field for over 30 years. She has managed The Johns Hopkins Tumor Registry since 1963 and in 1976 became the Manager of Oncology Data Operations. Ms. Kammer played a major role in the initial development of OCIS, and in 1979 she assumed her present position as Manager of Oncology Medical Information.

many objectives including providing a means of assisting with patient care while meeting the requirements established by the American College of Surgeons for a cancer registry, and complying with the American Association of Cancer Institutes (AACI) data set. In order to meet these diverse objectives, additional information was incorporated into the cancer registry core data set. The resulting system provided patient status, presentations, and clinical activity aids to assist physicians in the management of cancer center patients being treated by selected chemotherapy protocols.

As a result of this process, a more patient-oriented database was developed. This database would eventually serve as the foundation for future cancer center systems having extended clinical, administrative, and research objectives. Additionally, this cancer registry data system provided the institution with a working understanding of the operational management and clinical capabilities provided through such information in a cancer center setting.

Prior to the implementation of the CCPS, three phases of development were necessary. First, a comprehensive summary file of all patients from 1955 through 1975 was built. Although this file was not quite as complete as that for subsequent patients, it provided essential historical information for future studies. The second phase included the expansion of the system functions to support on-line edit and search capabilities. This phase included the implementation of an in-house computerized system with the capability of entering data directly into the database and querying the data for patient care and ad hoc studies purposes. The final phase encompassed the development of a more comprehensive computer-based data set with more system-oriented and patient-related capabilities. This provisional system immediately preceded the Oncology Clinical Information System (OCIS).

During these stages of development, the Tumor Registry evolved from a simple patient profile to an expanded data set, which complements patient care and research in the new Comprehensive Cancer Center at Johns Hopkins. The initial patient profile contained approximately 20,000 patient records. There are currently 45,000 patient records in the database, of which approximately 17,000 are under active annual follow-up. In 1987 over 3400 new patients were accessioned into the registry, encompassing both The Johns Hopkins Medical Institution and the Comprehensive Oncology Center (Figure 13). Close to 19,000 patients are actively followed by the registry.

The Tumor Registry has evolved from a one-person registry in 1955 to its present level of a staff of eight. While the OCIS can be viewed as the information backbone that supports the Oncology Center, the Tumor Registry is an integral part of that system as both a data provider and an information user. Data collected by registry personnel and data collected by clinical personnel are transparently available to all functions of the system.

Administratively, the Oncology Medical Information component of the Cancer Center is a part of the central administration services. Activities of this component include the Data Quality Unit, Oncology Medical Records Unit, and the Cancer Registry. Organizationally, the Tumor Registry is a function of The Johns

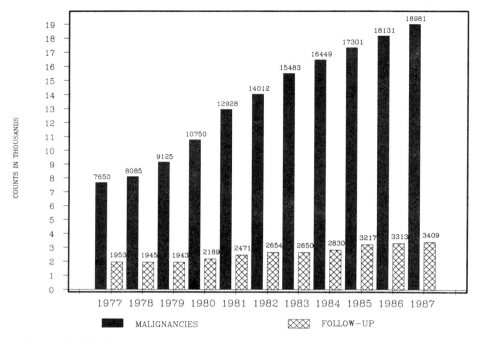

Figure 13. Number of new cases (malignancies) and total patient follow-up: The Johns Hopkins Hospital Tumor Registry, 1977–1987.

Hopkins Hospital's central administration that is carried out by the Cancer Center. Thus, the registry is responsible for collecting information on all cancer cases seen throughout the Hospital including the Cancer Center. Functionally, database maintenance and programming tasks are performed by OCIS staff under a joint agreement with the Hospital.

The data collection staff of the Tumor Registry performs such routine functions as case finding, data abstracting, quality control, coding, data entry, patient follow-up, and other assigned duties, such as ad hoc report generation. Patient identification begins when a document or computer listing is provided to the Tumor Registry staff through a variety of sources, including Admissions, and Pathology. Screening and selection of registry accessions begin with this procedure, and later decisions are made regarding the formal entry of the patient into the system. Factors influencing this decision are case reportability and department reportability, and whether the cases are on a consult only with no treatment or outside review only basis.

Once the decision is made to enter the case into the system, the available information is first verified against a centralized Hospital database containing all patient identification numbers and demographic information. The long-term database is a soundex patient identifier system developed by the Medical Records

Department to ensure correct and unique history number/patient name matches. After verification, the significant data about the patient is abstracted. This information is coded into a format termed a preliminary entry, which includes primary site, morphology, stage, pathology data, and other information that may be important in identifying the patient.

The case is maintained in a preliminary file for later completion. This preliminary file is maintained on line for immediate access by users, as well as in a manual form retained in a selective file. Within six months of this initial entry, the medical record is requested and the case is completed and entered into the computer system. The exception to this procedure is that Oncology Center inpatients are abstracted and entered into the system at the time of discharge.

The Oncology Clinical Profile (abstract) is completed manually by the abstracter and entered into the on-line system. A sample abstract is provided in Chapter 2, Figure 2. This procedure allows the abstracter to view all entries, identify any errors, and make immediate corrections to the database. A hard copy of the abstract is placed with the existing documents and, if appropriate, is then prepared for the quality control process.

The focal point of this process is to prepare the abstract. The abstract contains all the data needed to meet the requirements of the American College of Surgeons, support administration and research activities, and administer other oncology services. Its primary purpose, however, is to serve as the nucleus for Oncology Center patient summary. It provides essential information about the patient's disease in order to assist in clinical management.

The abstract file is a combination of coded information and free text within selected fields. The development of this type of profile was based on the needs of the Oncology Center physician staff to complement patient care. The basic contents of the profile are (1) demographic, (2) administrative, and (3) diagnostic information; (4) treatment; (5) medical history; (6) follow-up and end results.

At the request of physicians and administrative staff, it has been necessary in the past several years to develop a confidential section as part of the abstract. This suppressed information can be viewed only by authorized individuals and with the permission of the supervisor. Examples of information that may be contained under this section are psychiatric illness, family relationship to a staff member, AIDS diagnosis, and other predefined data.

As a component of the abstract, two systems currently exist to validate data. An on-line edit check system was developed initially as a spin-off of the Centralized Cancer Patient Data System (CCPDS), organized by the National Cancer Institute in the mid 1970s among comprehensive cancer centers. This procedure allows the abstracter to view all entries, identify any errors, and make immediate corrections to the database. The second portion of the quality control process of the abstract is a visual review of the abstract. This has functioned since the development of the computer system. This review was enhanced by a designated section of the abstract referred to as the administrative section (Figure 14).

The two primary reasons for the implementation of the quality control and edit check procedures were to ensure that the quality of data was valid and consistent,

```
ADMINISTRATIVE INFORMATION PRIMARY - 1
─────────────────────────────────────────────────────────────────────

ADMISSION DATE:      06/11/87        DISCHARGE DATE:
PRELIMINARY:  NO                     ACCS NO:   871498
PRELIMINARY CODER: BLL               DATE OF PRELIMINARY ENTRY:    07/24/87
ABSTRACTOR:    KDB                   DATE ABSTRACT COMPLETED:      01/13/88
FIRST DATA ENTRY ID:    KDB          DATE OF INITIAL GENERATION:   01/13/88
LAST DATA ENTRY ID:     KD           DATE OF LAST GENERATION:      01/14/88
QUALITY CONTROL COMPLETED:           REGISTRY FOLDER:    YES
```

Figure 14. Administrative information of the patient abstract: The Johns Hopkins Hospital Tumor Registry.

and to ensure that the case met the requirements for inclusion into the database. In addition to the on-line edit checks, it is possible to generate a report that captures all elements and identifies those items that require further verification for accuracy. This report can be generated on an ad hoc basis and be specific as to the individual abstracter who entered the case (Figure 15).

The visual review of the abstract is intended to detect cases that would not be reportable according to predefined criteria, and to detect inconsistencies in data collected in the text sections of the abstract data.

The quality control review provides the supervisor with a method of assessing the performance of the employees who perform the abstracting function and to use this information as part of the overall job performance evaluation mechanism. Errors are evaluated as major versus minor discrepancies.

Although cancer registry information use is limited in many hospitals, such information has been a primary data resource in The Johns Hopkins Medical Institutions. There are several factors that have influenced this high level of use. The first and foremost has been compliance with "individualization" of requests from the database. This is accomplished through an orientation of the users with the system and an explanation of the data available. Using this method has the advantages of providing education and streamlining the ultimate report request.

Second, with the continued development of more sophisticated information systems throughout The Johns Hopkins Medical Institutions, users have become extremely interested in having this information on line for a wide variety of purposes. As a result, the number of requests continues to increase. For example, the staff of the Surgical Pathology Department is provided with on-line review of existing physical, laboratory, and treatment information in order to facilitate better evaluation of surgical specimens.

Contacts are made annually with all internal departments, as well as with our affiliated institutions to encourage utilization of available cancer patient data. Many benefits are derived by the existence of the Tumor Registry. It is able to provide the Center and other requesters with comprehensive cancer statistics for

```
JOHNS HOPKINS OCIS                                              01/14/88


QUALITY CONTROL REPORT

HNO                      P#      EDCHKD                    VAL1      VA2

     PATIENT,NAOMI
       34346            1        A10  BLANK DAC - DATE ABSTR CPLTED
QC
       03436            1        D26  INVALID DDXDAT DAY
QC



     PATIENT,ANN
       74343            1        A10  BLANK DAC - DATE ABSTR CPLTED
       73434            1        T07  ADM,DDXI TXB RANGE>30
     01/22/79     03/03/79

JOB COMPLETED 5:50 PM
```

Figure 15. Quality control Edit Check Report: The Johns Hopkins Hospital Tumor
Registry.

patients diagnosed and treated within the institution in any specified year. The
Registry also enhances cancer patient management. A significant benefit is that
lifetime follow-up is effected for all patients diagnosed to ensure that they stay in
touch with the health care system. The data are available to identify patients at
risk for second malignancies and to stimulate interest in cancer prevention. The
database supports patterns-of-care evaluations both short term and long term as
required by both external and internal agencies.

Frequent requests are made by Oncology and Hospital administration for information to aid in resource planning and to evaluate the institution's experience
related to cancer patients. This can easily be obtained through the Tumor Registry database. Research has been enhanced by defining populations of specific
cancer patients for planned clinical and epidemiologic protocol development.
Information on cancer is available to support research by physicians, students,
health care providers, and organizations and to provide data for grant requests.
Valuable epidemiological data are available to identify common variables and
perhaps contribute to the prevention of this disease.

The information maintained by the Tumor Registry also enables the institution
to meet the American College of Surgeons requirements for accreditation of the
institution's cancer program. In addition, it provides information needed to meet
state and local requirements. Presently, The Johns Hopkins Hospital Registry
reports its new cancer cases to the Maryland State Cancer Registry. It is to be
hoped that the recent establishment of a statewide population-based cancer registry will assist with local primary and secondary cancer prevention activities.

In summary, the Cancer Registry has played a major role in defining data
collection and reporting activities that have been incorporated into the OCIS.
Today the Registry is an integrated part of the OCIS and shares in a synergistic

relationship with all data collection and utilization activities at the Cancer Center. It continues to serve a critical role in multiple areas within both the institution and the Cancer Center. Its role will grow with the other data utilization activities evolve.

System Operation and Administrative Services[8]

Introduction

This final section addresses some of the issues that relate to the computer support of the OCIS. Two factors are considered. The first deals with the methods used to protect the confidentiality of the patient information in the OCIS database; the second describes some special considerations that relate to the system's operation. The material in this section was prepared by the OCIS System Manager (A.W.S.), the Supervisor of Programming (F.M.), the Supervisor of Computer Operations (G.L.K.), and one of the original OCIS designers (B.I.B.).

Authority Control

Because the OCIS maintains a very large database containing sensitive patient data that are necessary for the efficient operation of the Oncology Center, special steps must be taken to ensure (a) data protection, that is, that the data are properly backed up to provide continued availability in the event of failures or catastrophe, and (b) data privacy, that is, that the data are guarded from unauthorized access. The former is accomplished by the rigid application of routine procedures, and this subsection addresses only the second issue.

A secure automated system requires three dimensions of control: control over the personnel, the facility, and the computer system. In a hospital system there is limited control over personnel and facility. All clinical workers are schooled in the sensitivity of patient data; they are taught how to retain the patient's confidentiality. Unlike a system that must control national secrets, however, no special screening of the staff is performed beyond that necessary to ensure that they will be effective members of the health care team.

---

[8]This section was written by Bruce I. Blum, Gary L. Kinsey, Farideh Momeni, and Alan W. Sacker.

Gary L. Kinsey joined the OCIS staff as a Data Coordinator for Hemapheresis in 1979. In 1981 he became Supervisor for Computer Operations. In 1987 he assumed his present position as Systems Programmer II.

Farideh Momeni, M.S., began work on OCIS in 1982 as a member of the clinical information component of the Johns Hopkins Biomedical Engineering Department. She joined the Oncology Center in 1985 as a programmer and assumed her present position of Senior Systems Programmer in 1989.

Alan W. Sacker joined the Oncology Center in 1976 and was initially a data coordinator/operator for OCIS. In 1978 he assumed a role as an applications programmer and participated in the early Phase I development efforts. In 1988 he assumed his present position as Systems Programmer III.

With respect to the facility, most areas must be left unsecured. Although many rooms are locked, the general hospital layout cannot prohibit visitor or patient access to all locations. Obvious exceptions include work areas such as the registrar's desk and the nursing control booth; here an unauthorized presence would be questioned immediately. During nonworking hours, however, a work area might be unattended. In this situation there would be no one to guard against the unauthorized use of a computer terminal. For example, it might be possible for a visitor to wander into the outpatient department in the early evening and experiment with a terminal.

Clearly, therefore, OCIS must have some means of authority control that can protect against accidental penetration of the system, that is, the review of private data by casual access. Nevertheless, it must be recognized that no hospital organization is designed to protect itself from a deliberate penetration of its security system by experienced and dedicated criminals. Any attempt to do so would be prohibitively expensive. Consequently, OCIS need not be concerned with all of the security attributes of, say, a national defense application.

There are a variety of techniques used in ensuring authorization to the data. The most common method is the use of a password during the sign-on process. The major difficulty with this approach is that it requires a log-on for each session. This involves casual users to remember their passwords. Moreover, because one would like the system to be available as a utility, a log-on prior to each session tends to act as a barrier to system use. These problems are often overcome by leaving the terminal in a logged-on state or by posting a common password for all to use. Both techniques violate the intent of the authority system.

In designing an authority system for OCIS the following goals were established:

The use of a terminal should be encouraged. Therefore, each terminal would provide access to all data that were normally available in that physical location. For example, in the 2 North unit, on-line access would be available to all data on 2 North patients; in the administrative areas, access would be available to the patients administrative (nonclinical) data.

Terminals should be identified by a location, which would indicate what data should be available and a time window of availability. For example, the outpatient terminals would not provide access to outpatient data after clinic hours.

Any terminal should be able to access OCIS. If the terminal did not already have a location-specific authorization level, then it would display the top-level menu (called the *universal terminal*) and demand a log-on with a password before performing any protected task.

Any terminal already logged on should provide access to any data in the system when the proper authority is given. This would be accomplished by testing each request against the authority of the terminal. If the request exceeded the terminal authority (as it almost certainly would in the case of the universal terminal), then the user would be instructed to log on. If authorized, processing would continue. When the processing was complete, the terminal authority would continue. When the processing was complete, the terminal authority would be returned to its earlier state.

Remote access and programmer access to OCIS should require additional levels of control.

Authority is established at the program (or function) level. This is a different philosophy from that used with most database systems in which individual files or attributes are protected. The designers felt that authorization according to how the data were to be used provided a finer granularity for control. Consequently, each program can have associated with it one or more authority levels. In general, it is sufficient to restrict the authority testing at the level of the menu programs that provide access to an associated group of functions. However, it is possible to associate a special authority with any individual program.

The authority codes are defined as a network. Each user or program may be given many authorities. For example, some codes might be:

Clinical data, view only (CD) or view and update (CDU).
Administrative data, view with (AFD) or without (AD) access to financial information.
Data coordinator special functions (DCSP).
Data coordinator assignment defined to be all the above, except for the access to financial information; for example, DC is defined as the set CDU, AD, DCSP.
SUPER, which provides maximum authority; that is, SUPER contains DC, AFD, . . .

A program may be given the authorities CD and AD which would require the user to have both authorities or an authority that includes both.

The OCIS System Manager is the person responsible for assigning authority codes to new users and to all programs. Log-on is initiated with a short public identifier, usually the individual's initials. This is followed by a prompt for a password. For the initial log-on, the user supplies the password. The password can be altered by the user at any time. Periodically, the unused authorizations are removed from the system. This approach to authority control has been in use since 1982, and it has been well received.

Computer Operations

In this final subsection we address some of the features that were incorporated into OCIS to support its computer operations. Because the system was initially developed in a period when computers were not a common tool in the delivery of health care, there was a limited demand for interactive displays. Moreover, because of limited funding, few terminals were available until the mid-1980s. Thus, OCIS was designed to be a paper-oriented system. It provided on-line access to clinical data, but this access was limited to special functions, such as the review of the morning hematology results. Also, because OCIS was developed well before there was any Hospital commitment to networking, communication with remote sites and computers had to rely on custom-crafted interfaces.

As a paper-oriented system, the daily operation was scheduled according to the need to produce and distribute data products. The key events were:

Plots and Flow Sheets. Plots and flow sheets had to be available in time for morning rounds and clinic opening. Drug doses were cumulated as a daily dose; processing, therefore, could begin only after midnight. By that time most outstanding clinical laboratory data had been reported, and little change to the database could be expected until the morning blood work was reported. Thus, the clinical database was updated each day during the early morning hours.

Daily Care Plans. The patient data had to be updated to indicate any deviations from the previous day's plan. This was done early in the morning by the data coordinators. Once the database was updated, the current day's plans could be produced and delivered to the units for the current day's orders.

System Backup. Each day the database was copied to backup disk packs.

System backup required a dedicated machine, but the first two activities were executed in parallel with on-line use. The first two activities were computationally intense and, given the limited OCIS computing resources, required several hours to process. Unfortunately, the running of computationally intense programs affected response time, and optional long runs, such as a Tumor Registry search, would be scheduled for the weekend.

To manage this standard production processing, a scheduler–stacker–spooler was developed, using both vendor-supplied and custom code. Routine jobs were identified along with the time at which they should be initiated. Requests for printed output were entered into the queue according to their priority. All clinical terminals were given the facility to enter requests for printed outputs. Because the computing facility had no local printers, all output requests were either picked up at the computer center or delivered.

The interfacing of OCIS with other systems introduced new problems. Chapter 6 has presented the issues from the perspective of the Pharmacy. Similar issues were raised with respect to the link with the Clinical Laboratory computer. Because OCIS was the only automated system that required access to the individual values in the laboratory reports, it was not reasonable to expect the Clinical Laboratory to modify its programs and provide access to this level. Consequently, OCIS was allowed to read only the automated form of the printed report and extract the data values. The obvious difficulties included matching patient identification, parsing the data after changes were made to the report format, dealing with text messages, and processing changes to previously reported values.

Because the conversion of the text report produced by the Clinical Laboratory into a value-oriented OCIS database was a time-consuming process, data transfers and updates initially were scheduled on a two-hour cycle. As the equipment was improved, this was reduced to an hourly cycle. Timeliness improved; nevertheless, there remains a lag between the time that a report is available on the Hospital system and the time it is available in OCIS.

When a link was established between the OCIS computer and the hematology laboratory located in the Oncology Center, it was possible to integrate the OCIS programs with the laboratory functions. These clinical data are available to OCIS users as soon as the data are recorded. As a result, on-line query using the OCIS Data function is the standard method of communicating the results of the hematology laboratory. Because of this use, the Data function is also used for reviewing the blood chemistry work as well.

A further system complication was introduced by the need to report clinical data in several formats, that is, vertical flow sheets, horizontal flow sheets, and plots. Because it is possible to have hundreds of data points per patient day and because a patient may have years of data available on line, some method was required to manage this diversity and, at the same time, provide acceptable response times. This was accomplished by replicating some of the data in formats that were suitable to the different reports. The normal storage of data provided very rapid access to the Data display and vertical flow sheets. However, the other formats proved to be more effective in displaying large amounts of patient data. Thus, during the evening update period, these secondary formats were partially regenerated to include new data and corrections to previously reported data. Although an individual patient's data could be updated on demand at a terminal, the practical consequence of this design approach was that the plots and horizontal flows were updated daily.

Clearly, there is nothing in the OCIS design that prohibits its use as an interactive system. The history of its development and the limitations imposed by its processing power combined to give the system a paper orientation. As noted already, the Data function is a very important part of patient management, and the discussion in Chapter 9 provides strong evidence that the system is used as an interactive resource. Nevertheless, most of its activities are supported in a paper-oriented manner. As is demonstrated in Chapter 10, an environment that has grown accustomed to interactive access for all functions may not find such a design satisfactory.

III
Evaluation and Future Directions

This section contains two chapters. Chapter 9 includes an evaluation summary and an overview of the future computing plans for the Oncology Center. Chapter 10 recounts an experience in transporting the OCIS system to another cancer center in the United States. The system has also been transported to a cancer center in Australia.

9
Evaluation and Future Directions
John P. Enterline

Over the past decade a dramatic rise in health care costs has placed a tremendous financial burden on society. This has led to a variety of cost containment efforts by governmental regulation agencies and third-party payers. As a result, there is a growing focus in health care management on efficiency, resource forecasting, and long-term strategic planning. In the future those organizations that can provide high-quality health care most efficiently will have the highest probability of success in a very competitive marketplace.

The majority of the cost containment activities in health care organizations will be highly reliant on efficient and timely information acquisition combined with effective decision-making tools. Modeling the objectives of medical information systems to support the corporate strategic plan will become a crucial element in an organization's ability to compete successfully. Managers and developers of medical information systems will be required to provide quantitative justifications for both developing new systems and maintaining existing systems. In this highly competitive environment, future support for individual information systems will be closely tied to an ability to document the development rationale, measure the resulting effectiveness, and communicate these elements to upper level management.

This chapter presents a variety of information that assists in quantifying the value of OCIS. Data are presented on the system's growth, efficiency gains, and effectiveness as perceived by its users. In an era where rapidly expanding and changing demands are placed on information systems, an existing system's potential to evolve and expand to fulfill new requirements is just as important as its ability to meet the requirements of the present. A true evaluation of OCIS must be based on both its present successes and its future potential. Thus current and projected development activities are described in the latter sections of this chapter.

Evaluation

Assessing the value of an information system in a totally quantitative manner is both difficult and controversial; in many instances it is impossible. This is particularly true in disciplines such as applied medical computing, where the information system is only one component in a continuously changing process. Determining long-term evaluation criteria and assessing efficiency gains in such an environment are very elusive. In most instances the true gains from such a system can be best expressed in subjective terms; the more objective elements that can be quantitatively measured represent only a fraction of the system's true value.

In this section a variety of both objective and subjective efficacy data are presented. Each of these data elements is but a partial measure or single view of the system's success. Baseline descriptive measures and subsequent changes in these measures over time do not prove that the OCIS has been either effective or ineffective. Measures of user perception can be biased by either a lack of vision or inflated expectation. Personnel efficacy gains are difficult to quantify in humanistic environments where increases in free time are used to improve the quality of service rather than to increase measurable performance. However, if all of the partial measures of success point in similar directions, the argument for a conclusion regarding the overall system's success is greatly strengthened. By all evaluable objective and subjective measures OCIS has been a success.

System Utilization

In environments where individuals are required to use computer systems, growth and utilization may not be directly related to the system's efficacy; it may simply be that more individuals are required to use the system. However, the users of OCIS are not required to use any of its clinical management functions in caring for their patients. Physicians can order patient charts and perform clinical management using the more traditional manual methods of data management and assessment. Nurses can maintain information such as transfusion and chemotherapy reaction results on local medical charts. Laboratory data can be obtained in hard copy and through telephone calls to the central laboratories. If OCIS were not perceived by its user population as a valuable tool for clinical data management, it would have experienced limited user interest and a small resulting growth.

A cross section of data elements that measure the physical growth in OCIS is presented in Table 1 for 1978 through 1988. OCIS has grown both in structure and function as a result of the direct demands and requirements of its user population. It has been a continuing management struggle to keep up with requests in terms of the system's power, user access, and additional applications. OCIS remains a growing and evolving system and is designed to respond to the requirements of its user population.

From 1978 through 1980, growth of the system was slow. It was a period of system development, and the population was restricted to those users who were essential to guiding and testing the basic system's capabilities. Chapters 1 and 3 provides a detailed description of the activities during this early Phase 0 stage of development.

Table 1. Oncology Clinical Information Systems Growth, 1978–1988

Year	On-Line Users	Daily Reports	Number of Terminals	Peak Users	Routines Developed
1978	10	0	15	10	†
1979	15	50	20	15	†
1980	20	100	30	20	†
1981	150	150	40	25	625
1982*	175	250	50	35	1388
1983	200	350	80	45	990
1984	250	425	90	50	1014
1985	300	500	110	60	737
1986	325	625	130	75	770
1987	400	750	175	80	820
1988‡	500	850	230	100	1000

*Operations expanded from 5 days per week, 8 hours per day, to 7 days per week, 24 hours per day; second PDP system added.

† Program development for Phase 1 system was not recorded.

‡ Estimated early Phase III growth by the end of 1988.

In 1981 the system went into true production and the number of users and terminals quickly climbed to 150 and 40, respectively. During the peak user period from 10:00 A.M. to 2:00 P.M. there were over 25 users concurrently logged into the system, many of whom were performing on-line database queries. This was the maximum on-line user load the OCIS could handle with a one-computer configuration. Over 150 user-requested reports were distributed daily throughout the Center, and the system operated 8 hours a day, 5 days a week. Development of the system continued as indicated by the number of new application routines written that year. There was an obvious requirement to increase both the on-line user capacity and the hours of operation.

In 1982 the Center added a second computer system and increased its staff, and hours of operation were expanded to 7 days a week, 24 hours a day. The on-line storage capabilities were increased fourfold because of the growing database necessary to meet user database requirements. Also, the integrated pharmacy system described in Chapter 6 came on line that year. The number of users that could be served by the system was doubled, and other system elements grew accordingly.

In 1984 the number of ports on the systems was expanded to 64 on each of the two computer systems to meet growing user demands for on-line terminal access. Although it was initially planned to purge data on deceased patients, the clinical faculty strongly requested that those data remain on line to assist in prospective clinical decision making. The retrospective patient data were also proving to be extremely valuable in meeting the needs of auditors from both third-party payers and clinical protocol review groups.

The two computers, however, were quickly becoming saturated with users during peak periods. Use of the system had gained popularity. It was apparent that

OCIS would soon be overloaded without either adding additional hardware or improving the system's ability to support an increasing user load. Although 128 terminals could be physically connected to the system, only 50 users could be logged into the system at any one time without dramatically degrading performance. Attempts were made to restrict access to critical users during peak times, and the number of unfulfilled requests for terminal connections climbed. System utilization statistics during peak periods continued to rise, as did the system's response time.

In 1985, Phase III expansion plans began for OCIS. Fortunately, during that year the interpretive MUMPS language used by the system became available in a compiled version. The conversion to this compiled version of MUMPS increased the CPU throughput over twofold and provided a grace period, which was essential in planning for a logical expansion of the system. With the increase in performance gained through compiled MUMPS, concurrent user access was expanded to over 100 ports for the 300 staff members with passwords to the system. The on-line storage was doubled again this year to accommodate both the ever-increasing number of data elements collected on each patient and the growing retrospective database.

Phase III expansion plans were submitted to the Hospital's central administration in 1986 and in early 1987 Phase III expansion efforts began. This phase of development will be described in detail later in this chapter. Today, 175 terminals and 20 of the Center's 140 PCs have connections to the OCIS system. Additionally, 40 users in other institutional computing facilities have network access to the system. Conversely, all terminals and PCs that are connected to the oncology data switch have the potential for accessing other institutional computing devices over a recently installed local-area network.

Demands for additional terminal and PC connections to OCIS and other computing resources continue to be strong. By the end of 1988 it is projected that within the Oncology Center there will be over 220 terminals and PCs having access to its computing facilities. This could easily climb to 280 by the end of 1989. Additional programmers are being recruited to address the present backlog of applications, and sufficient computing power has been installed to handle the anticipated expansion of the system over the next two to three years. On-line storage on the two production machines has been doubled again; each of the additional four recently added VAX computers matches the storage of the production machines. The recent expansion activities are described in greater detail later in this chapter.

Thus, there will be a new surge of growth in OCIS during the 1989–1990 time period. It should be emphasized that, although OCIS services are provided to users at no direct cost, users are not required to use the system and comparable data are available from other sources. The continued demand for additional applications and user access is a strong indication that OCIS has been a functional success, regardless of any cost saving and user perception components.

Personnel and Cost Savings

The initial purpose of OCIS was to provide an enabling mechanism for making clinical decisions in the timely manner critical to the optimal management of cancer patients. There was no direct intent to provide a mechanism for reducing personnel and other cost savings outcomes. No mechanisms were designed into the initial system to measure savings as a prospective outcome. Such evaluation mechanisms are presently being incorporated into the system.

Although savings in personnel and other costs can be estimated, many of the OCIS functions, such as the pharmacy system and the blood products system, have never been handled in a nonautomated manner. In fact, functions such as blood products monitoring could not be managed effectively without some form of computer-based system. Cost savings that can be quantified are discussed below for a variety of functions performed by OCIS. In general, these estimates on cost savings can only be made for activities that are mechanical in nature.

Direct cost savings are only one dimension of a health care system's operation. It is not possible to measure the time-saving benefit to physician, nursing, and other clinical support personnel, except in a nonobjective manner, as, for example, by the user survey described later in this chapter. It is impossible to place a value on the ability to make timely decisions in the treatment of critically ill patients. Also, it is difficult to place a quantitative value on the time spent in making a decision without including the quality of the resulting decision. Therefore, no personnel or cost estimates can be provided for the true function of the system, that is, that of enabling the quickest and highest quality treatment of cancer patients possible.

Pharmacy. Like many functions at the Oncology Center, the Pharmacy has always relied upon an automated environment. It was made an integral component of the OCIS system in 1983 and has followed a similar strategy of tailoring the system to meet user needs. In the oncology setting the Pharmacy is a major component in patient care, accounting for approximately 20% of inpatient charges. In terms of staff savings, it is estimated that it would take three to five additional personnel to provide the mechanical pharmacy functions supplied by OCIS. However, there are many additional cost and personnel savings that are more difficult to estimate. These include the ability to control protocol therapies and drug charge capture, as well as instantaneous quality control capabilities, and more. As discussed in Chapter 6, the advantages to automating routine pharmacy tasks are multiplied through an integration with other patient management functions.

Hemapheresis. One of the most critical areas in the treatment of cancer patients is the monitoring and proper use of blood products. Most aggressive cancer therapy regimens have a short-term and life-threatening toxic effect on the patient's blood and blood-making capabilities. This is also one of the most expensive single components of cancer treatment, amounting to over 20% of the inpatient charges. Thus, the efficient and effective use of blood products is critical to quality patient care and cost containment. As described in Chapter 7, it appears that, through the ability to quickly monitor a patient's blood requirements and response to selected blood products, it has been possible to achieve significant cost savings while providing higher quality patient care. It has been estimated that to perform tasks comparable to those achieved by OCIS, an additional 12 full-time staff members would be required. However, this is a spurious argument because additional staff could not replace the computer system's ability to monitor efficacy and make corrections to patient management in a timely manner. Such monitoring activities are essential to high-quality and cost-effective clinical care.

Third-Party Payer Reimbursement. One side benefit of OCIS is the assistance it provides with the documentation of procedures and tests that is required by third-party payer and clinical protocol auditors. This assistance is provided in two ways. The first is the production of procedure and test labels, which are partially filled out for physicians by the system. When procedures or tests are ordered, physicians sign an order label, which is affixed into the patients chart to verify the order. Second, the great majority of test results are received electronically and stored on OCIS indefinitely. This provides additional proof that not only was there a signed physician order, but that the test or procedure was actually performed.

It is difficult to quantify the savings by reducing third-party refusals to pay for undocumented tests and procedures. There is no way of estimating the percentage of payment refusals were the system not to assist with procedure documentation. Over the past several years, some third-party payers have ceased auditing care charges at the Center because of the extremely low rate of discrepancies with those charges. The overall audited charge rejection rate for the Oncology Center appears to be less than one-quarter of the general rejection rate for the Hospital. Additionally, many of the treatment regimens used at the Center have long-term admissions and are extremely expensive. These types of charges to third-party payers tend to have a much higher probability of receiving an audit than the smaller medical treatment charges.

Thus, it is probable that a significant savings is obtained through both the low charge rejection rate and the savings in personnel time necessary to respond to all types of audits. Whatever this cost savings, it is a total by-product of a data system that is considered to be essential for high-quality clinical management of patients.

Charge Capturing and Billing Monitoring. Because the system contains information on all procedures, tests, drugs, inpatient stays, and outpatient visits, it acts as a natural charge capture system for a great majority of the services provided to Center patients. In some instances charges from the Center are sent to Hospital billing components on computer tape; in other instances hard-copy charges must be generated to be reentered into Hospital billing systems.

While a great deal of personnel effort is saved through the charge capture capabilities of OCIS, a potentially more important capability is in monitoring whether these charges were actually billed. In multiple instances, data provided through OCIS have uncovered major errors in billing algorithms that have resulted in the recovery of substantial revenue for both oncology and other areas of the Hospital. Thus, OCIS acts as a form of independent verification and monitoring for billing mechanisms across the Medical Institutions.

General Administration. Today, OCIS is believed to result in considerable administrative cost savings by providing automated functions such as bed occupancy census, resource forecasting, and staffing projections. Not only do these automatic data-gathering and -monitoring tasks save on personnel time, but they also provide constant and extremely timely feedback on changes in the operations that should be further investigated. Examples of such temporal changes include occupancy rates, case mix, nursing level of care, demographic and geographic profiles of patients, and the use of ancillary support services. It is estimated that manual performance of the data-gathering and -monitoring tasks of OCIS would require at least two to three additional personnel by the central administrative component of the Center. However, the timeliness and completeness of these data would not be comparable to those provided through OCIS.

Another extremely important use of the OCIS database and associated computing facilities is currently under development. This use will encompass strategic planning, improved resource forecasting, and reduced patient care overhead. The emergence of reimbursement and cost containment mechanisms, such as prospective payment plans based on the diagnostically related groups (DRG) classification, will permit more efficient management capabilities to translate into significant cost savings and/or profits for health care facilities. The efficient "flow" of patients through a system structured to meet demands will not only result in cost savings but will also improve the patient's perception of the system. Thus, an efficient operation will result in both higher profits and increased patient attraction to a particular health care system. Such efficient operations will also act as a magnet for community physicians in terms of both data and resource availability. Proper information management and utilization will become even more important for both high-quality patient care and institutional viability in an increasingly competitive marketplace.

As described in Chapter 8, personnel at the Center are already developing methods to use OCIS data to forecast resource needs on the basis of past data and projected patient populations. These data are also being used to improve the definition of reimbursement categories specific to an oncology population. This will help to ensure proper prospective compensation from third-party payers. It is quite possible that OCIS will be as significant a strategic corporate tool in the future as it is a patient management tool today.

Conclusion. The primary intent of OCIS is to enable high-quality clinical care for cancer patients rather than serve as a direct cost-saving mechanism. The operating costs for OCIS is less than 3% of the total Oncology Center operating expenses, which compares favorably with other hospital information systems. However, it is difficult to compare costs directly, as the functions of hospital systems vary dramatically, and no system provides functions that are comparable to OCIS.

A quantitative case can easily be made for actual cost savings through the use of OCIS. It is apparent that the personnel, administrative, and reimbursement cost savings of OCIS easily pay for its one-million-dollar-per-year operating expenses. It is probable that systems with cost-saving capabilities similar to OCIS will soon be essential in most health care facilities. The inherent efficiencies of such systems will be required in a marketplace where cost containment combined with effective medical care will be the only means to succeed. However, there are no real objective measures of the true value of the system. The following section addresses the true value in the best means possible — user satisfaction with the system.

User Satisfaction and Perception Survey

A reliable measure of a system's success is the perception of its users regarding utility and unfulfilled requirements. To this end, two user surveys have been conducted among the clinical staff; additional surveys are planned for the future. The initial user survey was conducted in late 1984 after the Phase II porting of the system to a dual computer configuration and Standard MUMPS (see Chapter 3). This was felt to be a stable system with most of the central components in place and a critical mass of users who were familiar enough with the system to provide a valid assessment. After this survey, corrective actions were taken in response to survey results. A second user survey was conducted in mid-1988 prior to the implementation of initial Phase III functions, described later in this chapter. This second survey measured clinical users' perceptions of the OCIS. It also added questions intended to guide Phase III development activities in response to requested enhancements to the system.

A quantitative comparison of the users' response to the two surveys is not necessarily straightforward. For example, changes for the better could be due to either the users' familiarity with system functions or an actual improvement in the system's utility. Similarly, changes for the worse could be due to either the users' greater awareness of deficits in the system or greater expectations of system development. It should also be pointed out that in the time between the two surveys the microcomputer revolution took place. During the first survey there were approximately 30 PCs in the Oncology Center, whereas during the second survey there were over 140 PCs. In all probability, the population of the second survey was a more sophisticated user group than that of the first survey. Such factors are impossible to control in an analysis.

However, 90% of the questions in the two surveys were identical, and both instruments were pretested for their validity and reliability prior to being conducted. A comparison of selected questions from these two surveys is provided below. Also, user suggestions from both surveys are discussed. With this in mind, the results of these two surveys are contrasted and described below.

One measure of OCIS utilization is the frequency of system use by individual users in the population served. In the four years between surveys, the percentage of physicians that use OCIS on line more than once a day doubled from 34% to 68%, whereas the percentage that use the system less than twice a week fell from 35% to 16% (see Figure 1). A similar trend is noted among the nursing personnel and physician assistants (PAs). It is clear that nearly all of the clinical staff could be classified as frequent users of the OCIS in the 1988 survey. As the use of the OCIS system is not mandatory, the utility of this system appears to be evident. It is also clear that the increase in the number of users served by the system, terminal access to the system, system routine growth, and the number of daily reports, as described previously in Table 1, is accompanied by an increase in the individual use of the system. By these measures OCIS is a thriving and expanding system with a high level of user acceptance.

In the 1984 survey, the clinical staff members were asked to rate the usefulness of OCIS in the management of their patients. The percentage rating the system as excellent more than doubled in both the physician and nurse/PA groups in the intervening four years; while half the physicians and one-third of the nurse/PA population felt the system was excellent, 84% of each population felt that the system was at least good. As one might suspect, there is a significant relationship ($p < .05$) between increased knowledge of the system and the higher ratings of the system (see Figure 1). Although both the physician and nurse/PA groups report improved knowledge about OCIS functions, the increase has been slower among nurses and PAs; the percentage of Nurses and PAs reporting a poor to fair knowledge of the system was reduced from 77% to 45% over the period, while the percentage of physicians reporting poor to fair knowledge reduced from 63% to 29%. Both the lower usefulness and knowledge ratings of OCIS by the nurse/PA group are possibly a function of the greater staff turnover and indicate that training efforts should be increased among these personnel.

Another factor measured in each survey was additional functions required from information systems at the Oncology Center. In 1984 the most frequent request from physicians was to have better links between the OCIS database and existing PCs. Both the physician and nursing staffs indicated a strong desire for improved documentation and training for the OCIS functions. Also, there were high demands for additional training on PC applications such as word processing, spreadsheets, communication packages, and statistical packages. There were few suggestions regarding additional or improved clinical functions for OCIS. In the intervening four years, aggressive actions were taken with regard to PC connectivity and OCIS documentation and training.

In the 1988 survey, physicians and nurses had notably more sophisticated sets of requests from OCIS. The great majority of both groups would like terminal

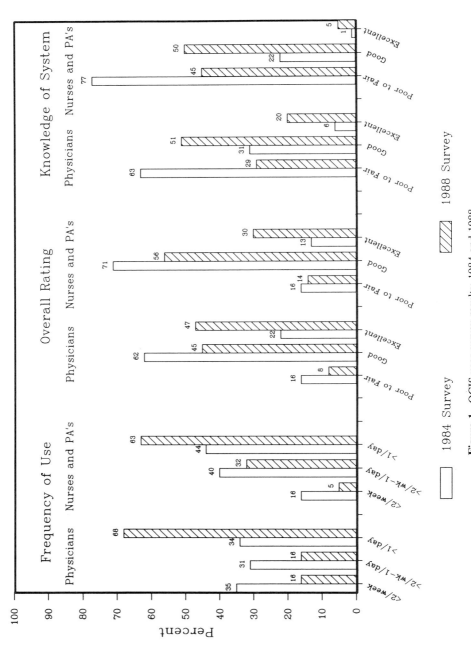

Figure 1. OCIS user survey results: 1984 and 1988.

access to other information resources at the Johns Hopkins Medical Institutions, such as a radiology report tracking system, an extremely fast clinical test results database, a pathology reporting system, and operating room schedules. Also, approximately 80% of both groups would like an on-line clinical imaging system to be developed on the inpatient floors. Over 80% of the physician population views the connection of the OCIS database and terminals with other institutional data resources as the number one priority of future development activities, whereas only 14% of the nurses viewed this as their first priority.

Nursing respondents indicated a strong need for additional on-line functions, such as nursing procedure documentation (70%), patient care plans (65%), discharge instructions (65%), and medication administration data entry (49%). Close to one-half of the nurses viewed such on-line nursing information as the number one development priority of OCIS; 18% of the nurses felt that additional OCIS training was the highest priority. The majority of both the nurses and physicians felt that better access to OCIS terminals would improve their use of the system; over one-third of the nurses felt that bedside terminals would improve clinical care, and another one-half felt that the idea had potential. Over one-half of the physicians indicated a need for access to a high-level statistical analysis package, and nearly 70% requested access to the institutional bibliographic retrieval systems. Approximately 40% of the physicians indicated a need for personal calendaring/meeting scheduling systems and electronic mail.

In summary, it appears that the user perception, utilization, and understanding of OCIS have improved dramatically between the 1984 and 1988 surveys. Further, if the types of additional functions required by users are any indication, the sophistication level of the OCIS user has increased dramatically during this time period.

Fortunately, the environment being instituted in the Phase III development activities will accommodate the types of demands that will be placed on OCIS in the future by its users. Both the present and future development plans for the OCIS are presented below. Specific development activities will be guided by the above survey results. Many of the above user requests have already been implemented.

Current OCIS Development

To the author's knowledge, there is no commercial equivalent to the OCIS system. The lack of comparable commercial products is echoed by the constant flow of individuals from other cancer treatment facilities who come to examine the OCIS structure and functions. Several institutions have chosen to adapt the OCIS directly to their environment, even though it is not presently a commercially supported product. The porting of OCIS to one such institution is described in Chapter 10 of this book. Other institutions are in the planning stages of developing systems that are comparable to OCIS in function but are structured to exist in a different computing environment.

Oncology Center users have significant requirements for new applications that are natural extensions of the OCIS database. However, technological advances in computing hardware, information engineering, and communications are moving at a rapid pace. The information systems component of the Oncology Center is restructuring its environment to ensure that full advantage can be taken of new technologies as they occur. A major emphasis in this development is to retain the proven reliability and effectiveness of the MUMPS-based applications without hindering development activities using newer state-of-the-art technologies.

The current OCIS development activities (Phase III) and associated rationale are presented below. Present development activities are categorized into application development, hardware and storage devices, and communications. It should be emphasized that these three areas are very interdependent. Future development strategies are described in the final section of this chapter.

Present Application Development

Personnel at the Center have indicated that a myriad of computing requirements still exist. Many of these requirements can be smoothly integrated into the present OCIS hierarchical database structure provided through MUMPS. Other user-defined needs are of a nature better handled by different tools and environments. The additional user-defined applications include

on-line nursing procedures, patient care plans, and discharge instructions;
bedside data entry and information access;
order entry for blood products, tests, and procedures;
charge capture integrated with Hospital's billing systems;
cross-clinic and consultation appointment systems;
clinical research data management, monitoring, and analysis;
enhanced resource forecasting and monitoring;
clinical image display and analysis systems;
ad hoc administrative and research query databases;
Center-wide electronic mail and document exchange;
higher level of office automation, including desktop publication, individual calendaring, and personnel scheduling.

A major emphasis in all future application development activities is the use of commercial products whenever practical. Although some of the user requirements, such as office automation, can be addressed through purchasing off-the-shelf software, a significant number of applications will need to be developed in-house. When in-house development is necessary, a focus will be placed on complying with industry standards. Significant efforts are being directed toward interfacing the MUMPS-based OCIS functions with non-MUMPS environments. When non-MUMPS application development tools are used, an emphasis will be placed on selecting viable and industry standard products.

As discussed in Chapter 3, OCIS was built using a locally developed environment called TEDIUM[1], which generates MUMPS programs and uses a MUMPS

---

[1]TEDIUM is a trademark of Tedious Enterprises, Inc.

hierarchical database. TEDIUM has also provided the data dictionary tools for controlling and maintaining the OCIS database and applications at a level presently not found in most commercial products. The hierarchical structure of a MUMPS database meets virtually all of the patient data management requirements. However, TEDIUM is not a fully supported commercial product, and it was never designed to interface with many of the new software tools and environments that are becoming available.

In order to meet the Oncology Center's expanding data management needs, it will be necessary to purchase and integrate development environments and applications that are not directly compatible with the present MUMPS environment. Since the mid-1980s there has been a great deal of industry focus and development in the area of relational database management system's (RDBMS) technology. Related to that development have been advances in local-area networks (LANs), other communication protocols, and modular growth over LANs through high-powered personal workstations. More recently, the Structured Query Language (SQL),[2] developed by IBM in the 1970s, has been accepted as the de facto industry standard query interface for RDBMSs. Technological advances in distributed database management, multinode updates with two-phase commits, referential integrity (triggers) at the database level, modular front-end/back-end network structures, and the use of standard network communications protocols make the RDBMS environment very appealing for new applications development. In practice, the relational database model is very attractive for queries that extend across patient populations, which are necessary for many research and management applications. Relational technology also has potential for applications requiring high-speed on-line transaction processing, such as appointment and order-entry systems.

Still, the hierarchical structure of MUMPS is favored for the majority of data management requirements in medicine that involve single patient queries. For most of the Oncology Center database applications, the MUMPS/TEDIUM environment is believed to be the most logical from a technical perspective. Even with these positive feelings about MUMPS, the Center is in the process of developing several new applications using RDBMS technology. Although MUMPS technically meets the Center's needs and it would be optimal to maintain a single database for all applications, the increasingly strong presence of RDBMS technology cannot be ignored.

The product that has been selected for the initial development of several applications is Sybase.[3] It is felt that this data management tool will provide the greatest long-term flexibility and allow for very modular expansion and growth. Not only does Sybase allow for distributed databases over high-speed networks, but it provides referential integrity at the database level. Ensuring referential integrity is potentially the largest component in the development and mainte-

---

[2]Structured Query Language and SQL are trade marks International Business Machines, Inc.
[3]Sybase is a trademark of Sybase, Inc.

nance of relational databases. Usually, this task must be performed directly by the applications developers, leading to potentials for data corruption and high long-term maintenance expenditures. These factors, combined with unusually high transaction speeds and industry commitment to Sybase, make it the product of choice.

In addition to developing new applications in the Sybase RDBMS, several MUMPS-based functions will be ported to test transaction speed. A major problem in using an RDBMS for medical data queries is the tremendous indirection in data access. While a hierarchical query on an individual patient may involve several pointers and two disk reads, the same query in a relational model could involve dozens of pointers and numerous disk reads. If Sybase can provide acceptable throughput for complicated OCIS queries, it is possible that many new OCIS applications will be developed using this tool. It will also open up the longer term prospects of using a single database to serve all oncology needs versus the dual database model described later in this chapter.

Hardware, Operating System, and Storage Technology

The reliance on a dedicated MUMPS-based operating system originated in an era in which computing hardware was very expensive. The ability of the MUMPS database environment to meet the OCIS applications requirements combined with its great efficiency on DEC's PDP[4] minicomputers dictated the initial system's configuration. However, the selection of a nonlayered operating system environment has greatly restricted the use of commercially available applications.

Versions of MUMPS are now available on many generalized operating systems, including DEC VAX/VMS,[4] IBM MVS,[5] MS-DOS,[6] and many UNIX[7] systems. These layered systems tend to trade off the MUMPS operating system's efficiency for the ability to communicate and coexist with other applications and environments. After several years of deliberation, in 1986 a Phase III development plan was implemented to initiate the gradual migration of the PDP/MUMPS-based OCIS system to a more modern layered operating system. This migration will allow the retention of all the code for existing MUMPS applications, while providing the capabilities of using other applications, databases, and programming languages.

As the underpinning of the development plan, a gradual migration from the PDP systems to the DEC VAX/VMS system was selected as the most rational, most cost-effective, and safest solution. The InterSystems' version of MUMPS, in which OCIS is written, is code compatible with the DEC PDP and VAX/VMS environments. InterSystems also provides network protocol software for dis-

---

[4]DEC, PDP, VAX and VMS are trademarks of Digital Equipment Corporation.
[5]IBM and MVS are trademarks of International Business Machines, Inc.
[6]MS-DOS is a trademark of Microsoft Corporation.
[7]UNIX is a trademark of AT&T.

tributed data access and updates between these environments. These factors allow a very controlled migration from the PDP to the VAX hardware environment. Additionally, the DEC VAX line of computers can support all of the functions required by the Center and serve as a natural interface with OCIS MUMPS-based data.

In 1987 the two PDP-11/70 computers that supported OCIS computational activities were replaced by two PDP-11/84 computers (see Figure 2). Even as this chapter is being written, the PDP environment continues to provide the most cost-effective means of supporting MUMPS-based applications. A direct migration to the VAX/VMS environment might have disrupted critical services to an unacceptable level; switching to a new operating system is best performed in a slow and methodical manner when critical functions are involved.

The two PDP-11/84 computers, however, can only accommodate approximately 100 concurrent OCIS users, and demands for services continue to grow. To begin migration efforts to the VAX environment, two MicroVAX 3600[8] computers have been installed and are being incorporated into the MUMPS/OCIS applications. The new VAX systems will be used primarily to provide additional computing power necessary to serve a growing user population, act as backup systems for the PDP configuration, and test the VAX/VMS systems' ability to handle the higher OCIS user loads anticipated in the future. They will also provide a gateway between MUMPS applications and other applications operating in a VAX/VMS environment and may support additional functions, such as Sybase front-end applications.

Additionally, a MicroVAX II is being used for statistical computing, mail, calendaring, and Sybase RDBMS front-end development. A MicroVAX 3500 has been installed to provide server (back-end) power for the Sybase RDBMS. The application front-end software for the Sybase server also can be run on personal workstations, such as the IBM PC. These two computers will be used primarily to develop and support the additional non-MUMPS-based applications required at the Center. All VAX/VMS computers are being linked through DECnet protocols using the DEC local-area VAX cluster (LAVC) approach over Ethernet. The PDP and VAX computers communicate over Ethernet using a proprietary communications protocol from Intersystems called Mnet.

Integration of the 150 Oncology Center PCs into this environment is being performed using Novell software, which permits microcomputers to join a heterogeneous network using DECnet and TCP/IP over Ethernet. A Gandalf Starport[9] has been selected as the central Novell network server for both terminals and smaller workstations such as IBM PC and Apple Macintosh[10] microcomputers. This Intel 80386-based Novell server can support up to 100 workstations. In addition, PC applications cards can be added to the server to allow any terminal connected to the Gandalf Starmaster switch to act as an IBM PC. Application cards

---

[8]MicroVAX is a trademark of Digital Equipment Corporation.
[9]Gandalf Starport is a trademark of Gandalf Communications, Inc.
[10]Macintosh is a trademark of Apple Computers, Inc.

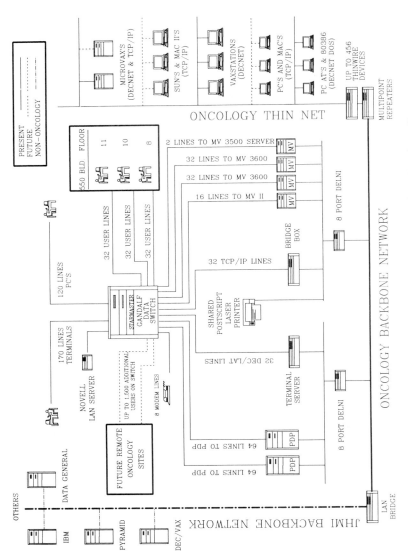

Figure 2. Present hardware and network configuration of the Oncology Center.

can be added for as many as 56 concurrent users and should support the needs of over 200 midlevel PC users. This will permit the integration of a wide variety of data servers with an equally wide variety of workstations and terminals.

The combined DECnet and Novel local-area networks will allow all processors and terminals to share the same applications environment, physical data files, and data backup mechanisms. PCs and other workstations can be converted into virtual terminals to use the processing power and storage of larger machines. Terminals can be converted into PCs and have access to the wide variety of applications software available in the MS-DOS environment. Larger machines can provide data-serving activities for smaller machines. Data storage and backup can be handled locally by the user or centrally by information system's personnel.

The majority of the very popular PC-based software has been ported to the VAX/VMS, Apple Macintosh, and Sun[11]/UNIX environments. The WordPerfect Office[12] product is being used as the hub for all office automation functions. This product can perform as a single system across heterogeneous computer equipment performing such tasks as multinode meeting scheduling and mail systems. Thus, users will have one homogeneous office environment. When available, the Sybase/Microsoft SQL Server[13] will be used for database management on the smaller machines. This server technology can act in total concert with the Sybase server on the MicroVAX 3500 allowing truly distributed databases across heterogeneous equipment.

All centralized data storage and backup activities are performed using extremely fast 760 megabyte, 5¼-inch Winchester drives from Maxtor, combined with removable drive technology from Trimarchi, Inc. Identical subsystems have been installed for both primary storage and backup on the VAX and PDP computers, and the Novell server. Identical controllers are being used on both the PDP and VAX machines, thus opening up the possibility for data sharing between these environments directly through the removable Winchester drives.

Each of the six minicomputers (two PDPs and four VAXs) have at least 1.2 gigabytes of on-line storage with two generations of removable Winchester backup. Storage capabilities will be doubled in approximately two years for minimal capital outlay. Optical storage devices are presently being investigated for addressing the growing demand for high-volume image data storage.

Communications

During the latter half of the 1980s, every year has been referred to as "the year of the local area network (LAN)." Real development in this area, however, has been very slow. Faster networks and standard network protocols are always just around the corner. In reality, faster networks will probably occur before standard network communication protocols, for example, the Open Systems

---

[11]Sun is a trademark of Sun Microsystems, Inc.
[12]WordPerfect Office is a trademark of WordPerfect Corporation.
[13]SQL Server is a trademark of Microsoft Corporation.

ONCOLOGY INFORMATION SYSTEMS

CLINICAL SYSTEMS

1. Oncology Clinical Information System
2. Radiology Reporting/Film Tracking
3. Pathology/Autopsy Report System
4. Anesthesiology Schedule System

SUPPORT SYSTEMS

5. WordPerfect Office/Word Processing
6. Welsh Medical Library
7. NCI/PDQ Protocol and Standard Therapy
8. Statistical Analysis System (SAS)
9. Modem Pool (Call In and Call Out)
10. JHMI Network Access

11. HELP

Enter Service Number:

Figure 3. User menu for accessing oncology and institutional resources through the Gandalf Starmaster data switch.

Interconnect Standard from the International Standards Organization. Even after standards for communications protocols have been established, it will take years for acceptance and migration. In the meantime, organizations requiring high-speed communications must adopt de facto standards such as TCP/IP, DECnet, XNS,[14] and SNA.[15]

There is a growing need to communicate both within the Center and with other areas of Johns Hopkins Hospital for activities such as cross-clinic scheduling, centralized registration, on-line charge capture, and electronic mail. The current development of communications capabilities at the Center incorporates a two-front approach (see Figure 2). An Ethernet backbone installed in the Center bridges to the main Hospital network, and all minicomputers communicate over this network. There has been a sizable expansion of twisted-pair capabilities for peer-to-peer and peer-to-host communications.

---

[14]XNS is a trademark of Xerox Corporation.
[15]SNA is a trademark of International Business Machines.

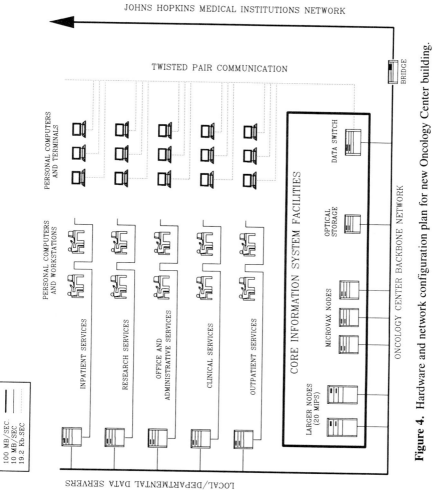

Figure 4. Hardware and network configuration plan for new Oncology Center building.

Concurrent with the PDP replacement, a Gandalf Starmaster data switch was installed to allow the virtual circuit connection of user terminals and printers with any of the Center's computing facilities and with the Hospital's Ethernet network. The 350 twisted-pair wire ports, which were incorporated into the initial building design in 1975, have been routed through this data switch and provide up to 19,200-baud virtual circuit access to hosts for both terminals and PCs within the Center.

This switch is also used to connect over 100 oncology users remotely located from the Center through a series of integrated statistical multiplexers and incorporates 64 terminal servers into the Ethernet network using either LAT or TCP/IP protocols. Both low-level and network-speed interfaces are provided for users through an additional 32-port network bridge and a high-speed filtering LAN bridge connected to the main hospital Ethernet network. Through this data switch, users have access to numerous computing resources throughout the institution, as well as within the Oncology Center (Figure 3). Users desiring high-speed access to host computers for their PCs and other workstations can connect to the Oncology network through the installation of thin Ethernet cable and appropriate interface devices.

The data switch also has 64-kilobaud capability and will act as a front-end or access point for the Integrated Services Digital Network (ISDN), when such a service becomes available during the next decade. Thus, communications efforts within the Center have been placed under central control, and there is room for significant growth and development in this area.

Future Development

Owing to the rapid growth at Johns Hopkins in both the areas of cancer research and oncology patient care, the Oncology Center plans to move into a new building in 1992. Thus, within four years all information systems applications in oncology will have to be available for use in a new physical environment when the move is made. A decade ago, the task of making such a move in an acceptable manner would have been enormous. Fortunately, two of the basic goals in evolving information systems standards are to provide the mechanisms for resource connectivity and modular growth. These factors will dramatically simplify the move of information systems functions.

Even without the planned move to a new building, a significant portion of the Oncology Center's long-term strategy would logically include moving existing OCIS MUMPS-based applications to hardware and operating systems that support modern computing standards. The planned move makes the implementation of a flexible information systems strategy even more important to the Oncology Center. Fortunately, computer connectivity can be designed into the new building in a manner that should make this necessary move transparent from an information system's user perspective (see Figure 4). Parallel operation of the old and new systems will be performed over a network between the two buildings. This

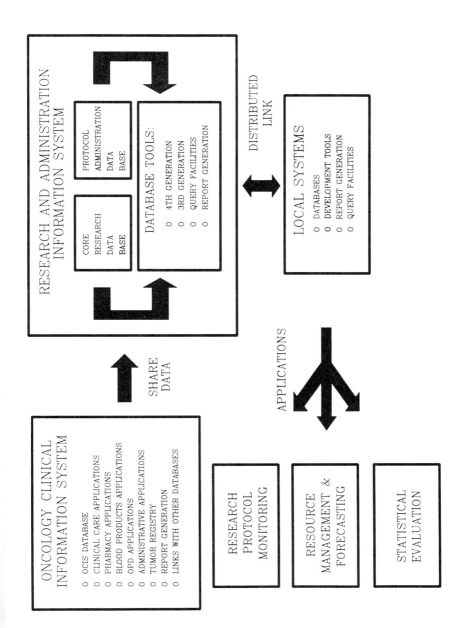

Figure 5. Dual database distribution model, clinical and research administrative systems.

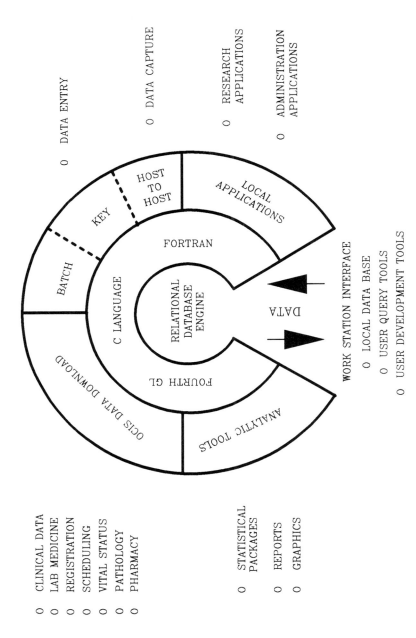

Figure 6. Relational database engine architecture for research and administrative systems.

move provides the Center with an opportunity to design a connectivity structure that matches its philosophy without a major building retrofit.

The basic hardware expansion strategy is extremely simple. There are some tasks in which massive power must be applied to a single task. However, if an application does not require enormous amounts of power to achieve acceptable single-task performance, systems designed in a modular manner can significantly reduce costs. Presently (1988), it is possible to network multiple CPUs to provide large amounts of power for many tasks, each of which requires only a fraction of the total. There is currently a fourfold difference between the power of microcomputer CPUs and those of minicomputers. There is a sevenfold gap between the fastest minicomputer CPU and those of the fastest mainframe.

The tasks performed within the oncology environment generally do not require enormous power—there are just lots of tasks that must share the same environment and data. Therefore, multiprocessor computers and networks to link computers will be the most cost-effective solution for the envisioned oncology environment. A modular hardware expansion will provide the necessary power for the least cost and greater long-term flexibility.

Additionally, the strategy must provide mechanisms to integrate the oncology computing environment with that being developed throughout The Johns Hopkins Medical Institutions (JHMI). It has become very apparent that data and functions that are essential to the Oncology Center are also essential to other areas in the JHMI. Following industry standards whenever possible provides the best probability for future integration with other systems not under the control of the Oncology Center.

The plan for integrating OCIS data with other applications involves both a dual database scheme and additional user and programmer tools to interface with this secondary database (see Figure 5). The secondary database will derive a significant portion of its information from the OCIS system. OCIS will continue to be used as the frontline clinical management tool for oncology patients. It will also function as a data collection front end for the research and administrative database.

The research and administrative information system will use a relational database engine (back end) with applications tools (front end) available from a wide variety of vendors on heterogeneous equipment (see Figure 6). This front-end/back-end strategy will make the modular expansion of computing power possible. The Sybase RDBMS engine (previously discussed) running on a MicroVAX 3500 computer should be able to support the data requests from over 200 concurrent users. The major expansion expense will be in adding individual workstations (front ends) as the system develops. The Sybase front end will be available for numerous workstations, including the IBM-PC/AT, the Apple Macintosh, and all VAX computers.

The primary concept of the Oncology Center information systems plan is to develop a uniform environment for linking heterogeneous computer equipment from a variety of manufacturers. Within the Oncology Center and throughout the

Hospital, computer equipment comprises and will continue to comprise micro-computers, minicomputers, and mainframes from multiple vendors, running under various operating systems and being used for a wide variety of functions.

The Oncology Center's strategy is to remain as homogeneous as possible in systems selection within the Center. This will make operations, management, communications, and general applications support functions extremely efficient. The strategy also includes currently available methods for high-level hardware and software integration with other Hospital computers. Future technological advances should allow nearly transparent systems integration with other areas of the Hospital and, potentially, with other similar treatment facilities throughout the world.

10
Implementing OCIS at the Ohio State University

Elizabeth E. McColligan[1]

Editors' Introduction

OCIS has been distributed to two other cancer centers for implementation. In 1984, the New South Wales State Cancer Council began to implement the system in Australia. They first sent some clinical staff members to observe the JHOC operations, and later a computer specialist (Parvis Ostovari) spent three months at JHOC. He had to learn MUMPS, TEDIUM, OCIS and clinical computing. At the end of that time, he took the various systems—about 6000 programs in all— back to Australia.

The system has been operational in the Prince of Wales Hospital, Sydney, for about four years. Its database contains information on some 2000 patients. It is called the Oncology Research Central Information System (ORCIS) in Australia, and it is described in a journal article.[2]

The second OCIS transfer is presented in this chapter. In this case the responsible person participated in the development of OCIS subsystems and was experienced in both of the development languages used: MUMPS and TEDIUM. The discussion covers the first year of conversion activity at Ohio State University.

Background

The Arthur G. James Cancer Hospital and Research Institute of The Ohio State University (OSU-CHRI) is a 12-story, free-standing building immediately adjacent to The Ohio State University Hospitals.

---

[1]Elizabeth E. McColligan, M.S., M.P.H., is Director of the Computer Center at the Arthur G. James Cancer Hospital and Research Institute of The Ohio State University, Columbus, Ohio.

[2]Terry J. Hannan and Michael Vincenz, Introduction of a Computer-Based Oncology Patient-Care System in a Teaching Hospital, *Medical Journal of Australia*, 148: 242–247, 1988. There also is a short paper in *Cancer Forum*, November 1987.

Construction of the OSU-CHRI began in July 1984, and it is scheduled to open in the first quarter of 1989. The 260,000 square feet of space includes an up-to-date Radiation Therapy Center on the ground floor. The Outpatient Department, located on the first and second floors, will be able to accommodate 100,000 outpatient visits annually. A sophisticated Bone Marrow Transplant Unit, consisting of 24 inpatient beds and modern treatment and research areas, will be located on the third floor. An ultramodern operating room suite, consisting of 6 operating rooms and equipped with intraoperative radiation therapy equipment, will be located on the fourth floor. The seventh, eighth, ninth, and tenth floors will house a total of 136 inpatient beds to facilitate the treatment of the 4800 inpatients expected to be admitted by the OSU-CHRI annually. The eleventh and twelfth floors provide approximately 26,000 square feet of basic research space.

The OSU-CHRI will support an interdisciplinary approach to the treatment of cancer and facilitate state-of-the-art cancer research. It is expected that most patients treated at the Institute will be on some type of research treatment protocol. The Ohio State University is currently recognized as a Comprehensive Cancer Center by the National Cancer Institutes and is a major contributor to the Southwest Oncology Group (SWOG). The Ohio State University also participates in other clinical cancer research protocols, including the National Surgical Adjuvant Breast and Colon Programs (NSABP), the Head and Neck Oncology Intergroup, the Gynecological Oncology Group, the Melanoma and Limb Perfusion Study Group, the Brain Tumor Study Group, and the Urological Tumor Study Group.

The Need for a System

The Bone Marrow Transplant Program (BMT) at The Ohio State University was begun in the summer of 1983 when Dr. Peter J. Tutschka joined the faculty. Dr. Tutschka had been at Johns Hopkins University prior to joining the faculty at The Ohio State University and was familiar with the OCIS system. Dr. Tutschka brought OCIS to the attention of the hospital's administration and Dr. Arthur G. James who had been lobbying for a Cancer Hospital and Research Institute for many years.

Dr. Tutschka appreciated the necessity of a clinical information system to assist with the data management needs of the BMT program. Although none was immediately available to him, there was a version of the Sloan-Kettering research data management system in use at OSU as part of the Comprehensive Cancer Center (OSU-CCC) program (see Serber). Although this system was unable to address many of the clinical information needs of the BMT program, it was decided to use this system for some of the emergent data management tasks. This is a MIIS-based system. It allows the user to define groups of data, up to 100 items per group, and provides for "repeated" items, such as laboratory tests, and nonrepeated "core" items.

The OSU-CCC system can store only one value per day for each of the repeated items, which is a limitation with respect to clinical management. Another limitation is that the data are stored by protocol. To get around this, a general "data" protocol was defined for all BMT patients. The system provides for the generation of basic flow sheets and allows searches of the database and the definition of aggregates, thereby facilitating the generation of statistics by diagnosis, protocol, and other user-defined cohorts. Finally, the system enables the definition of cohort files that can be transferred to more sophisticated statistical packages. All data must be manually entered and, as mentioned previously, only one value per day can be stored.

The first bone marrow transplant was performed in February 1984, and the BMT program began using the OSU-CCC system in a production mode by February 1986. Initially, data were entered on current patients, and eventually the backlog of data on patients who had been transplanted prior to 1986 was entered. In January 1988, when the conversion of the data from this system to OCIS occurred, the system had data stored on 125 patients.

Selecting a System

In early 1986, before the decision to go ahead and implement OCIS was made, a review of several other systems was carried out. These systems ranged from general medical-record-type systems, in particular, COSTAR (COmputer STored Ambulatory Record; see Barnett), PROMIS (PRoblem Oriented Medical Information System; see PROMIS Laboratory), and TMR (The Medical Record; see Stead), to systems developed specifically for Cancer Centers, in particular, WISAR (WISconsin Storage And Retrieval Data Management System; see Friedman), CDMS (Cancer Data Management System; see Horwitz), and CPIS (Clinical Protocol Information System; see Wirtschafter).

The general medical-record-type systems were considered too general because they did not provide any tools that would specifically aid in the clinical management of oncology patients, particularly with respect to protocol management. Of the oncology-specific systems reviewed, CDMS and CPIS were the most clinically oriented; however, both were much more limited in scope than OCIS. Although the primary focus of both CDMS and CPIS was the management of clinical protocols, OCIS was much more general in its orientation to managing clinical data for all patients, as well as having protocol management capabilities. It was decided that OCIS represented the most advanced system specifically developed for oncology patient management available at the time. We concluded that OCIS could provide most of the baseline functionality we required and would provide a solid foundation that would facilitate the development of an OSU-specific oncology clinical information system. Consequently, OSU-CHRI elected to install OCIS as a prototype on the BMT unit.

Installation History

The saying "ignorance is bliss" can certainly be applied to our notions of what would be involved in bringing the OCIS system up at the OSU-CHRI. As will be seen, the basic assumption that the system as it was written and functioning at the

Johns Hopkins Oncology Center (JHOC) could be easily ported to OSU-CHRI was not completely accurate. There were two basic causes for complexity in the system transfer.

When we decided to implement OCIS at the OSU-CHRI, we recognized that OCIS was not a turnkey system. We expected that there would be several modifications to be made and that many of the system dictionaries would have to be defined. However, we did not fully anticipate the magnitude or the level of complexity of the modifications we would be undertaking.

Our second underestimation is linked to the ever-present optimism of developers. It is known that the installation of a hospital information system can take 6 to 24 months, even when there are no programming changes. In our case, the author, working half-time on the conversion project, and one full-time programmer with MIIS experience expected to bring up and customize a 5000-program system with 1400 relations that ran on networked computers supporting 100-plus terminals. And we promised to have an operational product that supported a dozen terminals on a MicroVAX within a year. We did succeed, but as the last sentence suggests, it was a more difficult project than we had expected initially.

Standard Conversion Requirements

Every health care facility has local conventions and site-specific requirements. Vendors of clinical systems design their products so that they can easily accommodate these local demands. In the case of OCIS, the system was developed for internal use, and the transporters had to assume the responsibility for making the necessary changes. Because I had worked on a part of the OCIS and was familiar with the TEDIUM[1] development environment that was used, I was confident that many of these so-called routine changes would not be difficult to make. This section describes the expected modifications and our experience with them.

Patient Identifier. The patient identifier, or medical record number, is a seven-digit number at Johns Hopkins Hospital. At OSU it is a nine-digit number. Although this was a fairly straightforward modification, it was quite extensive. TEDIUM maintains a data dictionary that is used by all generated programs. To change the format of the history number (HNO) field primarily involved changing the element definition, which then was automatically reflected in the table definitions. However, the extensiveness was reflected in the fact that the element HNO is used as an index item in some 552 tables and as a data element in 53 tables. Therefore, I would estimate that more than half of the programs referenced these tables, and many made direct reference to the element HNO, either to its format or to check its range.

The range of the HNO at JHOC was used to categorize patients. Three ranges were used. Hospital HNOs were less than 8000000, numbers between 8000000

---

[1]TEDIUM is a trademark of Tedium Enterprises, Inc.

and 8999999 were used for outreach patients treated outside Hopkins, and numbers greater than 9000000 were "temporary" numbers used for preadmissions, etc. Medical record numbers at OSU are usually nine-digit numbers starting with 900 assigned by the Medical Records Department. However, medical record numbers may also be social security numbers or some other number assigned by Medical Records but not starting with 900. We chose to designate "temporary" numbers as those beginning with 999. As OSU does not have an outreach program at present, we did not need this category of medical record numbers.

This conversion modification was straightforward, but quite extensive. Fortunately, most of the HNO processing was performed by two input routines. However, some of the programs that had to make decisions based on the logical content of the HNO did so by using procedural code. As a result, it was decided that we would modify the registration and the two central patient identification routines initially, and we would review the need to alter other routines as we brought up each function. The initial modification required only several days. The remaining routines are still being modified, as the conversion is not complete and not all functions are active.

Clinical Laboratory Link. It was imperative that we establish a communication link that would permit the electronic transfer of laboratory data. This required writing routines on the laboratory system that would query the CHRI computer to determine which patients' data should be transferred and then search the laboratory system and transfer the resulting file to the CHRI system. Once the data are received, CHRI system reads the VMS file into a MUMPS global and then processes the data. Because the laboratory does not use unique laboratory codes (the laboratory code and specimen type are both required to uniquely identify a result), we needed to create and define a translation dictionary. This laboratory translation dictionary maps the laboratory code and specimen type into a unique Item Dictionary code. (The OCIS Item Dictionary provides mnemonic names, short names, formats, and the ranges for all test values, findings, drugs, etc., that are used in the clinical outputs, for example, in the plots and flows. Naturally, this dictionary is site specific.)

The laboratory transfer routines had to include procedures to hold the data in case the CHRI system was down and also to ensure that the data runs would be contiguous in case the laboratory system was down. This data transfer is done over an Ethernet link in a batch mode three times a day, 9:00 A.M., 3:00 P.M., and 11:00 P.M. Because of the load on the laboratory system and its inability to handle much of an additional processing load, this link presently only involves hematology, chemistry, and immunology data. University Hospitals' administration is presently considering upgrading the laboratory computer system, and it is our hope that we will be able to receive bacteriological (microbiology), blood banking, and surgical pathology data in the future. University Hospitals is also in the process of installing a fiberoptic network, which we hope will facilitate the real-time transfer of these laboratory data.

As one would expect, we also needed to write programs that would recognize errors, such as no item code defined, name mismatch, and comment field too long. The OCIS programs then were modified to allow data coordinators to review and correct the errors and reprocess the corrected data.

Dictionaries. As the reader may be aware, the OCIS implementation draws heavily upon dictionaries. Excluding the dictionaries used by the daily care plan functions, the pharmacy system, and the blood product management programs, there are over 100 standard dictionaries. Some, like the Item Dictionary, play a central role in most clinical processing; others, like the dictionaries of valid units and zip code–state combinations, are used only for input validation.

We are still in the process of redefining many of these dictionaries and continually updating others. Several crucial dictionaries had to be defined very early in the project. These included the Item Dictionary and dictionaries for flow-sheet and plot definitions, providers, diagnoses, reasons for admission, and protocols. The most extensive and time-consuming dictionary was the Item Dictionary and a related laboratory translation dictionary. As of the end of February 1988, our Item Dictionary contained approximately 1000 item codes. (650 laboratory codes, 50 clinical status items, and 300 medications.)

Help Message Updates. Another task that had to be undertaken was modifying the help documentation. TEDIUM manages the help messages as an extension to the data dictionary and program specifications; changing the data model definitions also changes the help messages that the end user sees. For us, customizing the help messages involved editing element descriptions, menu help messages, and internal program help messages. The main driver menus and generic variables (such as HNO) were updated initially, whereas the internal program help messages were modified as we implemented a particular function.

Menu and Report Headings. It goes without saying we had to replace all of "the Johns Hopkins Oncology Center" headings with "The Ohio State University". Although this was not a difficult task, it was time consuming and tedious. TEDIUM did help us somewhat with this modification in that many of the headings were stored in frames that are shared by many programs; a change to the frame is reflected in the output of all the associated programs. Unfortunately, some programs also used procedural code to augment the headings.

We decided to make modifications to only the frame programs initially and then to modify the individual routines, mainly report routines, as we brought up the various functions.

Data Conversion. The first phase of OCIS implementation was to use the system in a prototype mode on the Bone Marrow Transplant Unit. As mentioned earlier, data dating back to 1984 had been collected via a research data management system on 125 BMT patients. As a result, it was necessary to write routines that would allow us to transfer that database to the CHRI system and then load as much of the data as possible into the OCIS prototype database. This required yet another translation dictionary because items were stored by number on the research database. Although all of the repeated clinical data items, such as temperature and hematocrit, were added to the Item Dictionary, there were several core items that did not exist in the OCIS database. These items included the BMT unique patient number, a sequential number assigned when the patient is accepted for transplant; donor name and medical record number; and other BMT-specific data. As a result, we created a BMT-specific table consisting of 10 items. We also wrote routines to add and edit this table and modified other display routines so that if the patient is a BMT patient these data are displayed along with other general patient information.

Customizing OCIS for OSU-CHRI

In transporting OCIS to OSU-CHRI it was necessary to adapt the system's operation so that it would be "natural" to the CHRI users. Recall that OCIS was developed for JHOC as an internal product over a period of many years. Its users had grown with the system; many of the clinicians helped to define how that system would perform. Because OCIS was relied upon very heavily at JHOC, and because there was a large and stable body of users at JHOC, new OCIS users found it easy to accept OCIS "warts and all." Naturally, one could not expect this same willingness when introducing a new system to a new set of users.

Although OCIS is an on-line system, user interaction at JHOC, particularly with regard to the health professional user, was designed to manage the bulk of the clinical processing in a paper-oriented fashion. As a result, the system tends to have a batch mode approach to many functions. While the number of health professionals interested in an on-line clinical information system at OSU may not be so numerous as those at JHOC (especially since we are still in the prototype phase), those who are interested want to interact with the system directly and not via hard-copy reports or with the aid of a data coordinator. Although we recognize the need for data coordinators, we have taken the approach that the system should also support more direct physician and health care professional interaction. Part of this is due to the fact that the prototype users have had experience with a research data management system that gave them on-line access to data, permitted on-line report generation and listing, and was not strictly geared to hard-copy output.

Dictionaries. Physicians and other health care providers at OSU do not use a unique provider ID. (The Johns Hopkins Hospital has a central office that assigns unique IDs used throughout the institution for all clinical and administrative functions.) As a result, we modified the dictionary entry program so that these IDs are generated by the system and are only used for internal reference. The users of the system interact with the system via the provider's name.

Another difference in dictionaries involved the Protocol Dictionary. Health professionals at OSU were not accustomed to referring to protocols by their IDs, but rather by their short names. Although both the internal and SWOG protocols did have IDs, they were not generally used. In addition, the format of the protocol IDs differed, and so we had to modify the element definition and correct the programs that referenced the protocol ID. It was also necessary to modify several routines that displayed only the protocol ID so that they would display the short name in place of or in addition to the ID. This was a case of modifying the system to reflect what the health professionals were used to, a problem we encountered frequently and that has been responsible for most of the unexpected modifications.

Although the unit or location variable is stored in a dictionary, it was often referenced by the specific values used at Hopkins. For example, often a prompt was used that specified the various units at Hopkins. This was most often the case when selecting reports. This had to be changed so that the prompt did not specify the various units but only asked for a unit and then checked to be sure a valid unit had been specified by checking the dictionary.

Another minor modification that was used for several dictionaries was the use of an index option when prompting for a code. For instance, the format sequences used by the data entry and data coordinator staff were not always as mnemonic as one would like, and we found that often one had to go through several characters in the alphabet before the correct code could be identified. Our users therefore asked for an index option that could be used in addition to the character prompt to list through all of the possible codes quickly and in a more "user friendly" fashion. We also implemented this option in the Reason for Admission Dictionary, as well.

Preformatted Plot and Flow Updating. The general method that OCIS uses to update the preformatted flow sheets and plots is a batch mode approach. At various times, usually at night and after laboratory link runs, the unformatted clinical data are updated into the preformatted plot and flow files. There are three basic formats used by the OCIS clinical displays. One format contains the clinical data. This can be displayed in the Data format or the vertical flow-sheet format; these displays always contain the most current data. Because the plots and horizontal flow sheets present the data in a different sort order, the rapid production of output is managed best when the data are copied over into a format "close to" the display being produced, that is, the preformatted data. In JHOC, these displays are printed and seldom called on line; therefore, it is most efficient to update them infrequently or on demand. The on-demand update results in a response delay; displaying the preformatted data is immediate.

This design was not acceptable for OSU. We felt that the primary purpose of the system was to provide clinical data to the health care professionals in a meaningful way. If we were to have an acceptable system, we needed to be sure that the data being accessed by the health care providers were in the most convenient and useful format, flows and plots, and that the data were as up-to-date as possible. Therefore, we decided to rework the update processing. As we now process the clinical data, we record the date of the data in a new global called

REGEN. After all data have been updated in the basic OCIS clinical data table, we submit a background job that regenerates the preformatted flow and plot files from the earliest date in REGEN to the current date. In effect, we do the daily JHOC processing after each data update process.

Although this may not be entirely efficient from a computational point of view, it guarantees that the preformatted data are as current as possible. The overhead is not great at this point in time, but we are aware that this may have a negative effect on system performance under heavy loads. We plan to review the regeneration step so that only days that have actually been updated are regenerated.

Redesign of Flow-Sheet Format. Although OCIS has the ability to store multiple data values per day, only the first value of the day is shown on the standard horizontal flow sheet in both the on-line and hard-copy forms. We had the need to show all data values. In addition, the Medical Records Department required that the time associated with each data value and the normal ranges for the values be printed on the hard-copy flows. Because of character space limitations, we decided not to display the times or the normal ranges on the on-line flow, but the values are sorted by time, and we provide an option to look up normal ranges. Although we have the need to record normal ranges by age and sex eventually, we have decided to use the single-range scheme supported by OCIS at present. This is acceptable because we have opted to use the abnormal flag that is determined by the laboratory and sent with the result. The range stored as part of the Item Dictionary is used only as a reference and not to determine the abnormality of a data value. In the future we do plan to implement a more sophisticated abnormal range scheme based on age and sex.

Data Value Comments. Although OCIS has the ability to store comments with each data item, this feature was never used at JHOC and therefore was not fully implemented in OCIS. Our users felt that the comment field was essential, particularly in light of the fact that the laboratory routinely sends comments as part of the result. This required modifying many of the data entry routines and all of the clinical data display routines, both the unformatted data displays (Figure 1) and the flow sheets. It also required that a check be added to the plot routines: If the data value is not numerical, then look for another data value for that day until either a numerical value is found or there are no more data values for the day.

Other format changes were also made to the flow-sheet routines to satisfy both the additional requirements, as well as requests from the prototype users. There are two options available when requesting a hard copy of a horizontal flow: a flow with times and normal ranges, which makes use of a 132-column compressed print mode (Figure 2), and one with no times or ranges, which uses the standard 80-column print mode (Figure 3).

Refinement of Plots. With respect to the plot function, we found hooks for features that had been planned for in OCIS but had not been implemented. For instance, the plot definition routines allow for definition of an unlimited number

```
                                        CLINICAL DATA                    06/28/88

ITEMS FOR 02/19/88

LABORATORY
      .WBC        3.9*    7:25A    .RBC      2.67*   7:25A    .HGB       9.3*   7:25A
      .HCT       26.8*    7:25A    .MCV     100.2*   7:25A    .MCH      34.8*   7:25A
      .MCHC      34.8     7:25A    .PLAT      96*    7:25A    .MPV       7.5    7:25A
      .NEUT      55       7:25A    .BAND       0     7:25A    .LYM       32     7:25A
      .MONOS      7       7:25A    .EOS        5*    7:25A    .BASO       0     7:25A
      .META       1       7:25A    .MYEL       0     7:25A    .R1       PLTD    7:25A
      .R2        ANIS     7:25A    PTN        9.9*   5:55A    BUN        14     5:58A
                 2+
      GLUC       95       5:58A    CREAT      1.0    5:58A    NA        140     5:58A
      K           3.9     5:58A    CL        105     5:58A    CO2        24     5:58A
      UAPRN      STRW     9:00P    USPGR     1.018   9:00P    UPH        5.0    9:00P
                 CLR
      UPR        NEG      9:00P    UGL       NEG     9:00P    UKET      NEG     9:00P
      UBLD       NEG      9:00P    UBIL      NEG     9:00P    UWBC       2*     9:00P
      URBC       NONE     9:00P    UCAS1       1     9:00P    UCAS2       1     9:00P
                                             HYA                        WCST
      UCRYS      NONE     9:00P    UEPIS     FEW     9:00P    UEPIR     NONE    9:00P
      UMUC       NONE     9:00P    UBACT     NONE    9:00P    UAMOR     NONE    9:00P

NURSING INFORMATION
      TMAXO     102.2              PULSE     140              RESP       24
      BP SYS    130                BP DIA     80              BP<90       N
      WT        134                ITOT     2575              OTOT      1970
      UTOT      1970
MEDICATION
      BUSULO    296                BACTOT      2              IGV        39
      VANCOV   2000                LORAZV      2              MEPERV     25

          ANIS    = ANISOCYTOSIS
          CLR     = CLEAR
          HYA     = HYALINE CASTS
          NEG     = NEGATIVE
          NONE    = NONE SEEN
          STRW    = STRAW
          WCST    = WBC CASTS
```

Figure 1. Sample unformatted data display.

of items. However, the actual plotting routine only used the first two items. Because we chose to keep our hematology results, which come from the Main Laboratory, separate from the special Hematology Laboratory results, we needed to be able to plot a WBC from both the Main Laboratory and the special Hematology Laboratory as one item (There are separate WBC definitions in the Item Dictionary.) We also had the desire to plot more than two items on one graph. We have modified the plotting routines so that as many items as are defined will be plotted, but we have also put a limit on the plot definition of 10 items. Of course, we cannot have more than two scales, so the items must be correlated to a certain extent, and a plot could become difficult to interpret if too many items are selected; but we have left this to the user's discretion.

Data Entry Routines. OSU does not have an automated medication administration system, so we must manually enter the medications administered in the inpatient area and those prescribed in the outpatient area. The two most efficient ways to enter these data are as either a batched group or a formatted sequence. Because we had modified the way in which the formatted data were updated, this

```
THE OHIO STATE UNIVERSITY HOSPITAL                          MEDICAL RECORD NUMBER:
       COLUMBUS, OHIO                                       PATIENT NAME:
                                                            ADMISSION DATE: 02/08/88
STANDARD FLOW AS OF 06/28/88                                SERVICE:                    PAGE  1
   23 y.o.  WHITE  MALE
   ACUTE NON-LYMPHOCYTIC LEUKEMIA
---------------------------------------------------------------------------------------------------
|                         |  19 FEB 88 |  20 FEB 88 |  21 FEB 88 |  22 FEB 88 |  23 FEB 88 |  24 FEB 88 |  25 FEB 88 |
|  83H0268 ANLL BMT       |DAY  -7  |DAY  -6  |DAY  -5  |DAY  -4  |DAY  -3  |DAY  -2  |DAY  -1  |
|HEMATOLOGY---------------|---------|---------|---------|---------|---------|---------|---------|
|.WBC        5-10   K/CMM| 725A    2.9*730A  2.2*730A  2.2*800A  4.1*725A  3.9*750A  4.9*730A  4.3*
|.RBC        4.2-6.2 M/CMM|725A    2.67*730A 2.47*730A 3.53*800A 3.63*725A 3.23*750A 3.45*730A 3.59*
|.HGB        12-18  GM/DL|725A    9.3*730A  8.5*730A  11.7*800A 11.9*725A 10.5*750A 11.5*730A 12.1*
|.HCT        37-54   %   |725A    26.8*730A 24.7*730A 33.3*800A 33.9*725A 30.6*750A 32.3*730A 34.0*
|.MCV        80-99  CU U |725A   100.2*730A 100.0*730A 94.2*800A 93.4|725A 94.6*750A 93.7|730A 94.8*
|.MCH        27-31  PG   |725A    34.8*730A 34.4*730A  33.1*800A 32.8*725A 32.5*750A 33.3*730A 33.7*
|.MCHC       33-37  GM/DL|725A    34.8|730A 34.4| 730A  35.2|800A 35.1|725A 34.4|750A 35.6|730A 35.6|
|PLAT CT     150-400 K/CMM|  ...  |   ...  |   ...  |   ...  |   910P  115*  ...  |   ...  |
|.PLAT       150-440 K/CMM|725A    96*730A  79*730A  83*800A  81*725A  76*750A  116*730A  117*
|MPV         7.4-10.4 R/PL|  ...  |   ...  |   ...  |   ...  |   910P  7.0*  ...  |   ...  |
|.MPV        7.4-10.4 R/PL|725A    7.5|730A  6.8|730A  7.2|800A  7.3|725A  7.3|750A  7.8|730A  7.7|
|.RETIC OBS  .5-1.5  %   |  ...  |   ...  |   ...  |  800A  3.1|  ...  |  750A  2.2|  ...  |
|.RET COR            %   |  ...  |   ...  |   ...  |  800A  2.1|  ...  |  750A  1.6|  ...  |
|.NEUT       50-70   %   |725A   55|   ...  |   ...  |  800A  85|   ...  |  750A  85|   ...  |
|.BANDS              %   |725A   0|   ...  |   ...  |  800A  0|   ...  |  750A  0|   ...  |
|.LYMPH      25-40   %   |725A   32|   ...  |   ...  |  800A  11|   ...  |  750A  8|   ...  |
|.MONOCYTES  1-8     %   |725A   7|   ...  |   ...  |  800A  4|   ...  |  750A  7|   ...  |
|.EOSIN      0-4     %   |725A   A5|   ...  |   ...  |  800A  0|   ...  |  750A  0|   ...  |
|.BASOPHIL   0-2     %   |725A   0|   ...  |   ...  |  800A  0|   ...  |  750A  0|   ...  |
|.METAMYELO          %   |725A   1|   ...  |   ...  |  800A  0|   ...  |  750A  0|   ...  |
|.MYELO              %   |725A   0|   ...  |   ...  |  800A  0|   ...  |  750A  0|   ...  |
|.REMARK1            |725A   PLTD|   ...  |   ...  |  800A PLTDEC|  ...  |  215P TEXT 1|  ...  |
|.REMARK2            |725A   ANIS|   ...  |   ...  |  800A  POIK|  ...  |  215P  ANIS|  ...  |
|  NOTE              |       2+|   ...  |   ...  |       1+|  ...  |       1+|  ...  |
|.REMARK3            |  ...  |   ...  |   ...  |  800A  ANIS|  ...  |   ...  |   ...  |
|  NOTE              |  ...  |   ...  |   ...  |       1+|  ...  |   ...  |   ...  |
|PROTIME     9.5-12.5 SEC|  ...  |   ...  |   ...  |  755A  9.8|  ...  |   ...  |   ...  |
|PTT         23-35   SEC |  ...  |   ...  |   ...  |  755A  32|   ...  |   ...  |   ...  |
|QUANT FIB   170-375 MG/DL|  ...  |   ...  |   ...  |  755A  252|  ...  |   ...  |   ...  |
|FIBRIN DEG  0-5     TITER|  ...  |   ...  |   ...  |  805A  NEG|  ...  |   ...  |   ...  |
|CHEMISTRY ----------|---------|---------|---------|---------|---------|---------|---------|
|UREA        5-24   MG/DL| 558A  14| 615A  7| 709A  7| 802A  7| 606A  10| 648A  12| 640A  17|
| UREA               |  ...  |   ...  |   ...  |   ...  |  953A  10| 640P  12|   ...  |
| UREA               |  ...  |   ...  |   ...  |   ...  |  600P  9|   ...  |   ...  |
|GLUCOSE     65-115 MG/DL| 558A  95| 615A  99| 709A  101| 802A  96| 606A  138*648A  117*640A  104|
| GLUCOSE            |  ...  |   ...  |   ...  |   ...  |  953A  164*  ...  |   ...  |
|CREATININE  0.7-1.3 MG/DL|558A  1.0| 615A  .9| 709A  1.0| 802A  .8| 606A  .7| 648A  .9| 640A  .9|
| CREATININE         |  ...  |   ...  |   ...  |   ...  |  953A  1.2| 640P  .9|   ...  |
| CREATININE         |  ...  |   ...  |   ...  |   ...  |  600P  .8|   ...  |   ...  |
|SODIUM      136-146 MM/L| 558A  140| 615A  145| 709A  144| 802A  140| 606A  139| 648A  138| 640A  135*
| SODIUM             |  ...  |   ...  |   ...  |   ...  |  953A  140| 640P  136|   ...  |
| SODIUM             |  ...  |   ...  |   ...  |   ...  |  600P  135*  ...  |   ...  |
|POTASSIUM   3.7-5.3 MM/L| 558A  3.9| 615A  3.9| 709A  3.7| 802A  3.8| 606A  4.1| 648A  4.2| 640A  5.4*
| POTASSIUM          |  ...  |   ...  |   ...  |   ...  |  953A  3.9| 640P  4.2|   ...  |
---------------------------------------------------------------------------------------------------
```

Figure 2. First page of a sample compressed print flowsheet with times and normal ranges.

also meant we had to modify the data entry routines to reflect the update changes. In addition, since we allow comments to be entered along with a data value for every data item, we needed a way of entering comments efficiently. Because comments are only occasionally entered, it was not efficient to prompt for a data value and a comment for each item. Therefore, we adopted the convention that a semicolon (;) would separate the data value from the comment field.

As mentioned previously, our prototype unit had been using another research data management system and had certain expectations. One of the features of the

E.E. McColligan

```
THE OHIO STATE UNIVERSITY HOSPITAL                      MEDICAL RECORD NUMBER:
        COLUMBUS, OHIO                                  PATIENT NAME:
                                                        ADMISSION DATE: 02/08/88
STANDARD FLOW AS OF 06/28/88                            SERVICE:              PAGE  4
    33 y.o.  WHITE MALE
    ACUTE NON-LYMPHOCYTIC LEUKEMIA
---------------------------------------------------------------------------------------------------------------------
|                             | 19 FEB 88 |  20 FEB 88 |  21 FEB 88 |  22 FEB 88 |  23 FEB 88 |  24 FEB 88 |  25 FEB 88 |
|  83H0268 ANLL BMT           |DAY -7     |DAY -6      |DAY -5      |DAY -4      |DAY -3      |DAY -2      |DAY -1      |
|BLOOD PROD-------------------|-----------|------------|------------|------------|------------|------------|------------|
|TX RBC               UNITS|      ...    |      2|        ...  |      ...    |      ...    |      ...    |      ...    |
|TX PLAT PH           #PROD|      ...    |      ...    |      ...    |      ...    |      1|        ...  |      ...    |
|CHEMOTHER-------------------|-----------|------------|------------|------------|------------|------------|------------|
|BUSULFAN             MG PO|      296|        296|        296|        148|        148|        ...  |      ...    |
|CYCLOPHOS            GM IV|      ...    |      ...    |      ...    |      ...    |      4.47|      4.47|      ...    |
|ANTIBIOTIC------------------|-----------|------------|------------|------------|------------|------------|------------|
|ACYCLOVIR            MG IV|      ...    |      ...    |      880|        1320|      1320|        1320|      1320|
|BACTRIM TD           D-TAB|      2|        2|        2|        2|        2|        2|        2|
|CLOTRIMA             MG PO|      ...    |      40|        40|        10|        10|        40|        40|
|IMMUNOGLBN           GM IV|      39|        ...  |      ...    |      ...    |      ...    |      ...    |      ...    |
|VANCOMYCIN           MG IV|      2000|      2000|      2000|      2000|      1000|      2000|      2000|
|ANTIEMETIC------------------|-----------|------------|------------|------------|------------|------------|------------|
|DXMTHASONE           MG PO|      ...    |      8|        8|        ...  |      ...    |      ...    |      ...    |
|DXMTHASONE           MG IV|      ...    |      ...    |      8|        32|        32|        32|        8|
|DROPERIDOL           MG IV|      ...    |      2|        6|        8|        6|        8|        ...    |
|LORAZEPAM            MG IV|      2|        4|        ...  |      ...    |      ...    |      ...    |      ...    |
|P-C-PERAZN           MG IV|      ...    |      ...    |      ...    |      ...    |      25|        ...  |      ...    |
|ANTACIDS -------------------|-----------|------------|------------|------------|------------|------------|------------|
|MAALOX               ML PO|      ...    |      ...    |      ...    |      ...    |      ...    |      30|        30|
|ANALGESICS------------------|-----------|------------|------------|------------|------------|------------|------------|
|ACETAMIN             MG PO|      ...    |      650|        ...  |      ...    |      ...    |      ...    |      ...    |
|MEPERIDINE           MG IV|      25|        ...  |      ...    |      ...    |      ...    |      ...    |      ...    |
|ANTICONVUL------------------|-----------|------------|------------|------------|------------|------------|------------|
|PHENYTOIN            MG PO|      ...    |      600|        400|        400|        ...  |      ...    |      200|
|PHENYTOIN            MG IV|      ...    |      ...    |      ...    |      ...    |      500|        700|        ...    |
|DRUG LEVEL------------------|-----------|------------|------------|------------|------------|------------|------------|
|PHNYTN LEV           MG/L | 555A    9.9* 605A    7.7* 530A    9.9* 755A    7.8* 959A    5.7* 650A    9.0* 635A   13.0|

        ANIS   = ANISOCYTOSIS
        CLR    = CLEAR
        HYA    = HYALINE CASTS
        NEG    = NEGATIVE
        NONE   = NONE SEEN
        PLTDEC = PLATELETS DECREASED
        POIK   = POIKILOCYTOSIS
        SCAN   = SEE ELECTROPHORESIS SCAN
        SLT    = SLIGHT
        STRW   = STRAW
        TEXT 1 = TEXT-PLAT;DEC
        WCST   = WBC CASTS
        YEL    = YELLOW
```

Figure 3. Last page of a standard 80 column flowsheet showing list of abbreviations.

OSU-CCC system was easy data entry. Data entry on that system was similar to the formatted sequence data entry option in OCIS. However, one key feature that OCIS did not have was the ability to jump to various items in the sequence, including forward, backward, and to the end of the sequence. The lack of this feature in OCIS was a source of dissatisfaction to our prototype users. The slash mark (/) allows the user to get to the end of the list; a slash mark and a six-character Item Dictionary code allows the user to jump to that item in the sequence (Figure 4). The data entry time savings and the sense of satisfaction experienced by our prototype users was well worth the one day it took to rework these data entry routines.

```
BUN     - BLOOD UREA NITROGEN :                           :
GLUC    - GLUCOSE :                                        :
URIC    - URIC ACID :                                      :
CREAT   - CREATININE :                                     : /GLUC
GLUC    - GLUCOSE :                                        : 70
URIC    - URIC ACID :                                      :
CREAT   - CREATININE :                                     :
NA      - SODIUM :                                         : 140
K       - POTASSIUM :                                      : /
(A)CCEPT   (R)ETRY   (I)GNORE
```

Figure 4. Sample data entry sequence showing use of "/ " character.

Menu Reorganization. We have modified several of the main menus to accommodate the differences in the way the system will be used at OSU. Both the data coordinators' and the health care professionals' perspectives have been considered. We have changed menus to allow access by health care providers to some functions that were previously restricted to data coordinators. We allow health care professionals to define flows and plots and to enter certain data, such as protocol starts and events. Because we are just trying this feature out, we do not want to allow all health care professionals access to these functions at this time; we have restricted access to the BMT research nurse. To accomplish this, we simply added another level to the authority system. This new level allows greater access than the display of clinical data, but it is not so unrestricted as the data coordinators' level. The authority system feature in OCIS allowed us to do this quite easily without having to change all menus. We did create a new menu that consolidates these additional functions. We have also made minor changes to several other menus in an attempt to consolidate similar functions and facilitate easy access to other functions. Most of these changes reflect the difference in how the BMT data coordinator has utilized the system at OSU.

Report Format Customization. Although it was anticipated that the institution name would have to be changed on all reports, this was expected to be a rather minor modification, restricted to the frame specifications and the report driver routines that set up report headers. Again, we chose to make this modification function by function in the same way we are making the medical record number and help message changes. However, it turns out that a bit more customization was required in "sprucing up" the report formats. Many reports were found to be difficult to read in that much of the data ran together. Clearly, this was a matter of preference and did not alter the function of the system in a major way (Figure 5). We feel, however, that by addressing human factors issues such as this, as well as the data entry customization mentioned previously, we have probably enhanced the users' acceptance of the system and as a result improved its ability to convey information.

```
THE OHIO STATE UNIVERSITY HOSPITALS      MEDICAL RECORD NUMBER:
         COLUMBUS, OHIO                  PATIENT NAME:
                                         ADMISSION DATE:
VITAL SIGNS AS OF 06/30/88               SERVICE:                 PAGE  1

   30 y.o.  WHITE  MALE
   CML CHRONIC PHASE
```

CML RMT	DAY #	TEMPO DEG F	PULSE /MIN	RESP /MIN	BP MM HG	WT LB	IT01 ML	OTOT ML
04/05/88	4	...	...	...	...	233.8	4015	3110
12:00 AM		97	64	16	126/64	...	...	...
4:00 AM		97	68	16	134/90	...	...	...
8:00 AM		97.8	80	18	130/94	...	...	...
12:00 PM		98.6	78	20	134/90	...	...	...
:00 PM		98.8	80	20	140/98	...	...	...
8:00 PM		99.2	82	20	130/90	...	...	...
04/06/88	5	...	...	...	...	222.8	4390	4000
12:00 AM		98.2	68	20	160/90	...	...	...
4:00 AM		97.6	80	16	162/94	...	...	...
8:00 AM		98	84	20	144/88	...	...	...
4:00 PM		99	72	16	154/90	...	...	...
04/07/88	6	...	...	...	...	233.8	6280	4575
12:00 AM		98.8	84	16	144/84	...	...	...
4:00 AM		98.4	84	20	142/82	...	...	...
8:00 AM		97	100	18	130/73	...	...	...
12:00 PM		99	80	18	170/84	...	...	...
4:00 PM		100.2	88	20	160/60	...	...	...
8:00 PM		100.8	92	22	150/62	...	...	...
04/08/88	7	...	...	...	...	223.6	6075	3950
12:00 AM		100	92	24	142/68	...	...	...
4:00 AM		99.6	104	20	138/64	...	...	...
8:00 AM		99.2	84	20	142/90	...	...	...
12:00 PM		99.4	88	20	136/86	...	...	...
4:00 PM		99.8	80	18	128/86	...	...	...
8:00 PM		100.8	90	20	120/72	...	...	...
04/09/88	8	...	...	...	...	227.2	6414	4170
12:00 AM		100.2	96	20	150/86	...	...	...
4:00 AM		99.6	100	20	166/70	...	...	...
8:00 AM		98.8	92	16	136/78	...	...	...
12:00 PM		99.4	100	20	128/80	...	...	...
4:00 PM		99.8	88	20	138/82	...	...	...
8:00 PM		100.4	100	18	140/74	...	...	...
04/10/88	9	...	...	...	...	229.4	5674	5545
12:00 AM		101	100	16	150/74	...	...	...
4:00 AM		98.6	100	20	138/80	...	...	...
8:00 AM		99.2	96	20	158/88	...	...	...
12:00 PM		100	100	24	154/86	...	...	...
4:00 PM		100.2	100	24	148/88	...	...	...
8:00 PM		102.2	100	20	152/76	...	...	...
04/11/88	10	...	...	...	...	228	7091	4870
12:00 AM		102.6	110	22	144/70	...	...	...
4:00 AM		101.6	110	20	160/92	...	...	...
8:00 AM		101.8	104	20	178/80	...	...	...
12:00 PM		100.8	104	20	166/66	...	...	...

Figure 5. Sample of revised horizontal flowsheet format.

Planned Customization Activities

The effort described in the previous subsections is limited to the development of a prototype implementation that operates on a small computer for a single unit. It does not implement – nor would it be useful to implement – all OCIS functions. Plans for the future are to complete the conversion of OCIS functions that are of value in this Phase I prototype and plan for the implementation of a larger Phase II system. I close this section with a brief discussion of some of the planned changes to the prototype system.

Protocol-Directed Care (Daily Care Plans). We have not yet implemented the daily care plan function of OCIS at OSU at this time. However, we have given this function much thought. From this author's perspective, we find this to be the most interesting and exciting component of the system. We plan to make this component an area of emphasis for our system and hope to be able to develop some research projects along these lines. Specifically, we will initially be making modifications to this component so that it runs off the same Item Dictionary as the actual clinical database. At OSU the laboratory reports as part of each result both the battery code and the individual component test code. As a result, we will be able to verify the appropriate source of the result, the battery (CBC) or the individual result (WBC), or both. Because we also receive notification of pending results, we will be able to verify the laboratory tests that have been performed automatically without having to have the data coordinator manually verify laboratory procedures.

The other major modification we anticipate prior to initial use of the daily care plan is a more flexible order schedule. That is, we have a need to be able to order things more frequently than once a day, for example, vital signs or medications. Although we could accommodate this modification by simply printing the frequency of the procedure on the hard-copy care plan, we intend to develop a care plan that will function as a work list. We also would like to increase on-line use of this function in an attempt to get away from a hard-copy-based format and to promote more direct use of the daily care plan function by physicians and health care professionals. Our long-term research projects center around two main themes: (1) cognitive engineering issues, such as identifying what data are useful to the clinical decision-making process, and (2) human factors issues, concerned with how the data should be presented and what the system interface should look like.

Clinical Care Abstract. The other area of emphasis that we have targeted for further development is the tumor registry abstract. We plan to make the abstract more of a working clinical document, not only with respect to patient care but also from the clinical research perspective. We are developing a core of items that will serve as the basis for the clinical care abstract. We expect that many of these items are already part of the tumor registry abstract, but this core will be supplemented by a set of disease items and in some cases protocol and/or symptom-specific sets of items. We have not progressed far enough with this project to discuss the specifics, nor have we clearly defined the level of specificity we will use with respect to disease categorization.

Our goal is to attempt to develop an on-line clinical management record. This is different from an on-line medical record in that we are not attempting to capture all of the information contained in the legal paper medical record. Instead, we expect to organize and display on line the clinically relevant pieces of information contained in the paper medical record. Clearly, this is a controversial topic and will require a great deal of research and effort in identifying what are clinically relevant pieces of information. However, we are quite interested in how the clinician organizes and selects data, which is then used as a source of information in the clinical decision-making process. Our goal is not to replace either the decision maker or the paper medical record. We hope to develop a system that facilitates data collection and assimilation in order to provide information that can be used by the clinician in the decision-making process. We believe that part of this goal is not only to provide access to currently relevant individual patient information but also to develop and maintain a database that can also serve as a clinical research database.

Concluding Remarks

Earlier I mentioned that the conversion of OCIS to meet the needs of OSU-CHRI was more difficult than we had expected. Nevertheless, with very limited resources, we have achieved success. That we did so is a tribute to the installation team, the clinicians and administrators who supported us, and the power and flexibility of OCIS. I close this chapter with some observations that may be of value to others tasked with the installation of a clinical system, even if it is not OCIS.

TEDIUM's Influence

OCIS was implemented using a development environment that offered a higher view of the system implementation. Like OCIS, TEDIUM was an internally developed product, and it was very helpful for me to have been experienced in its use before the conversion effort began. Although we have encountered a few minor bugs in TEDIUM, definitely fewer than a dozen, there was only one bug that caused us any difficulty. This was more a matter of inconvenience than a real problem. Without going into any detail, the design of the system assumed that a certain class of program would not generate more than 10 MUMPS programs. For very large "entry" programs this became a problem, but we were able to find a simple workaround.

It should be obvious from the above discussion that without TEDIUM we would not have been able to implement the OCIS system at OSU. OCIS is not a turnkey system, and it requires a fair amount of customization to the environment. Clearly, we have chosen to make more modifications than those that were essential, but we still feel strongly that because of the magnitude of the changes, it would have required many more programmer years of effort to implement them if TEDIUM were not available.

Administrative Commitment

Adequate administrative commitment is essential to the success of a project such as this. The commitment must be of several varieties. The administration must recognize not only the need for an adequate level of resource support but also the OCIS dependence on other automated systems for its data. Resources must include hardware to support the project and, even more important, personnel support. An adequate programming staff is essential for a timely implementation of the system. If it takes too long to get anything functional, credibility is lost. Therefore, a phased implementation is the best method.

There must also be administrative support in developing links to the various other automated systems. Unless there is a single central information systems group, personnel from administratively separate departments may be assigned to work together in developing these system links. Therefore, it is essential that the project be supported by the central administration.

Our approach has been to get several basic components functional and in use in a prototype mode as soon as possible. This has allowed for user involvement at an early stage, and although it may have required additional customizations, we believe it has led to greater user satisfaction in the long run. We defined flow sheets, plots, and a link to the clinical laboratories as our initial basic functions. Since these basic functions have become operational, the users have been able to work with the system while further development proceeds in the glow of our increased credibility.

Project Summary

We have outlined several categories of modifications: the expected, the unexpected, and the anticipated. Some of the modifications were expected; for example, we did not think that the laboratory would report results in exactly the same way it did at Hopkins, and we expected to have to redo the laboratory link. It turned out that there were many more unexpected modifications than we had anticipated. This was partly influenced by the fact that an information system was already in use on the Bone Marrow Transplant Unit. More correctly stated, the unexpected modifications were mostly due to user sophistication and expectations of the system. What may be acceptable to the naive user becomes unacceptable as the user has had experience with other systems and learns that there are other (often better) ways of doing things. But most important, it should be recognized that, although OCIS can be successfully ported to another institution, it is not a turnkey system. In order to have it implemented successfully, the institution must have an adequate level of support both financially and administratively.

So far we have implemented the clinical data part of the system, including flow sheets, plots, and unformatted data displays and the summary function, which provides a general description of the patient, including diagnostic information, patient admission information, protocol information, and BMT program-specific data. We also have many of the census reporting capabilities functional and a few of the basic search functions. Within the next six months we intend to implement the microbiology (BACT) function, the basic daily care plan function, and the abstract/tumor registry function. We do not plan to implement the hemapheresis or the pharmacy component at this point in time. After the basic clinical functions are implemented, we will begin implementing the outpatient appointment and research data management functions. We will also be evaluating the system to determine what additional functions are required and begin work on the areas of research we have outlined previously, specifically the daily care plan enhancements and the clinical care abstract.

We are about halfway finished with the implementation of the basic clinical functions that are part of the baseline system. This has been accomplished in about 18 programmer months by one full-time programmer with various levels of support on my part, depending on what other tasks needed to be accomplished at the time. Clearly, my past experience with TEDIUM has been a major benefit, but my experience with OCIS had been limited primarily to the daily care plan. Our experience has shown that once the programming staff becomes proficient with TEDIUM, it becomes a tool with which any competent programmer can work more efficiently than with many other programming languages.

Clearly, OCIS and TEDIUM have provided a powerful and broad base from which we can develop a clinical information system to meet our needs. Unfortunately, the state of the art is such that no existing system can be immediately adopted without alteration. In our case we feel that the redesign and modifications we have made draw very heavily upon our ability to understand, develop, and implement a clinical information system tailored to the needs of the health professionals at The Arthur G. James Cancer Hospital and Research Institute, Ohio State University. Without OCIS, our job would be much more difficult and far more expensive; however, without this understanding, our job would be impossible.

References

Barnett, G.O., Justice, N.S., Somand, M.E., Adams, J.B., Waxman, B.D., Beaman, P.D., Parent, M.S., Van Deusen, F.R., Greenlie, J.K., COSTAR System, in *Information Systems for Patient Care*, B.I. Blum, Ed., Springer-Verlag, 1984, pp. 270–292.

Friedman, R.B., Enitine, S., Murray, G.M., Holladay, D., Steinhart, C.E., An Integrated Clinical Protocol Management System, in *Proceedings of the Third Annual Symposium on Computer Applications in Medical Care*, IEEE Computer Society Press, 1979, pp. 81–84.

Horwitz, J., Thompson, H., Concannon, T., Friedman, R.H., Krikorian, J., Gertman, P.M., Computer-Assisted Patient Care Management in Medical Oncology, in *Proceedings of the Fourth Annual Symposium on Computer Applications in Medical Care*, J.T. O'Neill, Ed., IEEE Computer Society Press, 1980, pp. 771–778.

PROMIS Laboratory, Representation of Medical Knowledge and PROMIS, in *Proceedings of the Second Annual Symposium on Computer Applications in Medical Care*, IEEE Computer Society Press, 1978, pp. 368–400.

Serber, M.J., Mackey, R. and Young, C.W. The Sloan-Kettering Information System for Clinical Oncology, in *Proceedings of the Fourth Annual Symposium on Computer Applications in Medical Care*, IEEE Computer Society Press, 1980, pp. 728–730.

Stead, W.W., Hammond, W.E., Straube, M.J., A Chartless Record – Is It Adequate? in

Proceedings of the Sixth Annual Symposium on Computer Applications in Medical Care, B.I. Blum, Ed., IEEE Computer Society Press, 1982, pp. 89–94.

Wirtschafter, D.D., Gams, R., Ferguson, C., Blackwell, W., Boackle, P., Clinical Protocol Information System, in *Proceedings of the Fourth Annual Symposium on Computer Applications in Medical Care,* J.T. O'Neill, Ed., IEEE Computer Society Press, 1980, pp. 745–750.

Index